SPORTS INJURIES

RECOGNITION AND MANAGEMENT

Third Edition

Edited by

M. A. HUTSON

Orthopaedic and Sports Physician,
Park Row Clinic, Nottingham

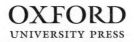

OXFORD
UNIVERSITY PRESS

Oxford University Press
Great Clarendon Street, Oxford OX2 6DP
Oxford University Press is a department of the Oxford University.
It furthers the University's objective of excellence in research, scholarship,
and education by publishing worldwide in

Oxford New York
Athens Auckland Bangkok Bogotá Buenos Aires Cape Town
Chennai Dar es Salaam Delhi Florence Hong Kong Istanbul Karachi
Kolkata Kuala Lumpur Madrid Melbourne Mexico City Mumbai Nairobi
Paris Sao Paulo Shanghai Singapore Taipei Tokyo Toronto Warsaw
with associated companies in Berlin Ibadan

Oxford is a registered trade mark of Oxford University Press
in the UK and in certain other countries

Published in the United States
by Oxford University Press, Inc., New York

British Library Cataloguing in Publication Data
Data available

Library of Congress Cataloging in Publication Data

Sports injuries: recognition and management/edited by M.A. Hutson – 3rd ed.
p.; cm. — (Oxford medical publications)
Includes bibliographical references and index.
1. Sport injuries. I. Hutson, M.A. II. Series.
[DNLM: 1. Athletic Injuries—diagnosis. 2. Athletic Injuries—therapy. QT 261 S7647 2001]
RD97.S72 2001   617.1′027—dc21   2001016275

ISBN 0 19 263271 x (Hbk)
0 19 263272 8 (Pbk)

Typeset by Expo Holdings

Printed in Great Britain on acid free paper by
Butler and Tanner Ltd, Frome

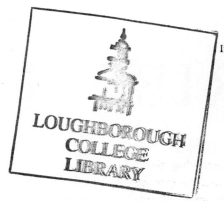

FOREWORD
HRH, *The Princess Royal*

As a competitive horse rider I have spent a great deal of time and effort worrying about the physical condition of my horse and trying to prevent injuries from either happening or getting worse. My own problems seemed less important. However, it is an inevitable consequence of sport, or recreational activity, that physical injury will intervene from time to time. Whatever the source of injury, the overall effect is to increase the demands made upon the medical profession.

Dr Michael Hutson has a background of general practice in which he developed his knowledge in orthopaedic and sports medicine and became medical officer to professional soccer and cricket teams in Nottingham.

Dr Hutson clearly understands the need for a greater background of knowledge of sports injuries by medical practitioners, particularly by physicians of first contact—the general medical practitioner and the Accident and Emergency doctor. Only by disseminating such knowledge into the general body of the medical profession will the requirements of the sporting populus at large be satisfied.

Fortunately, he is not alone as there are contributions from consultants in other medical disciplines who describe the recognition and management of more specialized problems.

The theme that underlines the purpose of the book is a *practical* approach to the problems of sports injuries. It should provide a valuable addition to the understanding of this increasingly important discipline, and it is a pleasure to be associated with it.

ANNE

PREFACE

The discipline of Sports Medicine has progressed slowly, but with more certainty over the last five years compared with the previous two decades. The development of exercise physiology, for instance, has been such that there are many texts of excellence available to the sports physiologist and clinician alike in his pursuit of a basic understanding of fitness and the body's response to various energetic sports and recreational exercise. However, the needs of the medical practitioner, who is concerned principally with the recognition and management of *injury* sustained during or as a result of sport, have been less well served. His overall requirement, notwithstanding the need for a satisfactory background knowledge of basic sciences, is for a greater clinical appreciation of the athlete's problems so that he may undertake both a principal and co-ordinating role. Inherent in these responsibilities is an awareness of the importance of early assessment of the severity of the pathological process in order to achieve maximal influence on healing, the relationship of the injury to the athlete's expectations regarding his future participation in sport, and recognition of the benefits of expert rehabilitation.

This book is not an encyclopaedia of medical conditions associated with sport. It is designed primarily for the clinician who requires a method of learning a suitable approach towards the musculoskeletal problems encountered in sport. Diagnosis, treatment, and rehabilitation of the most common, yet often inadequately treated, injuries are considered in some depth. Aetiological factors, particularly in overuse injury requiring some knowledge of biomechanics, are given due emphasis. A guide is given to the timely referral for further advice and to the role of the consultant in certain specialized fields. An attempt is made to define objectives for the sports physician and to outline aspects of his educational, managerial, and advisory responsibilities to the community.

The purpose therefore is for the text to be essentially a means of reference to complement the development of the practical skills required by the general practitioner with limited resources and facilities, the traumatologist in the hospital Accident and Emergency department, and the already established sports physician who requires greater in-depth information. As for the foreseeable future, specialists in sports injuries will come largely from the ranks of general practitioners, the more so as post-graduate degree courses in Sports Medicine are becoming increasingly available, it is understandable that the author has general practitioners in mind. However, both physicians and surgeons who have already developed specialist skills in disciplines such as orthopaedic surgery and rheumatology should find that the text provides information on those soft-tissue problems arising from sport that lie outside their principal field of interest or experience.

The 1995 text has been fully revised and updated. Basic principles will stand the test of time. However, over the last five years, there have been a number of improvements in investigative techniques and in some management strategies, and these have been incorporated in this edition. In particular, a more comprehensive section on MRI scanning is now included and the latest advances in specialized fields such as anterior cruciate deficiency are outlined. Additionally, a new chapter on Emergency Medicine in Sport, by John Sloan, a leading Accident and Emergency Medicine specialist, has replaced the chapter on First Aid in Sport.

2001   M.A.H.

ACKNOWLEDGEMENTS

The following are gratefully acknowledged for permission to reproduce figures.

Figs 1.1. and 1.8, T. Bailey Forman Newspapers Ltd, Nottingham; **Figs 1.2a, 1.5, 3.7a and b, 4.8b, and 5.10b**, B. Thomas, 19 Charnwood Ave, Northampton; **Fig. 1.2b**, The Associated Press Ltd, London; **Fig. 1.9**, T. Duffy, 83 Sutton Heights, Surrey; **Fig. 2.5**, Thomas Bond (Optometrist), 130 Melton Road, West Bridgford, Nottingham; **Fig 4.2**, E. D. Lacey, 16 Post House Lane, Leatherhead; **Figs 4.5, 5.3**, and **5.10a**, Supersports Photographs, Baslow, Derbyshire; **Fig. 6.9**, *The Times*, London; **Fig. 4.17**, Stark, H., Jobe, F. W., Boyes, J., and Ashworth, R. R. (1977). Fracture of the hook of the hamate in athletes. *J. Bone Jt. Surg.*, **59A**, 576; **Fig. 4.24**, Henderson, J. J. and Arafa, M. A. M. (1987). Carpometacarpal dislocation. *J. Bone Jt. Surg.*, **69B**, 213; **Figs 4.25, 4.27, 4.28, 4.38, 4.40, and 4.42**, Watson Jones (1982). *Fractures and Joint injuries*, 6th edn, (ed. J. N. Wilson). Churchill Livingstone, Edinburgh (Figs 4.27 and 4.28 modified from, London, P.S. (1967). *A practical guide to the care of the injured*. Churchill Livingstone, Edinburgh); **Fig. 4.41**, Stack, H. G. (1968). Mallet finger. *The Hand*, **1**, 85; **Fig. 6.21c**, T. Bailey Forman Newspapers Ltd. Nottingham.

CONTENTS

CONTRIBUTORS

M. J. ALLEN
Consultant in Sports Medicine
Leicester General Hospital
Leicester

N. J. BARTON
Consultant Hand Surgeon
University Hospital
Nottingham

D. B. L. FINLAY
Consultant Radiologist
Leicester Royal Infirmary
Leicester

J. L. FIRTH
Consultant Neurosurgeon
University Hospital
Nottingham

N. R. GALLOWAY
Consultant Ophthalmic Surgeon
University Hospital
Nottingham

M. A. HUTSON
Specialist Orthopaedic and Sports Physician
Park Row Clinic
2 Regent Street
Nottingham

F. R. I. MIDDLETON
Consultant in Rehabilitation and Disability Medicine
Spinal Injuries Unit
Royal National Orthopaedic Hospital
Stanmore

J. SLOAN
Consultant in Accident and Emergency Medicine
General Infirmary
Leeds

W. A. WALLACE
Professor of Orthopaedic and Accident Surgery
University Hospital
Nottingham

1 Introduction

M. A. HUTSON

Basic concepts

The primary requirement of medical practitioners who are consulted by patients injured during, or as a result of, sport is the establishment of an accurate diagnosis. Once a specific diagnosis has been made, a full assessment is predicated upon a knowledge of the aetiological factors associated with the development of injury, behavioural aspects, including motivation, and the standard of performance achieved. When underpinned by an appropriate level of knowledge of pathoanatomy and biomechanics, management of injury may incorporate a spectrum of treatment modalities prior to rehabilitation of the patient to a satisfactory level of fitness.

The theme throughout the text will therefore be one of *assessment and management*.

Assessment: history
aetiological factors
specific diagnosis
Management: treatment
rehabilitation

It is regrettable that within the clinical curriculum of the medical student, there is a very limited amount of time devoted to an introduction to the extensive field of orthopaedics and rheumatology. A paradox exists in that, although soft tissue problems of all kinds, encompassed by the specialities of orthopaedic (musculoskeletal) medicine and sports medicine, represent a high proportion of the work-load of doctors in general practice and in traumatology departments, there is little opportunity to hone the skills required for examination of the musculoskeletal system. Examination procedures will therefore be described in some detail in this book. In the past, the author has relied heavily on those basic procedures as laid down by, amongst others, James Cyriax in his *Textbook of Orthopaedic Medicine* (Cyriax 1982). Expansion in some directions, modification in others, and the addition of techniques such as ligament stress testing make it possible to build from basic orthopaedic medical principles in an orderly fashion, thus reducing the likelihood of diagnostic error from inadequacy of musculoskeletal examination.

Assessment

A basic knowledge of the biomechanical forces involved in specific sports is required. Track athletes run anti-clockwise both in their events and during training, so that asymmetrical forces continually are being applied to their lower limbs in particular. Javelin throwers may have an overhead style, or tend to sling; the forces applied to their shoulders and elbows are different in the two styles (Fig. 1.1). Tennis players may use a single- or a two-handed backhand, imposing different stresses upon the trunk and upper limbs (Fig. 1.2), and so on. Numerous examples are given throughout the text. These technical factors are particularly relevant when considering overuse injury.

An assessment of joint mobility some distance away from the site of injury is also included in the categorization of relevant aetiological factors. A squash player with a limited range of hip rotation, as a result of early degenerative disease, may develop low back pain when excessive rotational stress is transferred repeatedly to the lumbar spine. Weakness or tightness of one group of muscles acting about a joint similarly may result in injury elsewhere. Tight hamstrings for instance may be responsible for low back problems, or for muscle injury in compensating muscle groups.

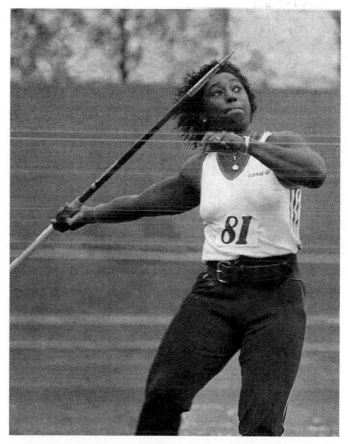

FIG. 1.1 Javelin throwers may have an overhead style or tend to sling: different forces are applied to the shoulders and elbows.

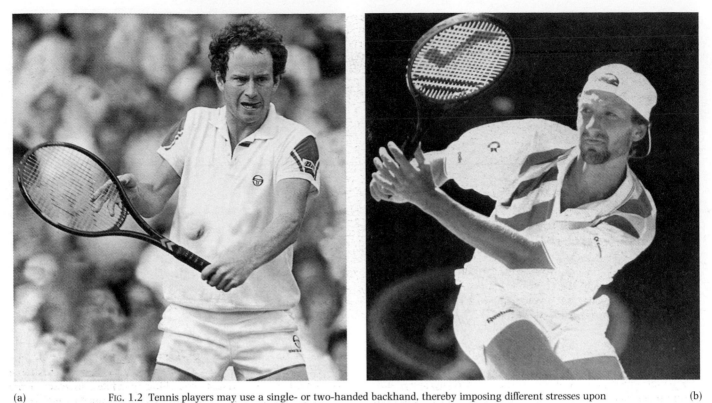

(a)   FIG. 1.2 Tennis players may use a single- or two-handed backhand, thereby imposing different stresses upon   (b)
the trunk and upper limbs: (a) single-handed backhand; (b) two-handed backhand.

These are simply a few of the factors that require identification for full assessment of the nature of the injury, and they will be explored in greater detail in the individual chapters which follow. Training schedules, behavioural characteristics, particularly the behavioural responses to pain, individual motivation, and ambition also need study. Although 'holistic' medicine enjoys much popularity at the moment, it has surely always been incumbent upon medical practitioners to develop a breadth of vision for every patient—a facet of their skills that they are trained in from the first weeks of the clinical curriculum in medical school. Sports injuries need no less perspicacity than other illnesses that are recognizably 'stress' related. When injuries in children are considered, the interrelationship between the expectations and ambitions of the patient, parents, coaches, and teachers becomes even more important.

The history given by the patient is often revealing. When injury is acute, particularly when extrinsic forces are involved, the direction of the externally applied forces should be established if possible. When injury is of a more chronic nature ('overuse injury', see p. 6) the history is quite different, as exemplified by the phases of discomfort experienced during the development of tendinitis:

(i)   discomfort (+ stiffness) after activity;
(ii) discomfort during the initiation of activity, subsequently improving ('run off') during further activity, and worsening afterwards;
(iii) discomfort worsening during activity, associated with functional impairment;
(iv) discomfort of sufficient severity to prevent activity.

Once a historical perspective of the symptoms and relevant background information have been gained, the establishment of a satisfactory diagnosis requires the application to the musculoskeletal system of examination techniques which previously may not have been used extensively or perfected by the majority of doctors. An appreciation must be gained of the importance of an examination routine that is founded upon sound orthopaedic principles, so that an *assessment of function* may be made. The moving parts require clinical appraisal according to the following code.

1. Observation.
2. Active movements.
3. Passive movements.
4. Resisted—i.e. isometric—muscle contraction (selective tissue tension).
5. Palpation.
6. Neurological and vascular examination.

The passive movements offer information on joint function and the integrity of the periarticular structures, and may be further subdivided into

- range of motion (around physiological axes)
- 'joint play' (movements not under voluntary control)
- provocative (stress) testing e.g. for impingement, for ligamentous competency, and for joint integrity.

The only compromise to this orthopaedic *medical* system of examination should be when, as a result of a history of acute trauma and the disposition of the patient or of the injured area, a fracture is suspected: gentle handling of the injured site may be followed by early X-ray, prior to more extensive examination

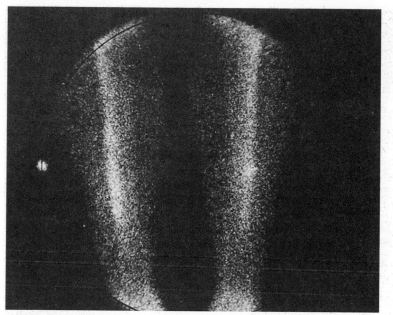

Fig. 1.3 Scattered increased uptake, representing recurrent physical stress, may be seen on bone scans in the lower limbs of long-distance runners.

procedures if appropriate (thereby conforming to the orthopaedic *surgical* system).

Further investigations such as X-rays, arthrography, ultrasound scans, bone scans, CT scans, MRI scans, haematology, etc., should be considered where relevant. Full assessment relies on an understanding that, just as there is a wider range of ECG changes in an athlete than in the non-sporting population, so 'abnormal' findings, such as are seen in X-rays of 'footballer's ankle' (marginal osteophytes and avulsion fragments (see Fig. 9.16, p. 165) or on bone scans of long-distance runners (scattered increased uptake in the bones of the lower limbs (Fig. 1.3), are simply a manifestation of recurrent physical stress. Interpretation must therefore be made with due care. This is no less important in magnetic resonance imaging—often considered to be the "ultimate" high-tech investigation—than in investigations that offer less resolution.

Management

Management of athletic injury requires substantially more than 'treatment' of an injured area. Patients need advice on a number of other aspects, including maintenance of overall fitness during recovery. They also require a prognosis. If physical treatment is desirable, it is necessary to have some knowledge of appropriate therapeutic modalities, and preferably a sound professional working relationship with the therapist of choice. It is erroneous to assume automatically that ice and ultrasound, for instance, cure all soft tissue lesions; more critical evaluation of the options is required before prescribing specific therapeutic regimes. A physical therapist needs, above all else, an accurate diagnosis. The therapist will probably have more experience in the usefulness of modalities such as effleurage, friction massage, laser therapy, etc. than the referring practitioner. However, it is incumbent upon the referring doctor to offer guidance, and thereby encourage suitable feedback of information on patients' progress.

Depending on the type, severity, and duration of the injury, it is often necessary for the patient to progress from the therapy room to the rehabilitation area, where progressive strengthening exercises and flexibility exercises may be performed. Isotonic, isometric, and isokinetic exercises all have their place; they should be combined with suitable stretching schedules. In view of the ready accessibility to many athletes of gymnasia and health clubs, in which sophisticated equipment is commonly available for both training and rehabilitation, it is increasingly important for progress to be monitored by the practitioner or therapist and for prescriptive exercises to be specific to both the injury and the sport. It is often forgotten that strengthening exercises which are performed primarily for specific muscle groups may impose stresses on other parts of the body—this is particularly relevant to the prevention of spinal injury during the rehabilitation of an injured limb.

Liaison with the coach or trainer should be considered to be an important aspect of both assessment and management. The coaches of athletes, particularly those in the younger age groups with considerable aptitude, may well be able to furnish useful information regarding the cause of injury which has not otherwise been disclosed; conversely, they need guidance on the reduction of specific forms of stress during the subsequent resumption of training. Occasions frequently arise when a telephone call to the coach of an up-and-coming tennis starlet, for instance, reveals the existence of abnormal biomechanical stress associated with faulty serving technique. Hyperextension of the spine on a tennis service (Fig. 1.4) or excessive forearm rotation on the forehand are not uncommon. Unless such information is presented to the physician, and flawed technique identified and corrected, recurrence of injury is to be expected.

Overall, the patient needs reassurance, whenever possible, regarding the likelihood of a satisfactory outcome, as his worst fears are not always overtly expressed. The parents of an adolescent with Osgood–Schlatter's disease often need a positive statement that the 'lump' is not a tumour, and likewise the patient with a thigh swelling from a rectus femoris tear (Fig. 1.5). These and other considerations will be explored more fully in subsequent chapters. In this branch of medicine, in which the frustration of injury is often compounded by a psychological 'low' secondary to inactivity, sympathetic understanding is required. Too many

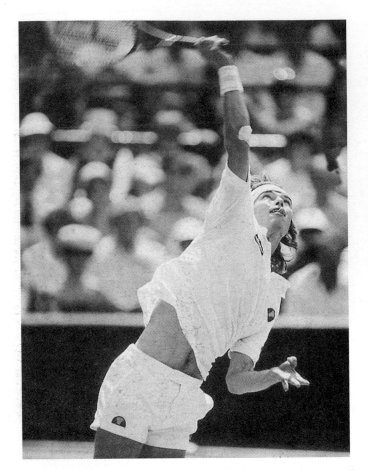

FIG. 1.4 The tennis serve may give rise to shoulder or spinal injuries if technique is faulty. In this illustration, the server avoids spinal hyperextension, having thrown the ball up correctly in front of his body.

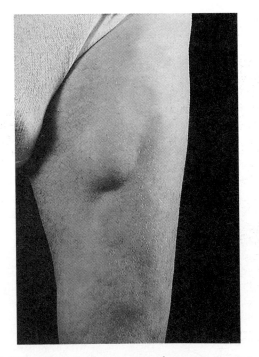

FIG. 1.5 Patients may need reassurance that a previous rectus femoris tear is not a tumour.

patients inappropriately receive a bland prescription for absolute rest, or an unhelpful reaction such as, 'I am not surprised that you have leg pain if you run seventy miles a week.' Patients, quite rightly, expect advice for injuries that have occurred in an era when recreation and sport are encouraged, not least by government-backed 'Sport for All' and 'Exercise for Health' campaigns. The abrogation by some members of the medical profession of their responsibility to provide a caring service on the grounds that sports injuries are 'self-induced' is unacceptable.

Sports medicine as a discipline has advanced steadily over recent years. In the UK, an Intercollegiate Academic Board of Sports and Exercise Medicine was created in 1998. This reflects the greater awareness of the need for Sports Medicine to develop as a consultant-led speciality service within the National Health Service. With the advent of the implementation of the proposals for the establishment of the United Kingdom Sports Institute in Sheffield and the proposed development of regional centres of excellence in sports medicine throughout the UK, it is to be hoped that an increasingly sophisticated and widespread service for those injured in sport will become available. It is anticipated, however, that doctors of first contact (in general practice and in hospital Accident and Emergency departments) will continue to take the brunt of an increasing work-load.

Features of soft tissue breakdown and repair

Acute inflammatory phase

When injury is sustained to the soft (connective) tissues, whether as a result of acute trauma or of repeated microtrauma, localized cellular damage results. In the early inflammatory phase, chemotactic agents are released from platelets and mast cells. These agents stimulate the migration of polymorphs (which are particularly active against pathogens) and monocytes (which develop into macrophages having a phagocytic function upon tissue debris). Degradative enzymes are released from a range of inflammatory cells. The concentration of the chemotactic agents appears to be dependent upon a raised intracellular level of calcium ions. Vasodilation and increased capillary permeability occur, mediated (at least in part) by prostaglandins (Anderson and Ramwell 1974). Interstitial oedema and frank bleeding into the tissues from the larger blood vessels are features of this early phase. During the inflammatory phase over the next few days, in the continued presence of macrophages, further chemotactic factors are released from within their granules: such factors stimulate the development of undifferentiated connective tissue cells into fibroblasts and endothelial and other mature cells.

If sufficiently severe, the inflammatory phase is responsible for the clinical features of erythema, heat, pain, crepitus, swelling, and dysfunction. The physical modalities of treatment described in Chapter 12 help alleviate the symptoms and the extent of the inflammatory process. Prostaglandin synthesis is inhibited by non-steroidal anti-inflammatory drugs (NSAIDs). Although it is conventional to think in terms of 'anti-inflammatory' treatment for acute soft tissue injury, the inflammatory phase is nevertheless essential to normal repair. Therefore modalities such as ultrasound may be considered more accurately to be 'pro-inflammatory' by stimulating mast cell activity, and *accelerating* the normal repair process (Dyson 1987). In chronic inflammatory conditions, however, it is more appropriate to remove the (overuse) inflammatory stimulus before the use of specific therapeutic modalities. However, despite relative, or even 'complete', rest, some chronic inflammatory conditions (such as plantar fasciitis and lateral epicondylitis) appear to be self-perpetuating. Stress reduction may then need to be combined with the more powerful anti-inflammatory activity of the injectable corticosteroids.

Proliferative phase

Within a few days of injury, the proliferative phase commences, thereby overlapping the late inflammatory phase. Fibroblasts form a connective tissue matrix and endothelial cells develop into blood vessels; the resulting highly cellular and vascularized tissue is known as granulation tissue. It is essential at this stage that the collagenous matrix is allowed to proceed to relative maturity without the imposition of excessive stress. In more chronic conditions, particularly in poorly vascularized tissue such as tendons, it may be useful to stimulate therapeutically the development of endothelial cells into capillaries. Extensive tissue destruction from the inflammatory phase or excessive fibrosis may sometimes develop, for example in chronic subacromial bursitis and Achilles paratendinitis, thereby creating the risk of permanent dysfunction.

Remodelling

The process of collagen maturation continues for some weeks and months thereafter. Collagen turnover is maximal in the early stages, when linear thickening may be palpable. The orderly deposition of maturing fibres presumably is dependent upon numerous factors, not least of which are the mechanical stresses to which they are subjected. Initial deposition may be somewhat haphazard, yet improved—that is, fibres are laid down in parallel—if the healing tissue is subjected to gentle stress, and is allowed to undergo a restricted amount of normal function. Noyes *et al.* (1974) have demonstrated the increase in wound strength related to mobilization rather than immobilization. Thus early gentle mobilization after connective tissue injury is desirable, and immobilization techniques are best eschewed unless absolutely necessary.

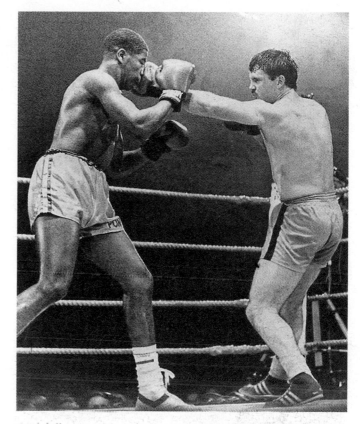

FIG. 1.6 Punching results in direct (extrinsic) trauma

Categorization

Injuries can be classified according to their nature or aetiology into

(1) trauma (acute)
(2) overuse (chronic).

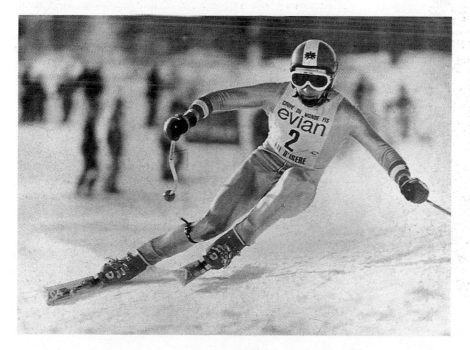

FIG. 1.7 The application of stress some distance from the injured site results in indirect (intrinsic) trauma: injury to the medial collateral ligament of the knee may occur while 'edging' during downhill skiing.

Trauma

Traumatic incidents occur suddenly, and can be considered to be *direct* (extrinsic) or *indirect* (intrinsic) in type. Examples of the former are direct blows to the body, for instance from the force of a cricket ball or as the result of an opponent's punch in boxing (Fig. 1.6), or direct confrontations with immovable forces, for example falling heavily to the ground. Injury to either the hard (osseous) or soft tissues may occur, and may present to the attendant medical officer, general practitioner, or traumatologist in the local Accident and Emergency department. In-depth analysis of fractures generally will not be undertaken in this book, though emphasis will be placed upon their recognition. Certain fractures—for example those to the wrist and hand— *will* be given further consideration, as early diagnosis and appropriate management, if necessary by referral for an expert opinion, are often required for good functional results.

Indirect trauma indicates the application of stress some distance from the site of injury, or not involving direct body contact (Fig. 1.7). The tissues involved may be muscular (rupture or 'pull'), tendinous (tendinitis, partial or complete rupture), ligamentous (sprain, partial or complete rupture), osseous (fracture), or cartilaginous. The latter may be divided further into injuries to articular cartilage (chondral) or to fibro- and hyaline cartilage, for example intervertebral disc injury.

Overuse

When describing the nature of overuse injury to patients, an analogy may be useful. Non-biological materials, such as aeroplane wings, have a fixed stress point, and, if they are subjected to a defined number of flights, fatigue fracture will inevitably result. Biological materials and organisms, on the other hand, may, with carefully graded incremental increases in stress, withstand the most enormous loads—for instance, the reputed forces as high as ten times body-weight in the Achilles tendon during running. Nevertheless if the application of submaximal stress has not been carefully graded, or there are adverse biomechanical factors, subsequent breakdown of the tissues results in *stress or overuse injury*. This may occur in any tissue, from bone (stress fracture) to bursa (chronic bursitis).

Whatever the cause or type of injury sustained, the response of the tissue is the development of inflammation. In some rheumatological conditions, the causative factor is known: bacteria, uric acid, and pyrophosphate crystals for instance. Tissue breakdown products resulting from repeated microtrauma are probably responsible for inflammation in overuse injury.

Tissue injury

Muscle

The musculotendinous unit comprises a contractile element (muscle) and a non-contractile element (tendon). Muscle fibres (muscle cells) contain hundreds of thousands of myofibrils, each composed of approximately 1500 myosin filaments and twice that number of actin filaments. The myofibrils lie in parallel, and are responsible for the striated appearance of muscle: contraction results from these filaments gliding past each other.

Muscle fibres are not homogeneous; several fibre types have been identified using histochemical and physiological tech-

Fig. 1.8 Myositis ossificans may result from direct (extrinsic) trauma. (a) In this instance, the proximal thigh muscles have been traumatized. (b) In this lateral radiograph of the femur, an area of myositis ossificans is well defined and contains bony trabeculae.

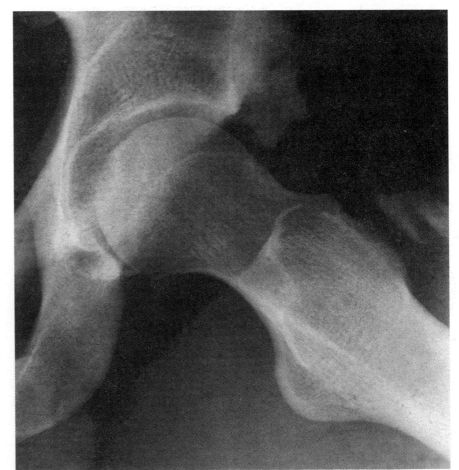

(a)

niques. Red type I (slow twitch or ST) fibres are well endowed with mitochondria, and thus with oxidative enzymes: they fatigue slowly, and are found in muscles with predominantly antigravity or postural function, such as the soleus muscle. White type II (fast twitch or FT) fibres are principally anaerobic, using creatine phosphate and anaerobic glycolysis for release of energy; they fatigue quickly, and are found in muscles requiring fast propulsive activity, such as the hamstrings and gastrocnemius muscles. Further analysis reveals that some type II fibres have relatively high potentials for oxidative metabolism, and these are labelled type II-A; others have a relatively low content of oxidative enzymes, and are called type II-B.

In addition to being a contractile unit, muscle acts as a shock-absorbing system; this is perhaps best illustrated by the automatic flexing of the knees that absorbs the shock through the legs when landing from a jump. Loss of shock-absorbing capacity (as in fatigued muscles) predisposes to injury (Chapter 11).

Muscle is capable of storing energy when preloaded by stretching. Muscle efficiency is enhanced when eccentric contraction (preloading) precedes concentric muscle contraction; viscoelastic energy initially is stored, and then released in this process, which is known as the 'stretch–shorten cycle'. The basis of athletic performance is the reliance upon eccentric contraction, with its inherent energy-storage characteristics. Thus activities such as running, jumping, racket sports, throwing, and kicking utilize the stretch–shorten cycle. By contrast, other types of exercise, such as swimming, rowing, and cycling, despite the fact that muscle groups are used rhythmically, do not have a phase of eccentric contraction; the recovery phase is passive (Shorten 1987). Storage of energy also takes place in tendon, which is a more compliant material and thereby has a much greater storage capacity. Overall, the capacity for elastic energy storage is greatest in muscle groups with long tendons.

Most muscle injuries result either from an excessive sudden demand for concentric contraction following eccentric contraction, or from excessive stretch during preloading. Sometimes unexpected (external) resistance to muscle contraction—for instance, kicking the ground or an opponent instead of the ball in soccer—is a causative factor. Although injury may occur anywhere in the contractile unit, the musculotendinous junction is a common site. A relatively minor injury may be referred to as a muscle 'pull' or 'strain'; more severe injury, in which capillaries are ruptured and intramuscular bleeding occurs, is known as a 'tear' or 'rupture' (partial or complete). Predisposing factors are as follows.

(i) *Immobilization*. Following disuse, there is a gross deterioration in the essential contractile and elastic properties, as well as in strength. Proprioception is also adversely affected, as the normal mechanism is dependent to a considerable extent upon normal function of the ST fibres in postural muscles. Immobilization by casting is thus eschewed as a therapeutic option as far as possible.

(ii) *Muscle imbalance*. This is particularly relevant to sprinters if the hamstring–quadriceps power ratios are disturbed. As a consequence of explosive hip flexion, the muscle antagonist (hamstrings) may be injured. Imbalance of the muscle components of the rotator cuff around the shoulder joint may be responsible for subacromial injury or glenohumeral instability.

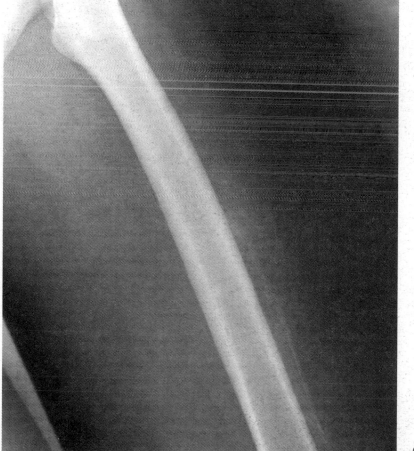

(b)

(iii) *Inadequate fitness*. Poorly trained muscles are prone to early fatigue, with loss of shock absorption. Statistics reveal increased incidence of injury in the last quarter of games such as rugby football as a result of muscle fatigue. Furthermore, training prolonged into fatigue may promote muscle imbalance. Flexibility is essential for the development of viscoelastic energy, and to allow efficient biomechanical joint function.

(iv) *Inadequate warm up*. Increased temperature should be achieved by graded 'limbering up' exercises which include long slow stretches. Amongst the effects on metabolism of raised temperature is an increased rate of muscle enzyme activity. Of additional significance in patients with established coronary artery insufficiency who undertake recreational (or therapeutic) exercise, a raised temperature delays the onset of ST depression.

'Warm down' and post-exercise stretching prevent over-rapid cooling. Removal of lactic acid is best achieved at 40–60 per cent of the previous level of activity.

Muscle may be injured by direct contusion (extrinsic trauma), or by overload when excessive tension is applied to a contracting muscle (intrinsic trauma). At a microscopic level, the initial biomechanical failure may occur in the interstitial muscle collagen lattice, although this view is conjectural (Medoff 1987). Fibre disruption occurs, with associated bleeding. Torn ends contract, and the defect fills with blood, subsequently becoming a clot invaded by fibroblasts and macrophages. If a complete tear occurs, dysfunction rather than pain is the predominant feature, and bleeding extravasates into the surrounding tissues. Partial tears may create a greater problem, as the developing haematoma may be 'intramuscular' (that is, retained within an intact fascia) instead of 'extramuscular' (when it escapes through a torn fascial lining, and is revealed as subcutaneous bruising, often some distance away). An intramuscular haematoma is more painful, and results in more protracted rehabilitation. Occasionally it becomes cystic and requires surgical drainage.

During organization, the intramuscular haematoma is gradually replaced by scar tissue. Although scar tissue remains inelastic, it may contract somewhat and become surrounded by hypertrophied muscle fibres, thus reducing the residual functional disability.

One complication of severe contusion by direct trauma is the development of myositis ossificans (Fig. 1.8). Ectopic ossification may be manifest radiologically within ten days, the most common site being the quadriceps femoris, though it does occur elsewhere whenever muscle is deep and adjacent to underlying bone. Numerous theories have been proposed for the development of bone within a muscle haematoma, including the migration of cells through damaged periosteum and crystalline calcification in necrotic tissue, leading subsequently to ossification. Whatever the cause, it appears to be a reaction by 'irritable muscle' to trauma, subsequently requiring a period of several months' rest to allow the bone to mature and contract. Of greater importance is the recognition of the risk of myositis ossificans, so that appropriate measures may be taken to prevent its onset (see Chapter 9: quadriceps injury).

Clinical assessment of muscle function involves four of the examination procedures previously described.

(i) Observation of wasting.
(ii) Passive stretching, invoked by passive movement of the joint(s) over which the muscle acts.
(iii) Resisted (isometric) contraction, thereby imparting information on muscle strength and, additionally (when contraction is painful), on torn fibres. Strength may be graded 0–5 on manual testing (see Chapters 2 and 5).
(iv) Palpation—specifically for tenderness, the presence of a defect, scarring, or a swelling.

The more significant muscle tears are dealt with in individual chapters.

Following an acute incident, the patient's subjective awareness of pain on movement, and the resulting relative disability, are usually effective in stimulating early rest. Reduction of bleeding and stimulation of the repair phase are mainstays of treatment. However, there is often inadequate realization of the importance during rehabilitation of the two Ss: *stretching* the inelastic scar formation, and *strengthening* the weakened muscle unit. The main reason that muscle injuries such as hamstring tears have such a bad reputation for recurrence is that training is resumed before 100 per cent elasticity and 90 per cent of muscle strength (compared with the normal leg) have been regained. Inadequate elasticity may have pre-existed and been a primary cause of the injury; muscle imbalance (either between the ipsi- and contralateral limbs, or between the involved muscle and its antagonist) should be detected and subsequently remedied during rehabilitation. An isokinetic dynamometer is a useful tool for such assessment (see Fig. 11.11, p. 203), and for use during the later stages of rehabilitation.

Tendon

Tendons connect muscle to bone, and are composed of blocks of collagen and elastin. These collagen fibres are highly ordered; their function is to withstand the distractive force associated with muscle contraction. Tendon is able to withstand approximately half the tensile strength of cortical bone, and twice the tensile strength of the associated muscle (thus muscle ruptures are more common than tendon ruptures). The basic pathophysiological cause for breakdown is the repetitive application of tensile forces beyond the biomechanical yield strength of the tendon (Medoff 1987). Although many *tendinopathies* are the result of overuse, some injuries, such as complete or partial rupture, are acute. Even so, an acute-on-chronic situation may arise. It is recognized that middle-aged sedentary males are at risk of rupturing their Achilles tendons when undertaking a sudden or unexpected burst of running; it is not always so readily appreciated that recurrent (chronic) stress in the experienced athlete may so undermine the tensile properties of tendon as to result in rupture. Sudden contraction of an already stretched musculotendinous unit may be the final provocative stress. The tensile strength of tendons may also be reduced by steroid injections, which should never be given into weightbearing tendons (see Chapter 12).

Since the musculotendinous unit acts as a united contractile structure, the clinical examination procedures in tendon injury are the same as for muscle injury. Although tendon may heal with conservative measures, there are circumstances (which are identified in the text) when a surgical approach is desirable, not least to allow more accurate approximation of the ruptured ends by evacuation of haemorrhage or granulomatous tissue.

Enthesitis is the term applied to a lesion that occurs at an enthesis—i.e. the teno-osseous junction. Examples of enthesopathies are lateral epicondylitis (tennis elbow), chronic adductor longus strain, and patella tendinitis (jumper's knee) (Fig. 1.9).

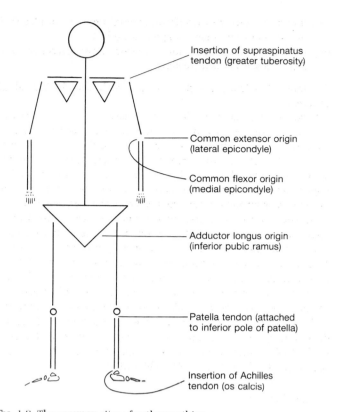

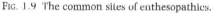

FIG. 1.9 The common sites of enthesopathics.

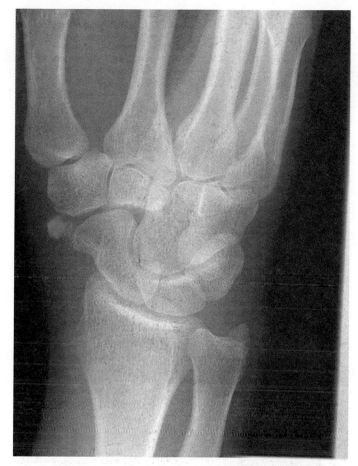

FIG. 1.10 Calcific tendinitis (of the flexor carpi radialis) may be acutely painful.

A *tendinitis* is normally secondary to overuse. It may occur in a tendon that is essentially healthy in other respects, or in one in which a central or focal degenerative process has taken place. Repetitive submaximal loading leads to recurrent microtrauma in the presence of a poor blood supply. Occasionally calcium hydroxyapatite crystals are deposited in a degenerate tendon: the resulting calcific tendinitis may be acutely painful (Fig. 1.10). MRI is a particularly useful investigative tool in the assessment of tendinopathies.

If the tendon has a sheath, a *tenosynovitis* may result from overuse: occasionally this may be crepitating, as in intersection syndrome of the forearm. If the tendon has a paratenon, a *paratendinitis*—for example, Achilles paratendinitis—may develop secondary to an underlying tendinitis, or be caused primarily by friction from extrinsic causes. A complication is the development of chronic paratendinitis, when the paratenon becomes progressively thickened, and may require surgical excision.

Ligament

Ligaments are composed primarily (70–80 per cent) of bundles of collagen, demonstrating a greater 'weave' pattern than tendons which have a similar structure. Ligaments are the 'static' stabilizers of joints, though the presence of elastin (3–5 per cent) allows some elongation under stress. At a certain stress level—the yield point—deformation of collagen fibres becomes excessive, with the formation of microtears and the loss of previous resting length. Frank rupture then occurs. Assessment of ligamentous competence is by stress testing in various positions of the joint. The clinical aspects of ligament injuries are considered in greater detail in the relevant chapters, as they are often assessed inadequately and therefore commonly mismanaged.

Important factors to appreciate following ligament injury are as follows.

1. Joint stability is created by ligaments (the primary or static stabilizers) and muscles (the dynamic stabilizers). A significant degree of ligament rupture may give rise to mechanical instability, incurring the risk of permanent functional instability—for example, ankle and knee ligament tears. Ligament injuries can be divided into three grades of severity:

(a) sprain (grade I), in which there is no macroscopic discontinuity;
(b) partial tear (grade II), in which some degree of joint laxity secondary to ligamentous insufficiency is recognized;
(c) complete tear (grade III), in which dislocation or substantial disruption of the joint occurs (Fig. 1.11).

2. The proprioceptive reflex is usually profoundly deranged as a result of disturbance to or disruption of the articular mechanoreceptors found in the joint capsules and ligaments (Wyke 1972). Specific rehabilitative exercises are required for restoration of function.

3. The capsule of the joint may be irritated, causing capsulitis or synovitis. Such a traumatic synovitis may resolve spontaneously, but it is sometimes prolonged, again requiring specific treatment.

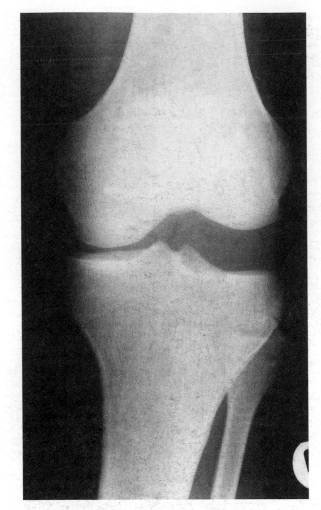

FIG. 1.11 A complete (grade III) tear of the lateral ligamentous complex of the knee is demonstrated on a varus stress test.

4. Capsular disruption may occur, resulting in substantial soft-tissue bleeding and oedema.

5. Intracapsular bleeding (that is, bleeding within an intact capsule) may take place—for instance, rupture of the anterior cruciate ligament, in which situation the resulting haemarthrosis must be recognized and dealt with by aspiration or washing out so as to reduce the severely irritating effect of blood on the synovium. A haemarthrosis may be suspected when a joint swells substantially within a couple of hours of the injury. A serous effusion, on the other hand, normally takes twenty-four hours to arise, and thus is usually recognized by the patient the following day. A haemarthrosis may develop in any joint; beneficial results of aspiration may be expected in such joints as the ankle, the elbow, and the interphalangeal joint of the hallux, as well as the knee. The immediate injection of steroid in appropriate dosage, once fracture or osteochondral injury has been excluded, should be considered. For aspiration, it is essential to have a sound knowledge of topical anatomy.

6. Disorganization of the parallel alignment of collagen fibres and bundles in ligaments occurs after immobilization (for instance in the management of ligament tears). Akeson *et al.* (1987) have summarized the *biomechanical and biochemical* effects as follows.

Biomechanical	(a) increased deformation with a standard load (greater compliance);
	(b) failure at a lower load and reduced energy-absorbing capability of the immobilized bone–ligament complex (at which destruction of fibres occurs).
Biochemical	(c) effects on collagen: reduced mass, increased turnover, increased degradation rate, increased synthesis, increased reducible collagen, and crosslinks.

Management strategies that are consequent upon exact diagnoses are outlined in the relevant chapters: the accepted procedure for grade I sprains is *early mobilization*, so that adequate function may be restored rapidly, often inside ten days. An important distinction in ligament injuries is between joint stability and instability, thereby determining the need for functional support during healing. The use of cast-bracing (hinged cast) techniques may be appropriate in the management of certain grade II/III lower-limb ligament injuries.

Joint

The capsular pattern

The soft tissue components of a joint are the synovium and capsule (strengthened by ligaments that have a close anatomical relationship). When a joint is injured or inflamed from whatever cause, its movements are restricted, initially from involuntary muscle spasms, in a *capsular pattern*. Capsular patterns vary from one joint to another, though they are identical from one person to another, and are described in the relevant chapters. The same pattern is produced by different stressors—for example, synovial irritation from a haemarthrosis, rheumatological conditions such as rheumatoid arthritis, crystal arthropathies, or osteoarthrosis (OA). In some conditions, such as adhesive capsulitis of the shoulder, the restricted movements are due to capsular contracture. If the passive movements are restricted in a *non-capsular pattern*, the possibility of intra-articular derangement arises; otherwise the periarticular structures are at fault.

Synovitis. A synovial reaction may be secondary to injury such as a ligament tear or a meniscus tear when it is associated with a serous effusion. Alternatively, a serous effusion, accompanied by synovial thickening, may be due to a rheumatological condition. Rheumatological screening is described in Chapter 10. Synovial irritation *per se* gives rise to the capsular pattern of restriction of movement. However, if synovitis is secondary to a mechanical derangement, such as a prolapsed meniscus or an intra-articular loose body, the signs resulting from the locked joint (a non-capsular pattern) will prevail.

Osteoarthrosis (OA). Degenerative joint disease should be included in the differential diagnosis when the capsular pattern exists from the fourth decade onwards. The hips and knees are predominantly affected following years of competition in contact sports such as soccer. Although less common, OA of the upper-limb joints may be secondary to previous fracture, or due to repeated joint-loading—for instance, from weight-lifting (see Fig. 4.5, p. 63).

Hypermobility

Although several terms are used in an interchangeable fashion, it is conventional to accept the following:

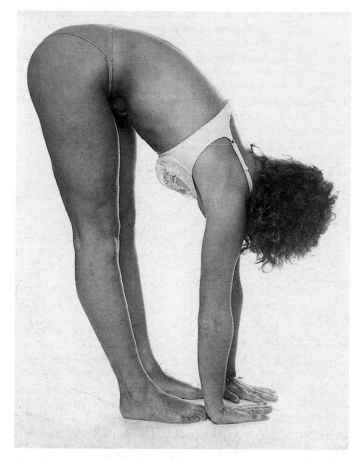

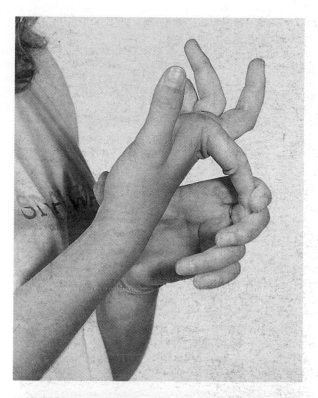

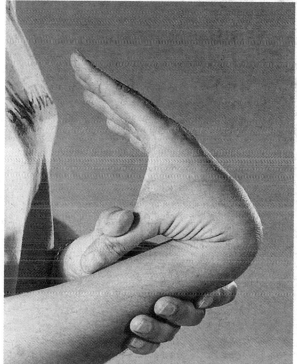

FIG. 1.12 Generalized joint hypermobility is associated with an increased incidence of injury and osteoarthrosis in later life.

flexibility refers to a joint's range of motion—that is, it is principally a function of muscle/tendon tightness;

laxity refers to joint distraction and shear—that is, it is a function of ligamentous competence;

hypermobility refers to generalized joint laxity (Fig. 1.12).

Hypermobility may be associated with connective tissue disorders such as Ehlers–Danlos and Marfan's syndromes. Even with no connective tissue disorder, it is clear that some individuals have an inherited joint laxity. Although, at first sight, this would appear to be beneficial in, for example, gymnastics and dance disciplines such as classical ballet, there is an increased incidence of injury and osteoarthrosis in later life (Nicholas 1970; Bird *et al.* 1978; Scott *et al.* 1979). Increased flexibility, resulting from training, may be best demonstrated by the ability to flex the spine and place the palms of the hands on the floor. Other hypermobile joints (for example, 'back-knee' and hyperextension of the elbows) would not appear to be due to training, and only result from genetic disposition or, in some cases, injury.

The Beighton and Horan (1970) modification of the Carter and Wilkinson (1964) index is often used (a score of 4 points or more indicates hypermobility):

1. Passive dorsiflexion of the little finger beyond 90°—2 points.
2. Passive apposition of thumbs to flexor aspects of the forearm—2 points.
3. Hyperextension of elbows beyond 10°—2 points.
4. Hyperextension of knees beyond 10°—2 points.
5. Forward flexion of the trunk with knees extended so that the palms rest flat on the floor immediately in front of the toes—1 point.

(Total = maximum = 9 points)

Hypomobility

The majority of acute traumatic incidents of all types give rise to local (or segmental) restriction of movement of the nearest joint: differentiation into articular and periarticular (soft tissue) lesions is made by the examination routine already described. The joint-play movements (Zohn and Mennell 1976)—that is, movements that are not under control of the voluntary muscles—perform a particularly useful role in the diagnosis and rehabilitation of spinal dysfunction. Peripheral joint dysfunction—that which is secondary to trauma or immobilization, for instance—also gives rise to loss of joint play.

Subluxation and dislocation

When distortion of the alignment of the opposing joint surfaces results from stress applied to a joint, subluxation occurs. Often this is transient, though it indicates weakness of the surrounding structures or abnormal biomechanical stress and therefore may be recurrent. When gross distortion of alignment takes place, dislocation occurs. This inevitably indicates rupture of the joint capsule, and possibly of the reinforcing ligaments. Apart from the sternoclavicular and acromioclavicular joints (in which reduction of subluxations and dislocations is not usually undertaken), manual relocation is necessary for a dislocated joint that does not reduce spontaneously. If ligaments have been disrupted, these must then be treated.

Bone

The application of force to a joint or limb may give rise to *osseous* injury, either at the point of impact or some distance away; hence the fractures that occur around the ankle on rotating the leg on a fixed foot, fracture of the scaphoid on forced dorsiflexion of the wrist, and fracture of the clavicle on falling on the outstretched hand. Although management of major fractures lies within the province of the orthopaedic surgeon, the simpler fractures, often not requiring fixation, are described in the relevant chapters. Guidance is also offered concerning the timely referral of injuries, such as hand fractures, which require particularly good functional results.

In children, fractures often occur at the *epiphyseal* (growth) *plate*, which is responsible for longitudinal growth of the bone, and is weaker than both ligaments and tendons. Of course, the presence of angulation suggests the presence of a fracture, possibly epiphyseal, and indicates the need for referral; the possibility of epiphyseal fracture should also be considered in the absence of significant deformity when a dislocation or even a sprain is diagnosed. Fractures involving the epiphyseal plate have been categorized into five types by Salter and Harris (1963). Separations usually heal satisfactorily unless there is vascular disturbance (for instance, at the upper femoral epiphysis, when avascular necrosis may occur). Fractures across the plate need careful assessment by an orthopaedic surgeon, as premature fusion and a shortened limb may result.

Traction injuries, sometimes termed traction osteochondroses, occur at the *apophyses*. These are a particularly common type of stress injury in the adolescent—for instance, at the tibial tubercle (Osgood–Schlatter's disease) and os calcis (Sever's disease): they result from overactivity. At some sites around the pelvis— for example, the anterior superior iliac spine, the anterior inferior iliac spine, the lesser trochanter, and the ischial tuberosity—the injury to the apophysis may be due to acute (indirect) trauma. Fracture separation of the apophysis takes place, and the injury behaves effectively as an acute muscle tear, which is its counterpart in the adult (Fig. 1.13). Rarely, a similar injury occurs at the shoulder, for example avulsion of the subscapularis attachment to the lesser tuberosity (Fig. 1.14).

Stress fractures result from the application of repetitive stress to bone. During endurance activities, bone increases in strength by constant remodelling. This response to loading may become inadequate, however. Two theories are propounded. In one it is suggested that, as muscles fatigue during repeated endurance activities, the subsequent loss of shock absorption results in the application of increased stress to bone. In the other, it is thought that repeated muscle activity itself creates increased stress on bone. Examples in weightbearing bones are commonly quoted— for example, femur, tibia, fibula, and metatarsal (Fig. 1.15; see also Fig. 10.10, p. 184). Stress fractures may also occur in non-weightbearing bones, such as the humerus in baseball pitchers and the ribs in rowers. They may also occur at epiphyseal plates—for instance, at the distal radius in gymnasts (Fig. 4.7, p. 66).

Bursa

Bursae are synovial lined sacs whose function is to reduce friction between tendon and bone, or between skin and bone. Direct, particularly repetitive, trauma may give rise to inflammation (bursitis) in the more superficial bursae—for example, olecranon bursitis, prepatellar bursitis ('beat knee'), and postcalcaneal bursitis ('pump-bump'). Alternatively, overuse of the overlying tendon (or tract) may result in a chronic bursitis due to excessive friction—for example, trochanteric bursitis and iliotibial tract syndrome. In some situations, the aetiology of bursitis may be multifactorial—for instance, the effects of rotator cuff degeneration and attrition under the coracoacromial arch on the development of subacromial bursitis (see Figs 3.7 and 3.8, p. 41). Bursae are also a common site of soft tissue inflammation in such rheumatological conditions as gout or Reiter's syndrome.

Cartilage

The articular surfaces of joints with a wide range of movement are composed of hyaline cartilage. Intervertebral discs and intra-articular menisci contain fibrocartilage. *Chondral injury* (involving articular cartilage) or *osteochondral* injury (also involving the adjacent subchondral bone) occurs after jarring or compression. Common sites are the ankle, knee, and elbow. There may be a history of acute trauma when an initial haemarthrosis (which may be unrecognized as such) is followed by recurrent pain and swelling as one articular surface impinges on another; there is a further possibility of loose body formation resulting in temporary locking of the joint (Fig. 1.16). An acute jarring injury to the ankle may cause an osteochondral fracture of the dome of the talus. During patella dislocation, an osteochondral fracture involving the posterior surface of the patella is to be expected (see Fig. 10.16, p. 187). Although there is dispute over the aetiology of *osteochondritis dissecans*, this condition, which commonly occurs in the teenager, may be due to recurrent compression trauma resulting in osteochondral fragmentation and separation. Frequent compression secondary to valgus strain is responsible for osteochondritis of the capitellum at the elbow in gymnasts and baseball pitchers (see Figs 4.3 and 4.4, pp. 60 and 62).

Articular cartilage is nourished by synovial fluid, which appears to be dependent upon joint motion for normal function.

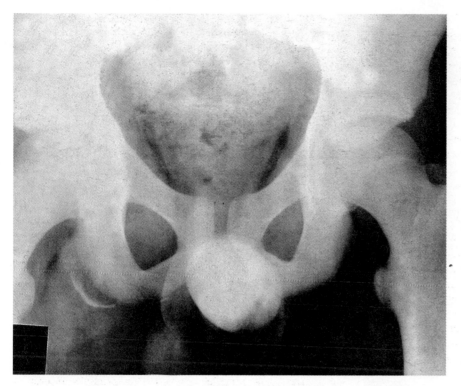

FIG. 1.13 Fracture separation of the ischial apophysis in an adolescent is equivalent to a hamstring muscle tear in an adult.

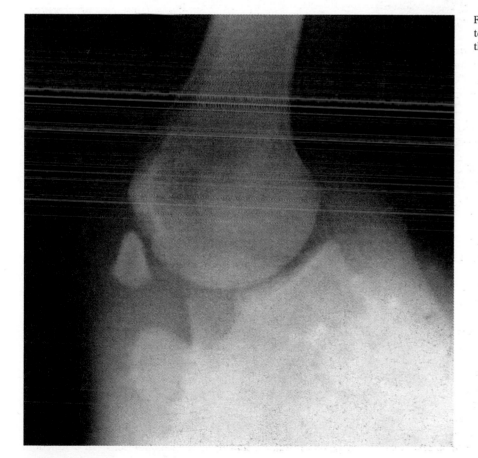

FIG. 1.14 Avulsion of the subscapularis attachment to the lesser tuberosity of the humerus is shown on this teenager's X-ray.

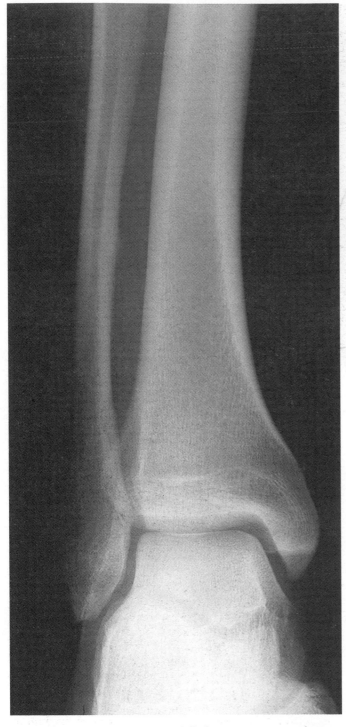

Fig. 1.15 Stress fracture of the distal fibula: a common type of overuse injury in the leg.

Degenerative changes, including erosions, may be seen in articular cartilage following prolonged immobilization.

Prolapse of an intervertebral disc occurs when the gelatinous nucleus pulposus herniates through a ruptured annulus. Previous stress changes will probably have already occurred at the disc, manifesting as small radial tears, so that the provocative traumatic incident may be apparently trivial or even not recorded at all ('the straw that breaks the camel's back').

Meniscus injury at the knee is considered in Chapter 7. The menisci which are present in other joints—for instance, the acromioclavicular and radiocarpal joints—may also be deranged by trauma.

Nerve

Nerve entrapment may result from overuse. Both the sensory and motor components of the larger-diameter myelinated fibres in peripheral nerves may be damaged by compression. A potentially reversible neuropraxia is the type of neuropathy found in the carpal tunnel and tarsal tunnel syndromes, in which entrapment occurs beneath an inflexible retinaculum. In other situations, such as compression of either the radial or median nerves in the proximal forearm of weight-lifters and rowers, entrapment results from muscular hypertrophy. Alternatively, direct pressure may be responsible for such conditions as 'handlebar palsy' (compression of the ulnar nerve in Guyon's canal at the wrist) and acute compartment syndromes in the lower leg, affecting either the deep or superficial peroneal nerves. Spinal nerve roots may be compressed by intervertebral disc prolapse, by lateral recess stenosis (as a consequence of bony hypertrophy) or from an inflammatory reaction within the spinal canal that is secondary to trauma or overuse (see Fig. 5.6, p. 92).

Aetiological factors in overuse injury

Aetiological factors *must* be sought in every case of overuse injury. They can be categorized as follows.

1. Inadequate training schedules:
   (a) intensity;
   (b) frequency;
   (c) overall loading;
   (d) associated physiological fitness characteristics.
2. Training surfaces, for example tarmac, tartan, flooring (sprung or otherwise), canted, uneven.
3. Equipment, for instance the suitability of footwear or protective devices.
4. Biomechanics:
   (a) technique;
   (b) joint mobility;
   (c) musculotendinous balance and adequacy;
   (d) inequality of limb length;
   (e) malalignment.
5. Growth factors in children, such as size by size rather than age by age matching in contact sports, bone–muscle length ratios.

Examples are legion, and will be described in the subsequent chapters. Liaison with parent, coach, or trainer is often necessary. Repeated reassessment may reveal clues not evident on the patient's first visit. Other evidence—derived, for example, from video recording or treadmill running—may be required. Examination of footwear or equipment, as well as the patient, is advisable. Examination of the musculoskeletal system some distance away from the injured site is mandatory; an obvious example in distance running, for instance, is the study of foot biomechanics (pronation, etc.) when faced with a presentation of low back or limb pain. Finally it must be remembered that slowly progressive pain may indicate more serious pathology. From time to time, osteoid osteoma presents in a fashion similar

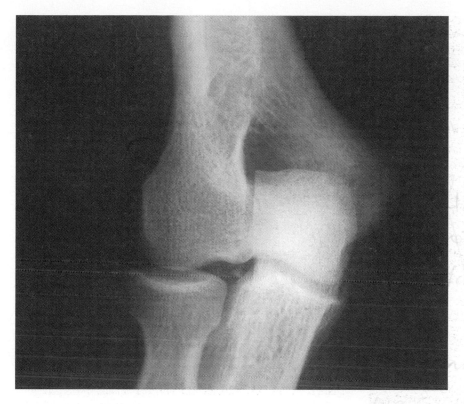

FIG. 1.16 A loose body in the elbow joint may give rise to recurrent pain, swelling (effusion), and locking.

to a stress fracture (see Fig. 10.14, p. 186); metastatic deposits may present as restriction of joint movement.

A 'philosophy'

An adequate history is important in orthopaedic and sports medicine. Cyriax taught that many diagnoses should be strongly suspected from the history alone. To balance this view, it is not unusual for atypical presentations to occur—perspicacity is required. Furthermore, the subjective description of pain has little discriminative validity: behavioural responses may be perceived as a better guide to disability. (It should be remembered however that disability is essentially behavioural, whereas "impairment" demands greater objectivity.). Frustratingly, in many overuse injuries there may be a paucity of physical signs; re-examination of the patient when the affected area is subjected to stress—for instance, measurement of compartment pressures in the lower leg immediately after exercise—may be required to establish the diagnosis. More refined investigations, such as CT or MRI scanning, may be necessary.

That there is an art to learning and to the practical application of knowledge is not an original concept. However, it is as applicable to assessment of sports injuries as it is in other fields. Just as the medical student attempting final MB understands the need for a sound written and practical examination technique to provide the examiner with evidence of his clarity of thought, so the practising physician requires the logical application of functional anatomy and biomechanics (allied to sports techniques) for the purpose of correct diagnosis and management. All too often these basic principles are forgotten. When the physician is faced with a history of localized pain, 'hands-on' palpatory techniques in the painful area are employed too often and too

rapidly without due attention either to history (the patient often supplies both diagnosis and aetiological factors if given the chance) or to the functioning both of the structure containing the lesion and of the musculoskeletal system adjacent to the lesion. Using by way of illustration the distribution of C5 pain, this is felt in the upper arm, particularly in the region of the deltoid insertion, and often radiates to the radial border of the wrist. Deltoid lesions may be incorrectly diagnosed (they are extremely rare), and useless injections given to the site of the pain. However, functional assessment of the cervical spine and shoulder will reveal the real *site* of the lesion, which may be found, for instance, in the neck, causing nerve-root pressure, or in the shoulder joint, causing referred C5 dermatomal pain. Given the opportunity, the patient may recall the neck stiffness and pain which had been temporarily forgotten when the presentation was of persistent arm pain. The pathological lesion may then be treated appropriately.

Furthermore, problem solving should relate to the likely sequelae if an injury should be misdiagnosed or mistreated. The simple (stable) ankle sprain, involving the lateral collateral ligament of the ankle, may give rise to greater problems from an overcautious approach that incorporates immobilization, thus increasing proprioceptive deficit, than from early mobilization; a discriminating functional assessment is a prerequisite (see Chapter 8). Although functional stability, provided by external or internal splintage, is required when acute bony or ligamentous instability is identified, early joint mobilization is still desirable. Bone has an excellent blood supply and therefore may be expected to heal well. However, management of the less well-vascularized soft tissues, particularly ligaments and tendons, requires sensitive judgement. The capsule, articular cartilage, and surrounding muscle react adversely to immobilization, while ligament requires suitable apposition if ruptured. Ligament heals in a more physiological fashion—that is, with parallel rather than haphazard collagen deposition—if the joint is allowed some degree of natural movement *during* healing: hence the frequent reference to cast-bracing techniques for the weightbearing joints of the lower limbs. In this way, muscle tone and articular cartilage nutrition are also maintained.

Overall, whatever tissue has been damaged, the desired primary objective is restoration of normal joint function.

The responsibility of the sports physician in advising and assessing potential participants in different sporting activities receives special attention in subsequent chapters. The popularity of certain endurance activities practised for aerobic fitness, such as long-distance running, is directly proportional to the incidence of overuse injury. The injuries sustained, however, are usually only temporarily disabling, and as far as is known do not appear to cause those degenerative joint conditions in the lower limb associated with years of participation in sports, such as soccer, which involve greater shearing forces. Endurance events such as marathon runs and competitive squash games place substantial demands on competitors' cardiovascular and other physiological resources: screening procedures, although considered contentious because of their time-consuming and often financially unrewarding nature, should be invoked whenever possible. Furthermore, sports physicians, in conjunction with sports associations, should be prepared to advise individuals and sports clubs on the inherent dangers relating to their particular sport. This responsibility extends to the provision of suitable first-aid facilities, and early management of injury advice to teachers, coaches, and trainers.

Prevention of injury is a major topic, which is explored in detail in Chapter 11.

References

Akeson, W. H., Amiel, D., Abel, M. F., Garfin, S. R., and Woo, S. L. Y. (1987). Effects of immobilisation on joints. *Clin. Orthop. Relat. Res.*, **219** (June), 28–37.

Anderson, N. H. and Ramwell, P. W. (1974). Biological aspects of prostaglandins. *Arch. Intern. Med.*, **133**, 30–50.

Beighton, P. H. and Horan, F. T. (1970). Dominant inheritance of familial generalised articular hypermobility. *J. Bone Jt. Surg.*, **52B**, 145–7.

Bird, H. A., Tribe, C. R., and Bacon, P. A. (1978). Joint hypermobility leading to osteoarthrosis and chondrocalcinosis. *Ann. Rheum. Dis.*, **37**, 203–11.

Carter, C. and Wilkinson, J. (1964). Persistent joint laxity and congenital dislocation of the hip. *J. Bone Jt. Surg.*, **46B**, 40–5.

Cyriax, J. (1982). *Textbook of orthopaedic medicine* Vol. I: *Diagnosis of soft tissue lesions* (8th edn). Baillière Tindall, London.

Dyson, M. (1987). Mechanisms involved in therapeutic ultrasound. *Physiotherapy*, **73** (3), 116–20.

Medoff, R. J. (1987). Soft tissue healing. *Ann. Sports Med.*, **3**(2), 67–70.

Nicholas, J. A. (1970). Injuries to knee ligaments, *J. Am. Med. Assoc.*, **212**, 2236–9.

Noyes, F. R., Torvik, P. J., Hyde, W. B. *et al.* (1974). Biomechanics of ligament failure II. An analysis of immobilisation, exercise and reconditioning effects in primates. *J. Bone Jt. Surg.*, **56A**, 1406–18.

Salter, R. B. and Harris, R. (1963). Injuries involving the epiphyseal plate. *J. Bone Jt. Surg.*, **45A**, 587–622.

Scott, D., Bird, H. A., and Wright, V. (1979). Joint laxity leading to osteoarthrosis. *Rheum. Rehabil.*, **18**, 167–9.

Shorten, M. (1987). Muscle elasticity and human performance. In *Medicine and sports science*, Vol. 25, *Current research in sports biomechanics*, pp. 1–18. Karger, Basel.

Wyke, B. (1972). Articular neurology—a review. *Physiotherapy*, **58** (3), 94–9.

Zohn, D. A. and Mennell, J. McM. (1976). *Diagnosis and physical treatment: musculoskeletal pain.* Little, Brown, Boston, MA.

2 Head injuries

J. L. FIRTH AND N. R. GALLOWAY

Intracranial injuries

J. L. FIRTH

With the exception of pugilism, head injury is not an intended objective in sport. As man is his brain, deliberate brain injury cannot reasonably be described as 'sport'. Head injury in sport is therefore unnecessary, and avoidable head injury is unacceptable. A primary objective in sport has to be to eliminate or minimize the opportunities for head injury. This does not have to detract from either the excitement or the enjoyment of sport. Indeed, they can be enhanced. However, it does require those responsible for and participating in sport to have an understanding of the nature of head injury.

Head injury mechanisms

Head injury is the injurious application of energy to the head. The key factor in head injury is brain injury. Brain injury requires the injurious transfer of that energy from head to brain. The three common injury mechanisms are head penetration, deformation, and acceleration.

Penetration

Penetration of the skull by missiles or sharp objects tears the meninges, the membranes covering the brain, and the brain itself, together with their blood vessels.

Deformation

Deformation of the skull causes brain percussion, compression, and mechanical distortion of the brain, as well as skull fracture, which may disrupt the meninges and strip the dura (the brain's tough outermost covering membrane) from the inner surface of the skull. Skull fractures may be 'undisplaced' or 'depressed'. In depressed fractures, shattered bone is driven into the head, reducing its overall volume, deforming and tearing brain and its covering meninges together with their arteries, veins, and the large dural venous channels, the venous sinuses.

Bleeding from these vessels leads to blood clot formation between the dura and the skull (extradural haemorrhage and haematoma). Expanding clots (see Fig. 10.21, p. 189) in their turn distort and displace the brain, and by so doing abolish its ability to control its own blood flow. This loss of local brain blood flow 'auto-regulation'—the phenomenon of cerebrovascular auto-regulatory failure or 'vasoparesis' (Sheinker 1944;

Langfitt *et al.* 1968; Bruce *et al.* 1981)—combined with a normal or raised blood pressure increases local cerebral blood flow (CBF), enhances local cerebral blood volume (CBV—the volume of blood in the brain at any one instant of time), and causes the brain to swell, compounding the danger posed by expanding clots. A rapid increase in intracranial pressure (ICP) follows within the inexpansile skull. Local brain swelling exacerbates pressure gradients within the head, accelerating brain shift from one side of the head to the other, or down through the tentorial hiatus (between the supratentorial compartment of the skull and the posterior fossa) and on down through the foramen magnum into the spinal canal.

Clots from bleeding in the posterior fossa displace both cerebellum and brain stem up through the tentorial hiatus and medulla and cerebellar tonsils down through the foramen magnum. Brain shift and moulding by being forced down through the tentorial hiatus or foramen magnum leaves the post-mortem appearance of 'coning' (Robbins *et al.* 1984).

Brain stem compression and distortion associated with coning produces a rapid deterioration of conscious level and death, if not immediately reversed. Coning of the medulla through the foramen magnum produces acute respiratory failure and death, often with little warning of impending disaster.

Management of coning is by rapid control of brain bulk, reducing the pathologically enhanced CBF by ventilation and hypocapnia (lowering the arterial paCO$_2$), shrinking the brain with the intravenous osmotic agent mannitol and the prompt surgical evacuation of the clot. Ventilation and clot evacuation are essential. To achieve this in time to save the brain and afford the individual a chance to enjoy their days again requires prior planning, preparation, clinical acumen, and determined, above all rapid, management. Time is the key. Literally a race with death.

The amount of energy required to fracture the skull and set in train these series of events is less than that required to produce unconsciousness (Gurdjian *et al.* 1950). In sport, therefore, any loss of consciousness associated with a head injury, however brief, indicates a significant head insult and a brain injury severe enough to lead to meningeal rupture, haematoma formation, brain swelling, and subsequent fatal deterioration. That this deterioration is reversible and death avoidable enhances the importance of conscious level as the key to head injury management in sport.

This is the basis of the first of the two classical sporting head injury scenarios. Head impact deforms the skull, percussing the brain and tearing meningeal blood vessels. An early recovery is made. The victim recovers, often to apparent normality, only to be overtaken by secondary deterioration as brain swelling complicates the expanding intracranial clot. The temporary improvement is the 'lucid interval'. It lulls all into the false assumption that improvement ensures recovery. The false sense of security given by that false assumption then wastes the very time on which the apparently recovering victim's life depends. Any individual who has been knocked out remains at risk until proved otherwise by continuous expectant observation in hospital.

In practice, the problem on the spot, in playing or sports fields, is that one cannot determine whether or not such a fatal train of events has begun. Conscious level is and has to be the cardinal sign. Its significance has always to be recognized. Once an alteration of consciousness has occurred, that individual merits careful observation in an establishment where appropriate intervention can be undertaken immediately and effectively should secondary deterioration occur. Of this, there can be no question.

Acceleration

Acceleration, the third of the three common head injury mechanisms, is still poorly understood. Debate on its effects has raged since the Paris Academy of 1766. This confusion is compounded by the fact that acceleration acts through a series of further, subsidiary mechanisms. They include:

(1) bridging vessel disruption;
(2) shear;
(3) cavitation.

The brain floats like a gelatinous mushroom in the cerebrospinal fluid (CSF) within the skull. The CSF is contained within the subarachnoid space between arachnoid (the second brain-covering membrane, within the dura) and pia mater (the brain's third membrane, its 'rind'). The brain is anchored imperfectly by its blood vessels and by arachnoidal ligaments, which traverse the subarachnoid space. This anchoring is tightest at the skull base and minimal over the outer surface of the brain. The cerebral hemispheres have considerable freedom of movement from front to back within the head (antero-posteriorly) and vertically along the axis of the brain stem (the 'stalk' of the mushroom).

The injurious force generated by acceleration in any one situation reflects the general equation:

$$F = ma$$

where F = the injurious force available to damage the brain, a = the acceleration associated with the accident, and m = the mass involved, often in sport the head itself.

Acceleration is the key to most sporting head injury. It is the rate of change in the velocity of the head (v) and commonly induced by violent deceleration by head impact. Speed is less important than the actual acceleration imposed ($\emptyset v/t$, the change of head velocity in unit time, where $\emptyset$ is the change in head velocity, and v, in the time during which that change occurs, t). Low speed, immediately halted by impact on a hard surface, can generate greater acceleration than the progressive deceleration from high speed of an individual cocooned in a vehicle with a properly arranged safety cage, occupant location

by five-point harness, helmet use, and airbags and/or cockpit geometry designed to stabilize the helmet and prevent head rotation on the body (adding further radial brain acceleration) whilst extending the time for deceleration during the impact sequence (and hence reducing $\emptyset v/t$ by extending t).

Bridging vessel disruption

Although embryologically 'impossible', aberrant blood vessels frequently run from the surface of the cerebral hemispheres to the overlying dura, traversing the subarachnoid and subdural spaces. These vessels may be arteries or veins. Firmly fixed superficially to the dura and the inner surface of the skull, they are also anchored to the mobile surface of the jelly-like brain. Sudden movement or acceleration of the head induces differential motion between skull and brain. A critical vector, which may not cause unconsciousness, can rupture such a vessel. Bleeding, which may be arterial, then produces a quickly expanding haematoma over the surface of the brain, deep to the dura. The expansion of such a subdural haematoma is rapid. Unlike an extradural haematoma (which has to strip the tough dura off the inside of the skull), subdural haematoma expansion is unhindered by any such constraint. It may follow apparently trivial head injury. Recovery from the immediate effects of head impact is short-lived and followed by rapid, early deterioration into coma and death. Subdural haematomas are more common in the elderly, but may occur at any age and are a plague of boxing. The 90 per cent mortality of acute traumatic subdural haematoma is staggering for a simple and easily treatable condition. They kill by the pace of their expansion, leaving little time for surgical evacuation. The speed of their development is accelerated further by disturbance of CBF and vasoparetic brain swelling. Management of such haematoma is straightforward: immediate ventilation and clot evacuation. However, success requires intervention before irreversible brain infarction has occurred. There is no time for delay. In practice, such simple but essentially rapid surgical intervention is rarely to hand. When available, it is all too often fatally delayed by failure of the attending medical team to recognize the priorities of the situation: ventilation and clot evacuation. Worse still, the victim's attendants may be lulled into a false sense of security by a transient improvement in conscious level or the apparently minor nature of the initial injury.

This produces the second stereotyped sporting fatality. The victim is knocked down, often with no more than an alteration of consciousness, an apparent bewilderment, or 'concussion'. Rapid descent into coma then follows, with prolonged on-the-spot efforts at 'resuscitation', when what is required is immediate ventilation to control brain bulk, combined with a burr hole in the skull to evacuate clot and reduce intracranial pressure ICP, then followed by full evacuation of the subdural clot and control of the bleeding.

In posterior fossa clots, hydrocephalus adds a further hazard. Upward displacement of the midbrain and cerebellum, by the clot, distorts the aqueduct, the narrowest part of the CSF circulatory pathway, and obstructs the CSF circulation. An eventually fatal build-up of pressure behind the obstruction enhances the need for speed once an alteration of conscious level occurs.

Bridging vessel disruption is also a problem in the brain stem. Here it is the long perforating arteries which are at risk. They run back from the basilar artery through the brain stem to the floor of the IVth ventricle. Under vertical acceleration along its long axis, the brain stem acts like a column of gelatin. Head acceleration is transferred to the outside of the column whilst its central core lags behind. Eventually, the core is accelerated, and when the outer surface of the column is halted with the rest of the head, the centre continues to surge along the axis of the previous acceleration, producing the phenomenon of brain-stem 'sleeving' (Lindgren 1966). The effect is to pull the long perforating vessels off their capillary beds. Multiple punctuate brain-stem haemorrhages occur. These are not invariably fatal. However, they give rise to a great variety of symptoms, sometimes with few accompanying objective signs, and are one component of the 'post-traumatic syndrome'.

Shear

Shear is well described by Holbourn (1943) and Stritch (1956, 1961, 1969). As a gelatinous structure under acceleration, the brain's internal complexity induces differential movement between adjacent components, and thereby shear, within the brain itself. The shearing forces so induced disrupt both nerve cell axons (the cells' long processes running within the brain and to and from spinal cord), small blood vessels, and dendrites, the multitude of fine connections between adjacent nerve cells which bristle out from each nerve-cell body. The resulting disruption, which may be cumulative with repeated head insult, can have a catastrophic effect on brain function, yet with little apparent, macroscopic (naked-eye) damage. This was a common finding in multiple, repeated head injury—the 'punch-drunk' traumatic encephalopathy of boxing and the 'lame brain' jockey of the days before a series of mandatory safety improvements (including the wearing of effective head protection to the British Standard Institute's then BS 4472 specification) were introduced to racing under Jockey Club rules (Allen 1976).

Cavitation

Under head acceleration, the gelatinous brain lags behind the skull. It behaves much as coffee in a cup when the cup is struck against a wall. Like the skull, the cup comes to an abrupt halt, but the coffee flows on, raising pressure adjacent to the point of impact causing the coffee to rise up the side of the cup, and to spill out of it. The rising fluid reflects the increased pressure induced under the point of impact. At the other side of the cup the coffee level falls as the coffee flows away towards the impact side. Oscillation then follows.

In the intact head, there is a sharp increase in local pressure under the impact point, producing a local percussion insult to the brain, the 'coup' injury of the French Academy. This may just bruise (contuse) or actually disrupt the brain substance. At the opposite side of the head, pressure falls acutely as the brain moves away. Pressure may fall below the tissue vapour pressure of gases in solution in the intracellular fluid in brain cells, in the extracellular space (which occupies 25 per cent of the brain's volume, between brain cells and their blood vessels), and within the blood vessels themselves. If the pressure drops sufficiently, bubble formation occurs, producing an explosive local decompressive lesion—the phenomenon of 'cavitation', opposite the impact site—the 'contre-coup'.

As a result of any one impact, acceleration insult can cause at least two severe injuries, one at, the other opposite to the impact site. In practice, a blow to the front of the head produces an impact, percussion, coup injury to the frontal poles of the brain and the tips of its temporal lobes. The associated fall in pressure at the back of the head is attenuated, damped by the ability of CSF to move up through the foramen magnum from the elastic spinal thecal sac. (Unlike the dura in the head, which is attached to the inner surface of the skull, the spinal theca covering the spinal cord expands and contracts within the spinal canal with every heart beat, part of the mechanism of the circulation of the CSF.) Frontal impacts therefore produce frontal injury. Brain substance may be blown down the nose, to appear as white material at the nostrils. Conversely, occipital impact injury produces little coup, percussion effect under the impact point at the back of the head, again due to the damping effect of the CSF, now moving out of the head through the foramen magnum. No such damping is available at the anterior end the skull. The contre-coup, cavitation effect on frontal and temporal poles of occipital injury is devastating. As a result, both frontal and occipital impacts produce frontal injury. Both may be exacerbated further by head rotation and radial brain acceleration. Blows to the side of the head—lateral, temporal impact—not only involve the thinnest and most easily fractured part of the skull, with enhanced risk of extradural haematoma formation from tearing of the underlying middle meningeal arteries, but also ensure coup and contre-coup insults to both sides of the brain.

Any head injury involves one or more of these primary mechanisms. In sport, the key is to *recognize the significance of unconsciousness or an alteration in consciousness. It is the threshold of disaster. Once crossed, the need is for speed. Time is now running out before disaster becomes reality.*

Secondary complications

To these primary insult mechanisms are added the secondary complications of intracranial haemorrhage and vasoparetic brain swelling. The latter is also the basis of the 'second impact syndrome (SIS)'. This is the rapidly fatal vasoparetic brain swelling which follows a second, usually trivial further head impact in those who have been knocked out yet allowed to return to the game.

Intracranial haemorrhage

Such bleeding has already been discussed. It may be extradural, subdural, or into bruised, cavitated and disrupted brain to form an intracerebral or intracerebellar haematoma. Such haematomas produce a generalized rise in intracranial pressure, focal brain distortion and shift, and are further complicated by brain swelling.

Brain swelling

As discussed above, post-traumatic brain swelling may complicate head injury on its own or in conjunction with an intracranial haematoma. The swelling is due to loss of the normal auto-regulation of CBF by terminal arterioles. This allows an increase in CBF, an enlarged CBV, and expansion in brain bulk.

Such loss of auto-regulation, or 'vasoparesis', may be induced by the impact itself or by brain compression and distortion by an expanding haematoma. In normal brain, auto-regulation maintains constant blood flow through each capillary bed, despite widely varying changes in systemic arterial blood pressure. Teleologically, with the skull having a fixed capacity, auto-regulation should be the most hardy of all physiological mechanisms. Sadly, one of the many fatal flaws in basic human design and function is that auto-regulation is easily abolished by any brain insult, including head injury.

In practice, loss of cerebral auto-regulation (vasoparesis) (Langfitt et al. 1968) is a major post-traumatic problem in its own right. In the past, only one in three of those who died of head injuries had a blood clot in the head (Miller 1979). The remainder died of raised intracranial pressure from the brain swelling caused by vasoparesis. This brain swelling can be controlled, if caught early enough, by manipulating the other mechanisms which control CBF—notably the brain's carbon dioxide (CO_2) response, the changes in CBF induced by changes in the arterial CO_2 level (the paO_2). Blowing-off CO_2 reduces brain blood flow and bulk. This requires ventilation, if necessary immediately by mouth-to-mouth respiration or by endotrachaeal intubation and mechanical ventilation. The significance of this is that *cardiopulmonary resuscitation should be available at any sports site where head injury may occur, and resuscitation should be part of the basic training of sports organizers, coaches, linesmen, umpires, and officials alike.*

The second impact syndrome, SIS (Saunders and, Harbaugh RE 1984)

Though the subject of debate (Cantu 1998a; McCrory and Berkovic 1998), this is a further manifestation of post-traumatic cerebral vasoparesis. The younger the player, the more likely it is to occur. It represents a hypersensitivity to a second head impact induced by a prior head insult. It may have a migrainous component. Typically, the victim is knocked out but makes a rapid, to all accounts complete, recovery. All are determined to play on, and do. A second head impact occurs, often apparently trivial, but catastrophic in outcome. The individual is either knocked out immediately or exhibits a paradoxical, inappropriately enhanced impairment for so minor an insult. Rapid deterioration then occurs and all attempts at resuscitation fail. Post-mortem examination reveals a grossly swollen brain. Death is due to raised intracranial pressure. Recovery, where achieved, has been associated with immediate ventilation once deterioration follows the second impact. That this has not been universally successful, as would be expected if vasoparesis were the only culprit, suggests that a second mechanism is also triggered by the first head injury. The adverse effect of youth and the often bizarre effects of post-traumatic vasospasm (cerebral blood vessels going into spasm rather than being rendered vasoparetic) in children makes a migrainous component likely, but this has yet to be confirmed. For the moment, recognition of the phenomenon and prevention are the only sure cure. Hence, *sporting policy is that an alteration of consciousness is a death warrant until proven otherwise. Leave the burden of proof to the hospital doctor.*

Other atypical neurological responses to sporting head trauma can occur, as detailed below.

Traumatic vasospasm
The interaction of migraine with head acceleration may produce bizarre symptoms, particularly in the young. Post-traumatic blindness is a terrifying condition in children. Every investigation is normal. A strong family history of migraine is the clue. Only when vision returns spontaneously, often several days later, can the true nature of the individual case be confirmed.

The concussion debate
'Concussion' is best defined as a transient, trauma-induced alteration of mental state that is not necessarily associated with unconsciousness (Kelly et al. 1991). In the literature, it is confused with traumatic coma in severe head injury (Cantu 1992). It may in some cases have a migrainous component or be reflex-based. Whether it is fully reversible is questionable. In practice, it indicates a significant brain insult, possible lasting injury, certain vasoparesis and a potential SIS candidate if exercise is resumed and head impact repeated before all symptoms and signs have cleared. In the author's view, 'concussion' represents a group 3 head injury profile (see below) with its associated hazard of secondary deterioration due to brain swelling, intracranial clot, or both. Rest, recumbency, hospital review, and continuous careful observation are indicated until normalcy is regained and all symptoms have settled.

'Reflex coma'
Facial impact followed by immediate collapse and convulsive movements during a rapid recovery phase is a regular feature of Australian Rules Football. A period of close observation, clearance of all neurological symptoms, and successful completion of a previously practised battery of psychometric tests is taken to indicate sufficient recovery to allow a safe return to the game, often within minutes. The SIS has not been a feature of a sport in which adult professional players are monitored neurologically and psychometrically. The convulsive movements are similar to those seen in critical basal gangliar perfusion and in military aviation during recovery from unconsciousness induced by head-to-foot acceleration in centrifuges (+Gz-induced loss of consciousness, GILOC). It is possible that the instantaneous loss of consciousness is triggered by the same brain stem mechanism that is thought to be responsible for instituting GILOC. The many questions raised by this phenomenon are of undoubted physiological importance. Exercise-induced hyperventilation on returning to a game in which all are continuously engaged at speed may induce sufficient hypocapnia to prevent vasoparetic brain swelling. Though a factor in the debate as to when, after brain insult, it is reasonable to return to sport, the Australian Rules' experience does not provide grounds for relaxation of the implacable attitude to sporting head insult expressed elsewhere in this chapter.

The post-traumatic syndrome
This is a rag-bag term often used to encompass a host of chronic physical, emotional, and psychological symptoms sometimes tinged by litigation. In the sporting world, the syndrome comprises a variable collection of symptoms without signs, each as unique as the individual afflicted. It is an area in which history is paramount. Patterns are discernible. It is important to recognize their origin, however bizarre they may seem. They arise from four principal injury sites:

- frontal lobes
- limbic system
- brain stem
- cervical spine.

The frontal lobes differentiate us from monkeys. They provide the massive reflex base upon which our emotions, personality, and our ability to live sociably in harmony with others depends. Frontal injury may persist as anything from a mild alteration of affect or personality, through humour failure, short temper and intolerance, to incontinence and total asociability. Limbic injury is reflected by continuing memory impairment. Brain stem symptoms, reflecting punctate sleeving injury, range from no more than vague unsteadiness through to vector-related vertigo. Cervical spine injury is both the commonest and the most frequently missed. Current fashionable, slouching, flexed, kyphotic, posture abuses the neck as well as the lumbar spine. Maximum instability is assured together with poor paraspinal tonic musculature and intervertebral discs maintained at the elastic failure boundary of their visco-elastic, hysteretic performance envelope. Athletes are often little better than the general population. Most coaches display little understanding of and less interest in spinal dynamics. All are cervical spinal disasters waiting for a place and time to happen. Cervical injury is maximized, recovery impeded, and chronicity promoted by continued cervical kyphosis: the sporting prodrome of later cervical spondylosis. The answer lies in symptom recognition, determined restoration and then maintenance of lumbar and cervical lordosis, the rebuilding of the tonic paraspinal musculature, and the adoption of habitual lordotic carriage—'Carriage' in the postural sense.

'Head injury is neck injury'
This dictum reflects reality (Schneider 1987) and all head injury should be presumed to be complicated by neck and cervical spinal cord injury until proved otherwise. Even in dedicated head and spinal injury units, neck injury may be difficult to exclude. The hazard that head injury poses to the neck is enhanced by the wearing of helmets and is maximal in the young.

Children are at particular risk from a combination of factors. The anatomy of the paediatric cervical spine with near horizontal facet joints, lax soft tissues, the carriage of a large head on a relatively small body imposing greater head–neck dynamic ratios, inexperience, poor balance, and reckless enthusiasm ratios mean that neck dislocation with spontaneous reduction is a constant hazard. They combine to ensure that apparently minor head injuries can cause cervical cord insult, yet without neck pain and with no more than transient sensory symptoms in limbs and trunk. *A child who complains of 'pins and needles' or any other symptoms in arms, trunk, or legs following injury should be assumed to have sustained a spinal cord insult with established spinal cord vasoparesis.* The child should be managed flat, with the neck stabilized until appropriate assessment can be made by a competent practitioner. In all cases of potential head and therefore spinal injury, the child should be questioned for any sensory or motor disturbance, however transient. Again presume cord injury until proved otherwise. It may be all too tragically obvious if the child or athlete is rendered immediately tetraplegic. However, they may report symptoms of spinal cord percussion, often with no more than transient weakness or 'pins and needles' (paraesthesiae), which are then ignored, the child being allowed to continue standing or even competing until spinal cord infarction occurs

The spinal cord is rendered vasoparetic by percussion, exactly like the brain. To compound the hazard, the sympathetic system running within the cervical spinal cord is damaged, rendering the individual 'sympathoparetic' and no longer able to maintain normal blood pressure. If the initial symptoms are not reported, or are unsought, overlooked, or dismissed, the result is secondary, delayed spinal cord infarction. The cord microcirculation is deprived of its ability to auto-regulate and maintain spinal cord blood flow at low blood pressures. The cord itself suffers

irreversible stroke due to the reduction of its blood supply and obstruction of its venous drainage as the ischaemic cord swells within its tight dural envelope. The individual is left tetraplegic, paralysed in all four limbs and unlikely to be able to breath adequately, adding further insult to the spinal cord. The window of therapeutic opportunity has very nearly closed by this stage. Recumbency (lying horizontal) and stabilization to optimize cord perfusion, ventilation to exploit the CO_2 effect on the cord circulation, mannitol to reduce ischaemic oedema, and steroids within 45 minutes of insult may yet reverse the situation, but are rarely instituted in time. The best treatment remains recognition of the hazard and its prevention. As in prevention of head injury in general, so in neck injury prevention is the first priority. When that has failed and head and actual or potential neck injury has occurred, then presumption of an unstable spinal cord injury is mandatory. One-third of spinal cord injuries are complete and irrecoverable from the moment of injury, but two-thirds are not and can recover if further damage and secondary ischaemic insult is avoided. The greatest care has therefore to be exercized in moving, observing, and transporting head and spinal injuries because of the probability of further spinal cord insult by the injudicious or thoughtless distortion of an unstable neck or spine. Horizontal management with neck stabilization and ABC—Airway, Breathing, Circulation—is obligatory.

Secondary injury
Whilst mechanical injury to the spinal cord is easy to understand, much attention is being paid to episodes of hypotension and hypoxia adding further additional injury to the initial brain injuries and their complications. That these occur is indubitable. They pose an additional challenge to maintain continuous optimized care in serious head injury and emphasize the immediate and continuing importance of ABC from the moment of injury onwards.

Tertiary problems

A further series of complications provide a 'third row' to the scrum of complications of head injury. They may be early or late. They include the following.

(i) Hydrocephaly: acute hydrocephalus in posterior fossa lesions, late post-traumatic hydrocephalus, and the phenomenon of post-traumatic encephalopathy and cerebral atrophy which may be difficult to distinguish from a treatable hydrocephalus.

(ii) Epilepsy: seizure on head impact, the exacerbation of a prior epileptic trait or later epilepsy in cerebral contusion, haematoma, and skull fracture.

(iii) CSF leakage in basal skull fractures with CSF rhinorrhoea—CSF running down the back of the nose—with later infection, i.e. meningitis

(iv) Infection: either early or late from the injection of infected material at injury, or the infection of subsequent intervention.

Cerebrospinal fluid rhinorrhoea and hydrocephalus

CSF leakage (tasting like sea water dribbling down the back of the nose), infection, and hydrocephalus are beyond the scope of this chapter and properly the business of the hospital doctor. That they have been excluded before a return to sport is made is the reasonable concern of the sporting discipline and their medical attendants and advisors. Exclusion is part of the clearance back to participation by personal physician or specialist review. That clearance is essential before flying. CSF leak may be accompanied by air entry into the head and the formation of an aerocoele, the effects of which can be exacerbated by ascent to altitude (typically to a cabin altitude of 8000 feet in commercial airline practice). Air in the head can be excluded by a simple horizontal ray lateral X-ray of the head. Any suggestion of CSF leak, hydrocephalus, or air in the head (aerencephaly) warrants neurosurgical review.

Post-traumatic epilepsy

'Epilepsy' is the likely spontaneous recurrence of seizure in an individual. That individual can in every other way be normal and meritorious, like Alexander, Julius Caesar, or Napoleon, engaging normally and competitively in sport. Epilepsy can be caused, exacerbated, or elicited by sporting head injury. It does therefore merit consideration. A family history of epilepsy or febrile convulsions under the age of five years doubles the risk of post-traumatic seizure should head injury occur. A past history of seizure enhances the likelihood of seizure complicating sport, usually on relaxation after effort. Someone subject to seizures should consult their neurologist before engaging in contact sports. All should know the essential management of convulsion: clear and maintain the airway. If there is no question of head and neck injury they should be rolled into the recovery position and the patency of the airway maintained until recovery from the seizure occurs. Exercise should not be resumed until the individual's general medical practitioner is satisfied that it is safe to do so.

Post-traumatic epilepsy may be:

(i) 'Immediate' or impact epilepsy: immediate seizure-like movements on head impact is not uncommon. They are a feature of Australian Rules Football, where they merit special attention. In general sporting practice, they indicate a significant brain insult and that the conscious level threshold for major mischief has been exceeded. Despite this they do not introduce a significant risk of later post-traumatic epilepsy.

(ii) 'Early' post-traumatic epilepsy: seizure at any time following immediate impact during the first week following injury. Such early epilepsy indicates a 25 per cent chance of later post-traumatic epilepsy.

(iii) 'Late' post-traumatic epilepsy: epilepsy related to a head injury but occurring more than one week from insult. This is similar to late-onset epilepsy in the general, non-traumatic population. It implies a risk of further seizure of at least 16 per cent and potentially an up to 65 per cent risk of long-term epilepsy. The risks of late post-traumatic epilepsy are increased by several risk factors associated with the head injury itself.

1. Early epilepsy (25 per cent late epilepsy, as above).
2. Clinically significant intracranial haematoma (30 per cent).
3. Depressed skull fracture (6–66 per cent). The range of risks posed by a depressed skull fracture is due to the influence of four further factors

   - the occurrence of early epilepsy,
   - focal cerebral hemispheric signs,
   - a demonstrated tear in the dura covering the brain, and
   - a post-traumatic amnesic interval (period of lost memory following injury) of more than 24 hours (Jennett 1975).

Post-traumatic encephalopathy

The term 'post-traumatic encephalopathy' (PTE) covers a number of evils. Strictly, it is a post-mortem, pathological diagnosis and the result of multiple, repeated head injuries with widespread shearing damage to the brain. Clinically, it is an alternative term for 'punch-drunkenness' in boxers and the 'lame brains' once seen in professional jockeys after a career of falls (Foster et al. 1976). It is also used to describe incomplete recovery from severe injury. Each individual case needs careful evaluation to exclude a remediable cause, of which post-traumatic hydrocephaly, due to a late CSF resorption block at the arachnoidal level or from basal CSF cistern occlusion, is amenable to CSF diversion or 'shunting'.

The present concern for medical advisors and selectors alike is whether a previous head injury places a particular individual at enhanced risk of later PTE. Head injury is cumulative, but the literature is scant, and one is often faced with the denial of enthusiasm by questionable good sense. The primacy of intellect in present society and economics has to bias decision and advise on the side of caution and the pursuit of other laudable aims.

Prevention

This litany of potential disaster emphasizes the first law of head injury—'Prevention is better than cure'. All sports disciplines need to review their practice continuously, to define the present incidence and risk of head injury, and to develop their sports either to exclude or at least to minimize these risks. Sadly, accidents may still happen despite every best endeavour.

Protection

The second law of head injury is therefore—'If you can't prevent, protect'. The place of head protection should be reviewed carefully and appropriate head protection worn at all times when the individual is at risk. A cavalier attitude to head injury is inappropriate in today's world, where all have to live by their brains. Likewise, an irresponsible attitude to prevention and protection is likely to not only to bring sport into disrepute—as with American College Football when it was nearly banned by law for the slaughter occasioned in the days of Theodore Roosevelt's presidency—but also to attract the attention of lawyers well practised in the extraction of punitive damages from those ignoring simple precautions (Davis and McKelvey 1998).

Major strides have been and continue to be made in head protection (Firth 1994). Where a discipline is such that head injury remains a major hazard, then full advantage should be taken of present progress, such as the wearing of protective helmets to the British Standards Institution's PAS 015 in riding. No specifications are perfect, but they reflect the state of the art and are therefore the minimum acceptable in sporting activities.

In sport, no head injury is necessary; all head injury is potentially preventable, and therefore any head injury has to be unacceptable. To be effective, protective helmets have to form one unit with the head and skull at impact. Any relative motion between helmet and head may actually exacerbate injury and degrade the helmet's protective performance. Most helmets have an outer shape to provide aesthetic appeal, either a 'hide' or, in riding, 'silk'. Within this is a hard smooth shell to prevent skull penetration and deformation and to facilitate the sliding of the helmet along surfaces so as to extend the period of deceleration. Within this 'shell' is an energy-burning, acceleration-attenuating 'liner'—either an air gap or a 'buffer' material which dissipates energy as it deforms, extending the time of the deceleration. An air gap is a time-honoured solution to the requirement for energy dissipation, but it depends for its effectiveness on a very precise relationship between head and shell, with accurate separation of both by a critical margin. This must be checked every time that the hat is put on. Buffer materials act by absorbing energy by their own progressive deformation or destruction. They have made possible major improvements in helmet performance. However, once deformed, the buffer's effectiveness is destroyed and the helmet has to be replaced. It will no longer protect from acceleration if subjected to a further insult. Within the buffer or air-gap zone is the 'harness', 'cradle', or suspension, which provides the interface between head and helmet. It has to fit snugly, firmly, comfortably, and coolly. It has to ensure that the helmet remains in place under any condition of acceleration, head movement, and impact. It must not be displaced axially or in pitch, roll, or yaw. To maintain head helmet geometry under acceleration usually requires a four-point fixation system, with a chin strap. Stabilization forwards and backwards in the sagittal plane conventionally requires two fixation points: one on either side of the head, four in all. Simple two-point chin straps, even incorporated in complex 'full-face' helmets, still allow helmet loss or separation in violent conditions of head pitch and sagittal plane radial head acceleration, a persisting hazard in motor cycle racing. In single-seat, Formula 1 motor racing, the only satisfactory arrangement to date has been to position the body accurately within a safety cage, using a five point harness and arrange the helmet–cockpit sill geometry to allow vision over the sill during normal racing operation but voluntary or involuntary arrest and stabilization of the helmet on and by the sill margin in case of an accident. This maintains both head and helmet position, extends the head deceleration interval and, thereby $\partial v/t$, by progressive destruction of the fuselage about the safety cage. Finally, radial brain acceleration and cervical spine insult are minimized by prevention of head flailing about the stabilized driver's body. Similar measures have been adopted in aerobatic aircraft, but helmeted head stabilization remains a major challenge in many disciplines.

The basic requirements for helmet systems are that they should be:

(1) aesthetically attractive, so that all will want to wear them;
(2) mechanically and dynamically effective;
(3) comfortable, cool, and of light weight;
(4) easily, effectively, and conveniently secured, removed, and stored
(5) not liable to exacerbate other injury, for instance to the cervical spine, nor introduce new hazards of their own (Firth 1985).

That these criteria can be met was demonstrated in the commercial introduction of motor cycle 'space helmets'. The success of this basic design as a fashion object can and should be emulated in other sporting disciplines where head protection is appropriate, particularly in horse-riding. Any device should comply with the appropriate published British Standards Institution, European, US or Australasian specifications to ensure minimum protective performance.

Management strategies

The First Law is to PREVENT. If this fails, the Second Law is to PROTECT. If this also fails, the Third Law is to PREPARE for head and spinal injury, that is, prudent preparation following appropriate assessment of the potential for head injury and disaster posed by each sporting discipline. Given such preparation, then careful management can minimize or exclude the secondary and later effects of the head injury, should such an accident occur. In effect, the Third Law of head injury is 'Prepare for the worst, work for the best'.

Having failed to prevent the head injury and then to protect the brain, initial assessment is the basis for subsequent successful head and cervical spinal injury management. All head injuries must be supposed to have an unstable cervical spinal injury until proved otherwise. The immediate problem is the infinite combination of head and cervical spinal injury mechanisms available in head injury. The very variety of head injury presentation and development creates confusion. Hippocrates noted the poor correlation between initial injury and outcome. A trivial injury can kill. Yet a severe initial insult does not guarantee death or a poor outcome, given good management.

Head injury severity

Though head injury is common in sport (MMWR Morbidity and Mortality Weekly Report 1997), serious brain injury is less so. Its comparative rarity ensures that most medical practitioners will be inexperienced in immediate management and assessment when the need occurs. The first practical problem following a blow to the head is to assess its significance. This may or may not be obvious.

'Significance' in head insult is best considered as any external sign of head injury and whether sufficient energy has been transferred from head to brain to cause actual brain injury. A significant brain injury is indicated by any neurological symptom or sign.

Head injury is 'serious' if sufficient energy has been transferred to the brain to render that individual unconscious, even if only for a moment, or if his mental state is left anything but normal. To be conscious requires the satisfactory function of all parts of the brain. *An alteration in conscious level is the best indication of a disturbance of the brain, that disturbance being itself significant.* A disturbance of consciousness, however minor or transient, indicates sufficient energy to fracture the skull and a severe brain insult. That degree of insult is more than sufficient to cause bleeding within the head, to induce auto-regulatory failure (vasoparesis) with brain swelling, and to render that individual a candidate for SIS.

No one remembers being unconscious. Unconsciousness is accompanied by a longer period of amnesia (loss of memory) both before and after the injury: the pre- and post-traumatic amnesic intervals. The latter is considered to extend until the restoration of continuous memory. It may later be used as an indicator of the severity of that brain insult. Pre-traumatic amnesia of up to ten minutes is commonplace and may represent disturbance of the initial 'electrical' phase of memory. A longer pre-traumatic interval probably indicates structural brain damage. That many report being 'knocked out' is the result of rationalization, fantasy, and hearsay leading to often quite misleading reconstruction.

Differential diagnosis

Altered consciousness is not infrequent in sport. Unless the incident is actually observed, an open mind for the differential diagnosis is prudent. This includes:

- sleep, fatigue and exhaustion
- hypotension, faint and dehydration
- hypoxia, pneumothorax
- hypoglycaemia
- hyperpyrexia
- intoxication, either metabolic, electrolytic, or drug-induced
- reflex, GILOC in aerobatics.
- seizure, epilepsy
- narcolepsy (abnormal, day-time somnolence)
- fugue (psychiatric)
- intracranial catastrophe
- trauma, head injury, associated spinal injury.

Immediate assessment

Because head and spinal injury go hand in hand, assessment is best made of the whole nervous system. As in all medicine, subsequent successful management depends on the initial assessment. This is based on the following:

(1) history to exclude the differential diagnosis, and to establish the mechanism of injury and progress since;
(2) examination

In practice, where airway, breathing, circulation and cervical spine are the priority, the *history* may have to be brief and expanded later. Yet, however brief, one needs to know the following:

(1) circumstance and detail of injury;
(2) potential for head penetration, deformation, and acceleration, together with that for an associated neck or spinal injury;
(3) unconsciousness, still present, recovering, or recovered?
(4) occurence of other neurological symptoms or signs, including arms and legs.

The *immediate needs* are as follows.

(A) Airway. Ensure that it is clear, get it clear and keep it clear.
(B) Breathing. Is it present and adequate? If not, commence mouth-to-mouth ventilation.
(C) Circulation and cervical spine. Check there is a pulse and keep the head and neck straight.

In practice:

(i) Lie the victim flat on their back with head, neck and spine moved as one and neck stabilized.

(ii) Again, check ABC; stop bleeding points.
(iii) Establish the airway, pulling the jaw and tongue forwards.
(iv) Commence mouth-to-mouth ventilation and external cardiac massage if adequate breathing or circulation is not demonstrated. With the patient flat, the cerebral circulation is likely to be adequate if there is a carotid, radial, or femoral pulse, provided that venous outflow from the head is not obstructed.
(v) If ABC is satisfactory and the patient cooperative, check whether they can move feet and fingers, legs, arms, and shoulders voluntarily and record what they can and cannot do. If not cooperative, check what they are moving (feet, legs, hands, arms, shoulders). Again record for the vital guidance of the hospital team.
(vi) By this stage, one can define conscious level accurately. It will be apparent whether or not the victim opens their eyes, makes any noise or moves. These three—eyes, mouth, and movement—provide the most reliable means of recording and communicating conscious level status yet devised: the Glasgow Coma Scale (Teasdale and Jennett 1974). Putting numbers on these three features is not easy. In the heat of the moment, most doctors cannot remember the scoring. It is sensible to carry a scoring table (Table 2.1) whenever you might encounter injury, certainly on any and every sporting occasion.

Table 2.1. Glasgow Coma scoring of conscious level

Score	Motor (M)	Conversation (V)	Eye-opening (E)
6	Obeys commands	–	–
5	Localizes pain	Orientated	–
4	Withdraws from pain	Confused	Spontaneous
3	Abnormal flexion	Inappropriate	To speech
2	Extends	Sounds only	To pain
1	Nil	Nil	Nil
Total	(M+V+E) =		

The score is assessed every five minutes and recorded against time. This can be complemented by a limb motor assessment to cover the actual or potential accompanying spinal cord injury. In spinal cord injury, one is concerned for the weakest movement. Power of foot, leg, hand, arm, and shoulder movement is best recorded using the Medical Research Council (MRC) motor power (muscle strength) scale (Table 2.2).

Table 2.2. MRC movement power score

Score	Movement at joint
5	Normal
4	Strong but not normal
3	Weak but can overcome gravity
2	Movement but not against gravity
1	Movement detected
0	No movement

If one has a simple observation sheet available, so much the better. An example is given in Table 2.3.

Table 2.3. Observation sheet

Name										DoB or Age			
Home address and telephone													
Date	Place												
Time and details of accident & injuries													
Observer's name and contact number													
↓ Score Time →													
Motor (M)													
6 Obeys commands													
5 Localizes pain													
4 Withdraws from pain													
3 Abnormal flexion													
2 Extends													
1 Nil													
Conversation (V)													
5 Orientated													
4 Confused													
3 Inappropriate													
2 Sounds only													
1 Nil													
Eye opening (E)													
4 Spontaneous													
3 To speech													
2 To pain													
1 Nil													
GCS Total													
Pupil size (right, left)													
Limb power (R & L, MRC)	0–5: normal = 5, against gravity = 3, detectable movement = 1, none = 0												
Shoulders													
Arms													
Fingers													
Legs													
Feet/toes													

Using 'R' and 'L' for arms and legs, a single table can be used for both sides. For the pupils, just draw large, small, or equal rings for the pupil size.

The importance of such observations, backing up the history of the injury, for the direction, speed, accuracy, and success of subsequent management cannot be over-emphasized. The above details are the essential minima for any formal reporting form. Such forms can be expanded endlessly, but, to be useful, they have to contain at least the above.

(vii) The other vital signs, pupillary reaction as well as size on each side, heart and respiratory rate, blood pressure, and temperature can be added as time and space allow (Table 2.4). They will be contained on the Ambulance sheet.

One or more of these signs will change with the onset of coning at the tentorial hiatus and distortion of the brain stem.

Table 2.4. Other 'vital signs' for observation sheets, if space allows (see Appendix)

Time →									
Left pupil									
Right pupil									
Heart rate									
Respiratory rate									
Blood pressure									
Temperature									

This indicates a critical situation at the 'Piccadilly Circus' of the head. The first pupil to enlarge is usually on the same side as the clot and brain swelling causing the cone. Where there is either no scanning available or time is running out, this is a vital indication as to which side requires the first burr hole to start evacuating the blood clot and lowering the raised ICP. Any major brain shift at the tentorial hiatus or foramen magnum will be reflected in a change in one or more of these signs. Once conscious level is lost and without ICP monitoring, they are the only indicators of the terminal stage in the head and that the last chance of saving life has been reached. In sporting head injury, the aim is to have got the victim to hospital well before this stage. However, if the activity is taking place far from hospital back-up, either in time or space, a full form incorporating all the above elements is warranted. Most can be filled in without any equipment, other than a pen and a watch. Any ambulance will have a blood pressure machine and a thermometer.

Risk status

The assessment of risk is eased if it is based on conscious level once the individual is horizontal, with the neck stabilized, ABC established, and an assessment of limb motor function made. Immediate risk is now indicated by conscious level trend. Once two observations have been made, risk is easier to determine.

Progress following head injury falls into one of seven groups, each with its distinctive conscious level trend, each based on improvement or deterioration following the first and subsequent assessments (Table 2.5 and Fig. 2.1).

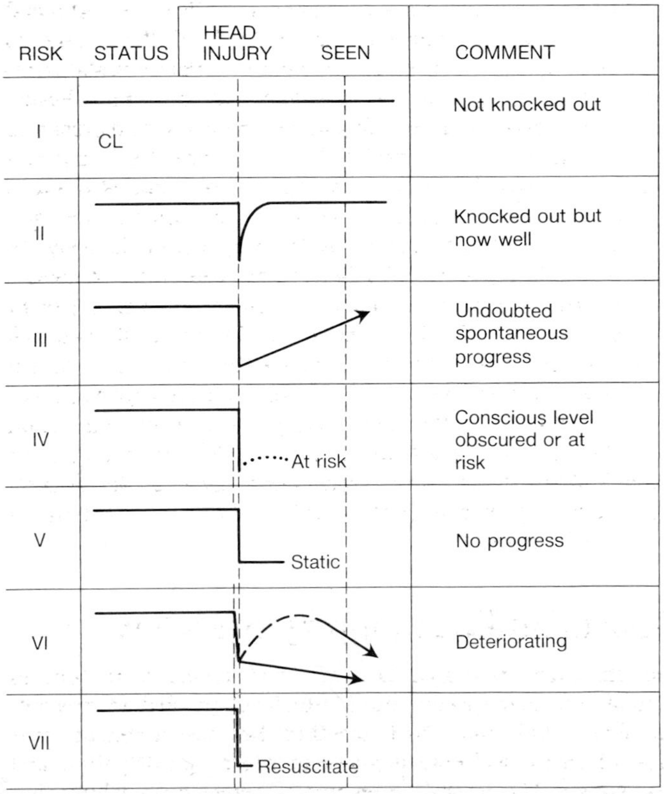

Fig. 2.1 Head injury groups in terms of changes in conscious level between two observations separated in time.

Table 2.5. Risk groups based on serial assessment.

Risk group	Conscious level profile	Significance
1	Subject to head insult but not knocked out.	Neurological symptoms? If not, unlikely to require assistance.
2	Was unconscious, but has recovered and appears normal by time of assessment.	Potential for intracranial mischief remains. May suffer secondary deterioration. Neurological symptoms? Observe. Hospital.
3	Was knocked out, still suffering impaired or altered consciousness, though undoubtedly improving.	Recovering, may deteriorate, ABC, observe as 2. Hospital.
4	Difficult to assess because of epilepsy, other injuries sustained or other treatment in progress.	At risk of every intracranial mischief until proved otherwise. ICP monitoring required. Hospital.
5	Conscious level remains static.	Should be improving, the natural history of recovery following head injury. No improvement means intracranial clot, brain swelling, or both.
6	May have improved initially but is now deteriorating.	Will die from intracranial clot, brain swelling, or both unless ventilated and clot excluded.
7	Required resuscitation following head injury.	Whole-brain vasoparesis is guaranteed. Immediate ventilation and clot exclusion required.

Management

Based on risk status, all groups need ABC, initial assessment and recorded observation.

Groups 1–3 need careful observation to ensure that improvement is maintained and that secondary deterioration from swelling, clot, or seizure does not occur. *Return to exercise after being knocked out or 'concussed' is foolhardy.* It is the best way to swell a vasoparetic brain, accelerate intracranial haemorrhage, and elicit the SIS.

Group 1 should be made the responsibility of a responsible adult who can observe them for more than 24 hours.

Groups 2–7 are at risk of the full panoply of post-traumatic complication and merit hospital review.

Group 4 may need intracranial pressure monitoring.

Groups 5–7 require the immediate control of brain swelling and the exclusion or removal of intracranial clot.

Positioning

Head and spinal injury are best managed with the patient horizontal, the airway cleared and breathing, and circulation maintained. However, the supine position means that they require continuous supervision. ABC cannot be disregarded without hazard to their airway. If there is no question of head injury and the integrity of the spine is undoubted (as after a spontaneous seizure), the airway can be protected by rolling the individual into the recovery position. This is inappropriate in the circumstances of sporting head and neck injury. Head, neck, and shoulder position must be kept neutral. If ABC prove inadequate, then restoration and maintenance of the airway, mouth-to-mouth ventilation, and external cardiac massage have to be instituted immediately. Likewise, the essential, repeated assessment of the individual's conscious level and limb movements is difficult in the recovery position.

'Minor' head injury

Where severe injury is present, the ABC requirement and the need for rapid transport on a spinal board to hospital is obvious. 'Minor' head injuries present their own difficulties (Sturmi *et al.* 1998). There may be real uncertainty as to whether or not the conscious level was disturbed. A child or adult under stress may not complain of neurological symptoms, that is of sensory or motor involvement of limbs and body, unless specifically asked for them. Caution is the key and a high index of suspicion prudent. If the individual is obstreperous, uncooperative, anti-social or aggressive, this behaviour is itself a sign of frontal lobe injury and reason enough for hospital review. When the individual appears normal, well, and determined to continue the game, the touchstone is altered consciousness. If consciousness was disturbed, then the risk of secondary neurological deterioration can be presumed until such a risk has been judged as remote after an appropriate interval by properly qualified medical review.

Return to sports after head injury

Though the sporting ethic is to 'press on regardless' in the heroic manner, this otherwise commendable attitude is foolhardy following head injury. Opinion varies as to return after head injury (Cantu 1998b; Sturmi *et al.* 1998). Given the touchstone of an alteration or loss of consciousness, several principles apply in considering when it is reasonable to play or compete again:

(i) Early post-traumatic epilepsy may occur at any time during the first week after being knocked out or appearing 'concussed'. It is unwise to risk brain insult during that period. Two weeks without symptoms is the minimum; a month is prudent.

(ii) Being knocked out indicates sufficient skull deformation to cause actual skull fracture. Arterial healing cannot be relied upon for at least 10 days. Neurosurgeons are not happy about intracranial vascular repair until at least six weeks. The skull takes as long as the femur (thigh bone) to heal and fuse. Unaided, the femur cannot be relied on to bear weight for at least six weeks; three months in competition.

(iii) The incidence of intracerebral haemorrhage into areas of brain contusion is maximum at ten days; hence the concern over return to competition during the first fortnight following brain insult.

(iv) The return of cerebrovascular auto-regulation (recovery from vasoparesis) cannot yet be established with certainty by non-invasive means. Trans-cranial Doppler (TCD) may mislead. A full week, preferably a fortnight, following the cessation of all headache and post-traumatic symptoms is the minimum which can be relied upon.

(v) Time and circumstance indicating the cessation of risk of SIS are debatable. It is unlikely to be less than that the 7–14 days for vasoparesis.

(vi) Persisting symptoms merit neurological review.

(vii) Repeated head injury, the effects of which are cumulative, but may not yet be obvious to the victim or a lay observer (MMWR Morbidity Mortality Weekly Report 1997), also merits neurological review.

Table 2.6. Return to sport after alteration of consciousness:

Test	Requirement
History (the most sensitive and subjective test)	Personal integrity. No symptoms, no headache. No specific abnormality
Examination	No physical or neurological signs. No objective anomaly
Investigation (where appropriate)	No abnormality on appropriate testing.
Medical advice:	GP letter: safe to return (the minimum requirement)
Expert review	Opinion from a specialist, if there is doubt.

In practice, the individual should be barred from a return to games or competition until formally assessed by a medical practitioner who is prepared to accept responsibility for the consequences. Once knocked out, even if feeling well, the sportsman or sportswoman should, at least, remain in the care of a responsible adult and their general practitioner informed. Return following two weeks' freedom from symptoms (Table 2.6) and with a letter from one's usual GP is a reasonable minimum. Skull fracture raises this to six weeks.

Communications and cover

An on-site, qualified, practised, well-organized and motivated medical team with ambulance back-up is the ideal. Whether this is practicable depends on the occasion. At least two ALS (Advanced Life Support) trained individuals on site with telephone communications is a reasonable aim. Providing ABS and spinal care are available on the scene and the means to summons an ambulance are to hand, immediate hospital management is available at most Accident and Emergency departments. However, organizing further investigations and preparing for the removal of intracranial clots takes time. CT (computer assisted tomographic) head scanning may be required to guide further care. Prior warning allows staff and scanners to be prepared and operating theatres to be freed-up and made ready. To a degree, this is possible after head injury using the ambulance radio network. How much better it would be if sporting event organizers prepare for the worst and establish prior liaison, well before an event, with the Accident and Emergency department within whose catchment area the event is being organized. For an event of any size, this is mandatory. Lines of communication can then be established and a plan of disaster management agreed. Without such prior arrangement, opportunities to minimize head injury complication will be lost and questions of neglect of care raised.

Sports and head injury overview

Despite every best intention and endeavour, head injuries remain a bane of sport (Cantu 1996). Though head injuries outnumber spinal injury 10:1, together they cast a shadow over the otherwise welcome increase in sports' participation and enjoyment. The hazard varies widely between disciplines, but none are immune. Consideration for head injury has therefore to be a factor in:

- selection, where the individual's own history is the best guide—based on present symptoms, past history (previous head injury, neurological conditions, seizure or febrile convulsions, migraine), family history (seizure, head injury, neurological conditions, especially migraine), sporting, and social history to date—with examination and a letter from their own GP if in doubt
- training
- tactics
- equipment
- development of the discipline to reduce hazard yet enhance enjoyment and competitiveness
- arrangements for assessment should head injury occur and for management if it does
- criteria for returning to the individual sport after head injury

Hopefully, this chapter will be of assistance in addressing these issues.

References

Allen, W. M. (1976). Letter: brain damage in jockeys. *Lancet*, **1** (7969), 1135–6.

Bruce, D. A., Alavi, A., Bilaniuk, L. *et al.* (1981). Diffuse cerebral swelling following head injuries in children. The syndrome of malignant brain oedema. *J. Neurosurg.*, **54**, 170–8.

(BSI). British Standards Institution. (1998) PAS 015. *Protective helmets for equestrian use.* BSI, London.

Cantu, R. C. (1992). Cerebral concussion in sport. Management and prevention. *Sports Med.*, **14** (1), 64–74.

Cantu, R. C. (1996). Head injuries in sport. *Br. J. Sports Med.*, **30** (4), 289–96.

Cantu, R. C. (1998a). Second-impact syndrome. *Clin Sports Med.*, **17** (1), 37–44.

Cantu, R. C. (1998b). Return to play guidelines after a head injury. *Clin. Sports Med.*, **17** (1), 45–60.

Davis, P. M., and McKelvey, M. K. (1998). Medicolegal aspects of athletic head injury. *Clin. Sports Med.*, **17** (1), 71–82.

Foster, J. B., Leiguarda, R., and Tilley, P.J. (1976). Brain damage in National Hunt jockeys. *Lancet* **1** (7967), 981–3.

Firth, J. L. (1985). Equestrian injuries. In *Sports injuries: mechanisms, prevention and treatment* (ed. R. C. Schneider, J. C. Kennedy, and M. L. Plant), pp. 431–49. Williams and Wilkins, Baltimore.

Firth, J. L. (1994). Equestrian injuries. In *Sports injuries. Mechanisms, prevention, treatment.* (ed. Fu, H. U., and Stone, D. A.), pp. 315–31. Williams and Wilkins, Baltimore.

Gurdjian, E. S., Webster, J. E., and Lissner, H. R. (1950). The mechanisms of skull fracture. *J. Neurosurg.*, **7**, 106–14.

'Hippocrates'. Cited in Knight, G. and Rains, T. J. H. (eds). (1971). *Bailey and Love's short practice of surgery.* p. 376. H. K. Lewis, London.

Holbourn, A. H. S. (1943). Mechanics of head injury. *Lancet*, **2**, 438–41.

Jennett, W. B. (1975). *Epilepsy after non-missile head injuries* (2nd edn). Heinemann Medical, London.

Langfitt, T. W., Marshall, W. J. S., Kassell, N. F., and Schutta, H. S. (1968). The pathophysiology of brain swelling produced by mechanical trauma and hypertension. *Scand. J. Clin. Lab. Invest.*, **Suppl. 102 XIVB**.

Lindgren, S. O. (1966). Experimental studies on mechanical effects in head injury. *Acta Chir. Scand.*, **Suppl. 360**.

McCrory, P. R., and Berkovic, S. F. (1998). Second impact syndrome. *Neurology*, **50** (3), 677–83.

Miller, J. D. (1979). Intracranial mass lesions. In *Neural trauma* (ed. A. J. Popp *et al.*), pp. 173–80. Raven Press, New York.

MMWR Morbidity Mortality Weekly Report (1997). Sports-related recurrent brain injuries—United States. **46** (10), 224–7. See also *J. Am. Med. Assoc.*, 1997 277 (15), 1190–1 From the Centers for Disease Control and Prevention. Sports-related recurrent brain injuries—United States.

Robbins, S. L., Contran, R. S., and Kumar V. (eds). (1984). *Pathologic basis of disease* (3rd edn), pp. 1374–7. Saunders, Philadelphia, PA.

Saunders, R. L., and Harbaugh, R. E. (1984). The second impact in catastrophic contact—sports head trauma. *J. Am. Med. Assoc.*, **252**, 538–9.

Schneider, R. C. (1987). Football head and neck injury. *Surg Neurol.*, **27**, 507–8.

Sheinker, I. M. (1944). Vasoparalysis of the central nervous systems. A characteristic vascular syndrome. *Arch. Neurol. Psychol.*, **52**, 43–56.

Strich, S. J. (1956). Diffuse degeneration of the cerebral white matter in severe dementia following head injury. *J. Neurol. Psychiatr.*, **19**, 163–85.

Strich, S. J. (1961). Shearing of nerve fibres as a cause of brain damage due to head injury. *Lancet*, **2**, 443–8.

Strich, S. J. (1969). Pathology of brain damage due to blunt head injury. In *Late effects of head injury* (eds A. E. Walker, W. F. Covaness, and M. Critchicy), pp. 501–26. Charles C. Thomas, Springfield, IL.

Sturmi, J. E., Smith, C., and Lombardo, J. A. (1998). Mild brain trauma in sports. Diagnosis and treatment guidelines. *Sports Med.*, **25** (6), 351–8.

Teasdale, G. and Jennett, W. B. (1974). The Glasgow Come Scale. *Lancet*, **2**, 81–4.

Appendix

Basic head and spinal injury observation chart

Name							DoB or Age					
Home address and telephone												
Date	Place											
Time and details of accident & injuries												
Observer's name and contact number												
↓ Score Time →												
Motor (M)												
6	Obeys commands											
5	Localizes pain											
4	Withdraws from pain											
3	Abnormal flexion											
2	Extends											
1	Nil											
Conversation (V)												
5	Orientated											
4	Confused											
3	Inappropriate											
2	Sounds only											
1	Nil											
Eye opening (E)												
4	Spontaneous											
3	To speech											
2	To pain											
1	Nil											
GCS Total												

Limb power (R & L, MRC: 0–5: normal = 5, strong but not normal = 4, can overcome gravity = 3, clear movement, but not against gravity = 2, detectable movement = 1, no voluntary movement = 0)

	Shoulders											
	Arms											
	Fingers											
	Legs											
	Feet/toes											
Vital signs												
	Left pupil											
	Right pupil											
	Heart rate											
	Respiratory rate											
	Blood pressure											
	Temperature											
Treatment/notes												

Ocular sports injuries

N. R. Galloway

The importance of ocular sporting injuries has been underestimated in the past, perhaps because such injuries are not very common in ophthalmic practice and they are therefore quite rare in general medical practice. To some extent, the problem has been unmasked in recent years by the virtual abolition of perforating eye injuries following road traffic accidents. This has come about with the introduction of seat belt law and public education concerning drinking and driving. Likewise, the incidence of industrial injuries to the eyes has diminished over the past century due undoubtedly to the introduction of preventive measures. By contrast, eye injuries in sport have been increasing, and to discount them is to ignore the sometimes devastating effect such an injury can have on an individual. Quite often, the severity of an eye injury is not apparent at first glance or without proper microscopic examination, and delays in referral may occur as a result. The prompt treatment of a perforating eye injury can be sight-saving but, in spite of prompt treatment, the results of surgical management are not always satisfactory and often amount to preserving what remains. Nevertheless, all these injuries are avoidable or preventable, and perhaps the next few decades will see their gradual disappearance as greater public awareness and better preventive measures are introduced.

The incidence of eye injuries

Most eye injuries during sporting activities probably never demand medical attention. They are discounted at the time and resolve without any permanent damage to the eye. Out of the many various injuries, which are seen in eye casualty departments in the UK, only 2.3 per cent are due to sport. The sporting injuries though have a much higher chance of being admitted to hospital. This shows that although significant eye injuries in sport are uncommon, they can be relatively serious. It is interesting to note that in 1968, 4.2 per cent of eye injuries admitted to hospital in the UK were related to sport. In 1988, the figure had risen to 25.1 per cent and in 1989 a figure as high as 42 per cent has been estimated. (McEwan 1989)

In the absence of a national reporting system for eye injuries sustained in sport, accurate statistics are not available in this country. Numerous attempts have been made to assess the problem in other ways, such as by the inspection of hospital records or through surveys conducted by means of questionnaires sent to practicing ophthalmologists. A retrospective study of the records of those attending the Southampton Eye Hospital with various sporting injuries in 1978–79 is of interest. In this study, the number of playing sessions generating these injuries has been estimated by reference to the results of the 1977 General Household Survey, published by Her Majesty's Stationary Office in 1979. At that time the results indicated that

Table 2.7. Sporting causes of hyphaema, Sussex Eye Hospital, UK, October 1982–March 1984 (Gregory 1986)

Sport	No. of patients
Squash	3
Soccer	6
Badminton	7
Tennis	1
Rugby	1
Golf	1
Marbles	1
Total	20

squash produced the most injuries per playing session in the UK, as well as the greatest number of hospital admissions. The injury rate for squash was estimated at 5.2 per 100 000 playing sessions compared with 2.3 per 100 000 playing sessions for injuries from all causes (Barrell et al. 1981). Racket sports still account for a significant proportion of sports injuries throughout the world and apparently about half of all sporting injuries in the UK (McEwan and Jones 1991).

Hospital records can provide useful information concerning the more severe injuries. For example, a survey of the causes of traumatic bleeding into the anterior chamber ('hyphaema') seen at the Massachusetts Eye and Ear Infirmary from February to September 1980 showed that 45 out of 90 cases were due to sports injuries, and 'raquetball' accounted for the largest proportion of these. In an English series reporting sports injuries seen in hospital over a period of 18 months, 20 hyphaemata were recorded, and the various sports causing these are shown in Table 2.7. Squash and badminton were the main offenders, but the numbers of injuries from association football is noteworthy (Gregory 1986). In a more recent prospective study of eye injuries to an eye emergency department in Portugal, 72.6 per cent of the cases were due to football (Filipe et al. 1997), which is perhaps a surprising finding and a cause for some concern.

The inspection of hospital records does not always give a true incidence of the problem among either the general population or the population at risk. For this reason, one set of figures is not comparable with another. Organized sport is in a better position to provide accurate figures, and this has been especially true of ice hockey. Here a high and increasing injury rate was effectively reduced by preventive measures (Pashby 1985).

A useful database for showing trends in the incidence of sporting injuries of the eyes is that collected by the Canadian Ophthalmological Society. Table 2.8 shows a sample of this over the 20 years from 1972 to 1992 (Vinger 1994)

Table 2.8. Canadian sporting injuries from 1972 to 1992.(after Vinger 1994)

Sport	No. of patients
Hockey	1759
Ball hockey	27
Racket sports	997
Baseball	409
Golf	52
Skiing	31
Volleyball	27
Football and soccer	161
Basketball	31
BB guns	15
War games	57

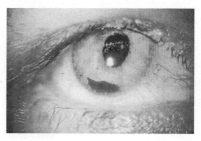

FIG. 2.2 Blood in the anterior chamber (hyphaema) following a cricket ball injury to the globe.

The incidence of eye injuries in boxing is worthy of special mention. The number of participants in this sport is relatively small, and reported statistics have not been as forthcoming as in ice hockey for example. It was reported in 1981 that retinal detachment was not a common occurrence in boxing (Whiteson 1981). This is contrary to the experience of individual ophthalmic surgeons, and indeed a questionnaire sent out to eye surgeons in the UK, which achieved a 50.35 per cent reply rate, gave a total of 38 cases of retinal detachment in boxers over the preceding five years (Elkington 1985). Even this figure, which is likely to be under-reported, suggests a higher incidence of retinal detachment than in the general population. In a different study, the routine examination of boxers with or without eye symptoms has revealed a surprisingly high incidence of signs of ocular contusion, and especially of lesions predisposing to retinal detachment (Giovinazzo *et al.* 1987). A more recent Italian survey involving 75 active and ex-boxers revealed evidence of eye damage, often asympomatic, in both professional and amateur boxers. There were three cases of retinal detachment (Vadala *et al.* 1997).

A different approach is to look at the reasons for removing eyes surgically. There has been a dramatic decline in the number of surgical enucleations over the past 20 years, but the small number of enucleations due to sporting injuries has not shared this decline. Many of these cases have been the result of 'BB gun' (air rifle or air pistol) injuries.

The mechanism of ocular sporting injuries

Racket sports in general involve playing with a high-velocity missile, which is small enough to squeeze through the bony orbital margins and contuse the globe of the eye itself. In tennis singles, as in badminton, injury is rare, but in doubles there is an extra risk mainly from injury from another player's rackeet. Playing at the net in tennis doubles has an extra risk of eye injury from the ball itself, and retinal detachments have been reported. Most squash rackets injuries are due to impact from the ball and occur as the player in front turns to follow his shot. He is then struck by the opponents next stroke.

In large ball sports, which involve fast-moving teams of players, injuries to the eyes occur less often from the ball than from physical clashes involving hands, elbows, or feet. In rugby and basketball, for example, injuries can occur from opponents' fingers during scuffles for the ball. The ball itself is too large to pass through the bony margins of the orbit but sometimes it may be distorted or a projecting lace may cause damage. A cricket ball might be expected to be too large and hard to contuse the eye, but this does sometimes happen perhaps because of the particular anatomical configuration of the injured player's eyes and orbits (see Fig. 2.2).

Ocular contusion

The mechanical results of direct contusion depend to some extent on whether the eyelids were open or closed at the moment of impact, as well as the size, speed, and weight of the missile. The squash ball, which measures 40 mm in diameter, is an ideal size for causing compression of the globe, whereas in the case of the larger tennis ball, some of the force of impact is cushioned by the surrounding orbital margin. Unfortunately, even a football may mould itself into the orbit and cause contusion of the globe, so that the larger size of the ball cannot always guarantee protection. Flying objects are most likely to contuse the eye if they are coming from in front or slightly down and out. This is because the nose and brow provide some protection. Some people's eyes protrude more (for example, very short-sighted people) than others, and this can be an additional risk factor. A high-speed missile may contuse the globe through the closed eyelids, but bruising of the eyelids often indicates that the eyes have been closed in time to avoid more severe damage. A squash ball may be travelling at more than 100 miles an hour and so can strike the eye before the blink reflex has had time to occur. In such cases, the cornea tends to be abraded, causing severe pain and photophobia. The more severe effects of such a contusion are due to distortion of the globe. The force of impact is usually upward and inward on the lower temporal quadrant. This causes stretching and tearing of the iris root, and may result in the rupture of tributaries of the major arterial circle of the iris. Typically, bleeding into the anterior chamber can occur with an associated iridodialysis or rip of the iris root (see Fig. 2.3). The blood in the anterior chamber forms a fluid level (a 'hyphaema') and this is a sign that specialist advice should be sought immediately. This bleeding may recur more seriously after two or three days in 10 per cent or more of such patients. (Wilson 1980).

If the force of impact is centred more posteriorly, then the retina may be torn (retinal dialysis). Such tears can go unnoticed until eventually the retina becomes detached, often after several weeks or months. These tears can be sealed by laser treatment if spotted in time, thereby preventing the retinal detachment. The distortion of the globe can also cause splitting open of the angle of the anterior chamber, or angle recession.

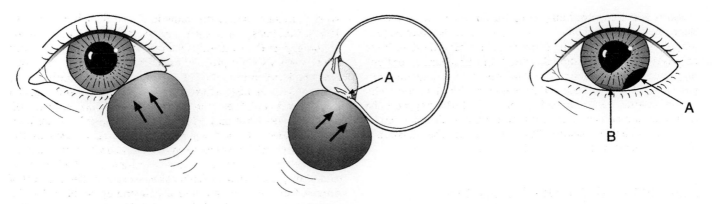

FIG. 2.3 The mechanism of ocular contusion. The figure shows how a squash ball can distort the globe causing a rip of the iris root. A = rip in iris root; B = blood in anterior chamber

This can affect the drainage of aqueous fluid from the eye with a consequent rise in intraocular pressure. If untreated, this in turn can lead to pressure atrophy of the optic nerve head (secondary glaucoma). Sometimes the sudden stretching produces small tears in the iris sphincter at the inner margin of the pupil, and as a result the pupil may be fixed and dilated. This of course can cause great concern if a head injury is suspected, but the diagnosis can be clarified easily by proper ophthalmological examination. Contusion of the eye may also cause posterior sub-capsular opacities in the lens, although these may take some days or sometimes much longer to develop. Bruising of the retina itself is seen as grey patches with multiple haemorrhages; this may have a serious permanent effect on the visual acuity if the fovea is involved. Distortion of the globe can cause ruptures of the choroid, seen with the ophthalmoscope as circumferential white crescents concentric with the optic disc. One final effect of contusion may be bleeding into the optic nerve sheath. After the impact, the patient finds that he cannot see out of one eye. The physical signs may be minimal, apart from the afferent pupillary defect, in spite of the fact that the eye is completely blind and usually remains so. After a few weeks, the optic disc becomes pale. Early decompression of the optic nerve may be helpful in such cases.

Effect on surrounding structures

It is perhaps surprising how often a contused globe is seen as an isolated injury but other injuries may mask the eye damage. Typically a larger 'missile', such as a knee or fist, may cause a 'blow-out fracture', in which the globe and orbital contents are forced posteriorly, causing fracture of the floor of the orbit and trapping of the inferior rectus muscle. The infraorbital nerve is usually injured, causing anaesthesia of the cheek, along with the other typical signs such as enophthalmos (posterior displacement of the eye), with diplopia on upward gaze. In the absence of a blow-out fracture, injury to the superior orbital margin may damage the pulley of the superior oblique muscle, thus causing diplopia by a different mechanism.

Ocular perforation

Perforation of the globe is usually caused by a sharp object, and the site of perforation is in the anterior segment of the eye. If the cornea is perforated, aqueous fluid escapes, and the iris shoots forward under hydrostatic pressure to plug the opening. A knuckle of iris may project through the wound, and on no account should this be mistaken for a foreign body by the first-aid attendant. Any perforating injury of the eye demands urgent surgical attention, because of the risk of infection and disruption of the intraocular structures. If the lens of the eye escapes damage, then the visual outcome may be very good, but once the lens is involved then a cataract inevitably forms. Cataract surgery may present technical difficulties in an injured eye, and even the best surgical result leaves the patient with no focusing power. This may be acceptable to the elderly patient who has lost focusing power through natural ageing but may be a handicap in the younger patient. If the perforation involves the sclera further posteriorly, then there is a high risk of retinal detachment.

It can be seen that a perforating injury is a serious risk to the sight of the eye, and may result in the need for repeated operations and time off work. Most people have heard of sympathetic ophthalmia, and are aware that the uninjured eye may become inflamed after a perforating injury. Fortunately, this is very rare indeed, and the risk is largely eliminated by careful reparative surgery.

Risks when there is pre-existing eye disease

Some people are at special risk when taking part in sport because they have had previous eye surgery. This applies after cataract and corneal graft surgery in particular. Subjects with high myopia have a thinner than normal sclera, and this can rupture more easily. They also have a higher risk of retinal detachment after injury. It must be remembered that some high myopes may have undergone refractive surgery, which in itself carries extra risks. Refractive keratotomy, a now largely super-seded treatment for myopia, is known to weaken the cornea and has been associated with rupture of the globe. Excimer laser treatment for myopia is probably much safer in this respect.

The patient with only one good functioning eye is at a greater risk of injury presumably because of the reduced field of vision and distance judgement. Such a patient also has much more to lose if an eye injury occurs. None the less, 'only eyes' are some-times blinded and it is very important that these patients are properly advised about the use of protective glasses and the suitability of different sports before such a tragedy occurs.

Sports which involve hanging upside down can cause a transient rise of the intraocular pressure, and this rise may be prolonged in patients with glaucoma or ocular hypertension. Yoga exercises that use the shoulder-stand and head-stand positions may increase the amount of visual field loss in patients with glaucoma (Rice and Allen 1985). Patients with glaucoma, who are on treatment with Timolol eye drops, and who happen to be endurance athletes can find that their exercise endurance can be reduced, probably because Timolol reduces the maximum obtainable heart rate (Atkins *et al* . 1985).

Injuries and particular sports

Squash and racketball are particularly likely to produce eye injuries. Retinal detachments from squash injuries seem to have a worse prognosis than spontaneous detachments (Knorr and Jonas 1996). Eye damage is less common where the players are separated by a net, as in tennis and badminton. Injuries are more common in tennis doubles and rare in singles. Soccer is at present responsible for more eye injuries than any other sport (MacEwan 1987). The problem is that the wearing of face protection would alter the whole nature of the game. Another problem is that an increasing number of these injuries are apparently deliberate. Some cases have led to successful prosecution. American and Canadian football involves a considerable amount of head protection, but injuries still occur from fingers penetrating the face mask (Helveston 1987).

The pattern of injury from ice hockey in Canada in 1972–73 showed 15 ruptured globes, 91 hyphaemata and 31 orbital fractures. Out of the 287 injuries, 20 caused total blindness of the eye. Such a severe toll prompted vigorous protective measures, which have proved effective. In 1983–84, there were only 124 reported injuries, and none of these were in players wearing guards. The average age of injured players rose over this period, reflecting the more regular wearing of guards among younger players.

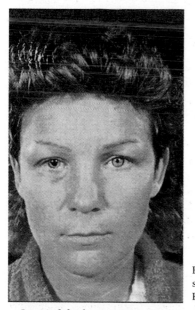

FIG. 2.4 The wicket keeper who suffered the eye injury seen in Fig. 2.2

Some of the less common sporting eye injuries have their own peculiarities. Hurling can cause severe injuries; the solid 75 mm ball has been the commonest cause of sporting injury in the West of Ireland, where the game is played (Lynch and Rowan 1997). Golf balls nearly always cause devastating injury to the eye on impact (Miller 1967), as do airgun pellets and darts. Dart injuries are a serious problem in children either as a result of a direct perforation from the point of the dart or, curiously, in the shape of damage inflicted by the tail of the dart when it is pulled out of the board (Cole and Smerdon 1988). Eye injuries still occur in cricket, but only when protective masks have not been worn. Fielders at short leg and silly mid off as well as the batsman and wicket keeper need to wear helmets. (see Fig. 2.4). Fishermen are not immune from eye injuries, which may be caused by penetration by fishhooks or by spears. The removal of a hook from an eye can pose a challenging problem for the ophthalmic surgeon (Bartholomew and MacDonald 1980). War games became increasingly popular in the 1980s. The aim is to simulate a military operation using body and face protection. Projectile weapons are used which shoot paint-filled pellets at high speed and produce an indelible mark on the opponent. Severe eye injuries have been reported in those who have spurned the use of face masks (Mamalis *et al.* 1990).

Eye protection and glasses in sport

Since about half the population need to wear glasses in any case, it makes sense that the lenses worn for regular sport

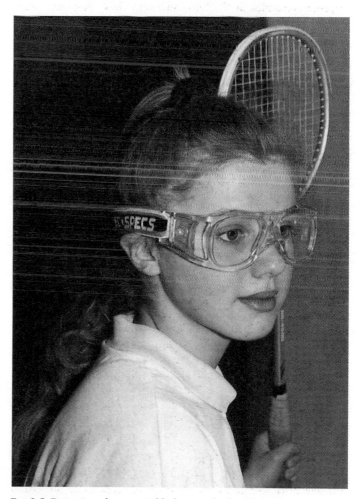

FIG. 2.5 Protective glasses suitable for squash players

should be made of the toughest possible material and yet be optically satisfactory. Polycarbonate is a modern plastic with excellent optical properties, and it has much better impact resistance than other types of glass or plastic. Figure 2.5 shows suitable polycarbonate eye guards which can be made up to the players prescription or they can be plain lenses. Studies have shown that experience is no protection in squash and rackets and open eye guards are of no use and may even contribute to injury (Easterbrook 1997). In North America the wearing of eye guards for sport is often mandatory. It has been claimed that the wearing of face guards by American footballers has caused a huge reduction in the number of facial injuries, whereas, by contrast, the current regulations for soccer prevent the use of any guards as they could themselves cause injury to the player.

When face guards are used, it may not be practical to wear glasses at the same time and, if a correction is needed, then contact lenses should be recommended. Contact lenses, especially soft lenses, can be worn for most sports and are usually preferable to spectacles in that they provide better all-round vision and do not mist up. They do not provide any protection to the eye from injury and they can sometimes make matters worse. On the whole though, the only significant problem with them is that they can be lost on occasions, and very rarely they can cause severe infections of the cornea. Even those engaged in aquatic sports can find contact lenses useful, but they do need to be cleaned especially carefully and there is an extra risk of losing them. It seems that parachute jumping provides extra problems in this respect!

Refractive surgery

Over the past few years, it has become possible to correct short-sightedness by laser treatment. In principle, the shape of the cornea is altered in a carefully measured manner by shaving off its surface. The treatment has become possible thanks to the development of accurate computer measurements of the cornea and the development of the excimer laser. Many shortsighted people (myopes) have found this beneficial for sport since the need for glasses may be eliminated. Not everyone is suitable for treatment and no one should have this treatment without careful consideration of the possible risks. At present, longsighted (hypermetropic) individuals cannot be treated satisfactorily; persons under 21 years or those with other eye problems should avoid such treatment. Before the advent of laser surgery, a technique of making radial cuts in the cornea known as radial keratotomy had been used to improve the uncorrected vision of shortsighted persons, but this has now been largely replaced by laser techniques such as PRK (photorefractive keratotomy) or LASIK (laser assisted in-situ keratomileusis).

First-aid management of eye injuries

When a sporting injury involves the eyes, the first-aid attendant should make a simple assessment of the vision. If the vision is impaired and cannot be cleared by blinking, then immediate referral for specialist treatment is essential. The examiner can test the field of vision by using finger movements in all four quadrants; if the examiner sees his or her own finger significantly before the injured athlete does, then referral is indicated. A near vision test card can be a helpful item in such circumstances. A simple test of eye movements, in which the athlete is asked to follow the examiner's fingers, may reveal damage that needs expert attention. The majority of suspected eye injuries demand prompt referral, but the first-aid attendant may be able to assist with the removal of foreign bodies or the replacement of a dislodged contact lens.

Many contact lens wearers can replace their own contact lenses if they have a small mirror, and such an item might be included in the first-aid kit, together with a pen torch and sterile cotton swabs. A hard eye-shield is another useful item; this is taped over the injured eye to protect it. The first-aid kit should also include a sterile eye irrigating solution. When a perforating injury of the eye is suspected, no further attempt should be made to examine the eye. A protective shield should be applied, and the injured person should be given nothing to eat or drink in case an emergency anaesthetic is needed subsequently.

Economics and prevention of eye injuries

Sports-related eye injuries should not be regarded as accidents; their epidemiology can be studied and the various factors causing them can be eliminated. Furthermore, the cost of these injuries to the country is far more than one might think, when the total hours of work lost and the total treatment costs are considered. It has been estimated that of the 1.6–2.4 million Americans who sustain eye injuries each year, 40 000 will be legally blinded in the injured eye. About one-third of these result from sport. The total annual cost of eye injuries to hospitals in the USA has been put as high as $200 million (Tielsch and Parver 1990).

The prevention of eye injuries involves firstly an estimation of the risk in any particular sport and then the application of suitable protective devices where necessary. Canadian ice hockey has been a model for the study of prevention of sporting eye injuries. In the early 1970s, eye injuries from this cause became a national problem, and public realization of this led to a change in ice hockey rules. Experimental work on masks led to the development of protective headgear. The Canadian Standards Association (CSA) published a standard for eye and tooth protection in 1977, and in 1981 the wearing of such CSA-certified masks was made compulsory for all Canadian minor league hockey players (Pashby 1985). This combination of measures—changes in the rules and the compulsory use of protective headgear—has resulted in a dramatic reduction of eye injuries and a probable saving of several million dollars annually.

In the USA, squash eye protection has been promoted since 1976, and in 1983 the US Squash Rackets Association became the first national body to require that eye protection should be worn by all participants in national championships. Since then, the USSRA has made the wearing of polycarbonate lens eye guards mandatory. Australia now has a standard for eye protectors in racket sports, but the matter is still under investigation in Britain.

References

Atkins, J. M., Pugh, B. R., and Timewell, R. M. (1985). Cardiovascular effects of topical beta-blockers during exercise. *Am. J. Ophthalmol*, **99**, 173.

Barrell, G. V., Cooper, P. J., Elkington, A. R., MacFayden, J. M., Powell, R. G. *et al.* (1981). Squash ball to eyeball; the likelihood of squash players incurring an eye injury. *Br. Med. J.*, **283**, 893–5.

Bartholomew, R. S. and MacDonald, M. (1980). Fish hook injuries of the eye. *Br. J. Ophthalmol.* **64**, 531–3.

Cole, M. D. and Smerdon, D. (1988). Perforating eye injuries caused by darts. *Br. J. Ophthalmol.* **72**, 511–14

Easterbrook, M. (1993). Eye injuries in sport: prevention and cure. *Can. J. Diagn.*, 77–89.

Elkington, A. R. (1985). Boxing and the eye: results of a questionnaire. *Trans. Ophthalmol. Soc.* UK., **104**, 898–902.

Filipe, J. A., Barros, H., and Castro Correia, J. (1997). Sports related ocular injuries. A three year follow-up study. *Ophthalmology.* **104** (2) 313–8.

Giovinazzo, V. J., Yannuzzi, L. A., Sorensen, J. A., Delrowe, D. J., and Campbell, E. A. (1987). The ocular complications of boxing. *Ophthalmology* **94** (6), 587–96.

Gregory, P. T. S. (1986). Sussex Eye Hospital sports injuries. *Br. J. Ophthalmol.* **70**, 748–50.

Helveston, E. M. (1987). Football. In *sports ophthalmology* (eds L. D. Pizzarello and B. J. Haik), ch. 4, 59–62, Charles C. Thomas, Springfield. IL.

Knorr, H. L. and Jonas J. B. (1996). Retinal detachments by squash ball accidents. *Am. J. Ophthalmol*, **122** (2) 260–1.

Lynch, P. and Rowan, B. (1997). Eye injury in sport: sport related eye injuries presenting to an eye casualty department throughout 1995. *Ir. Med. J.*, **90** (3) 112–4.

MacEwan, C. J. (1987). Sport associated eye injury: a casualty department survey. *Br. J. Ophthalmol.* **71**, 701–5.

MacEwan, C. J. (1989). Eye injuries: a prospective survey of 5671 cases. *Br. J. Ophthalmol.* **73**, 888–94.

MacEwan, C. J. and Jones, N. P. (1991). Eye injuries in racket sports. *Br. Med. J.* **302**, 1415–6.

Mamalis, N., Monson, M. C., Farnsworth, S. T., and White, G. L. (1990). Blunt ocular trauma secondary to 'war games'. *Ann. Ophthalmol.*, **22**, 416–8.

Millar, G. T. (1967). Golfing eye injuries. *Am. J. Ophthalmol.* **64**, 741–2.

Pashby, T. (1985). Eye injuries in Canadian amateur hockey. *Can. J. Ophthalmol.*, **20** (I), 2–4.

Rice, R. and Allen, R. C. (1985). Yoga in glaucoma. *Am. J. Ophthalmol.*, **100**, 738.

Tielsch, J. M. and Parver, L. M. (1990). Determinants of hospital charges and lengths of stay for ocular trauma. *Ophthalmology*, **97**, 231.

Vadala, G., Mollo, M., Roberto, S., and Fea, A. (1997). Boxing and the eyes: morphological aspects of the ocular system in boxers. *Eur. J. Ophthalmol*, **7** (2), 174–80.

Vinger, P. L. (1994). The eye in sports medicine, vol. 5, ch. 45, 1–94, In *Duane's clinical ophthalmology.* (eds W. Tasman and E. A. Jaeger) Eye protectors for sport. In *Sports Vision* Easterbrook, M. (1997). (eds D. F. C. Loran and C. J. MacEwen), ch. 5, 68–87. Lippincott-Raven, Philadelphia, PA.

Whiteson, A. L. (1981). Injuries in professional boxing. Their treatment and prevention. *Practitioner*, **225**, 1053–7.

Wilson, F. M. (1980). Traumatic hyphaema. *Ophthalmology*, **87**, 910–19.

3 Injuries to the shoulder

W. A. WALLACE AND M. A. HUTSON

Basic anatomy and biomechanics

The shoulder is a complex anatomical area which allows the arm to be moved in a number of directions to position the hand for either everyday or sporting activities. The design is superb, and is arranged to allow the maximum amount of both power and fine control to the movements of the arm and hand. Unfortunately, because of its generous range of movement, it is potentially a very unstable joint, and this may lead to considerable problems when the soft tissues around the shoulder are injured.

There are four different 'joints' in the shoulder region, all of which contribute to arm movement: the glenohumeral or true shoulder joint; the acromioclavicular joint; the scapulothoracic joint; and—perhaps the most important joint—the subacromial joint. This last joint has only become appreciated in recent years, but is the one most likely to give rise to pain from the shoulder—particularly in athletes. Then there is the sternoclavicular joint, some distance from the shoulder, which anchors the shoulder girdle to the chest wall and may also sustain a number of sports-related injuries.

The *glenohumeral joint* (Fig. 3.1) is rather like a ball (the humeral head), sitting on a shallow saucer (the bony glenoid). The saucer is deepend by both the glenoid labrum—a fibrous structure in some ways very similar to the meniscus in the knee—and the capsule of the shoulder joint, which provides some flexible restraint to the joint. Superiorly the humeral head is held down by the long head of biceps, which passes from its origin at the superior pole of the glenoid over the top of the humeral head and anteriorly downwards into the bicipital

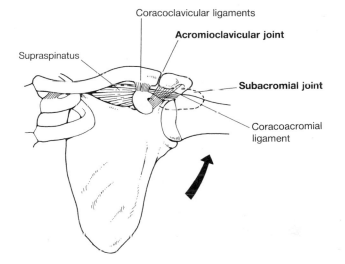

FIG. 3.2 The aromioclavicular and subacromial joints are demonstrated.

groove between the greater and lesser tuberosities of the humerus. Surrounding the humeral head and holding it in place is the rotator cuff, composed of four different muscles. Anteriorly is the subscapularis and superiorly the supraspinatus—both muscles becoming tendinous before reaching their insertions into the lesser and greater tuberosities of the humerus, respectively. Posteriorly lies the infraspinatus, which is muscular right up to its insertion, and the teres minor, which is very thick indeed. The difference between a tendinous insertion and a muscular insertion is important with regard to both injury and treatment. Injury to the supraspinatus will behave more like an Achilles tendon injury, while the infraspinatus will react to injury in a similar way to a torn hamstring or gastrocnemius muscle.

The *acromioclavicular (A-C)* joint (Figs 3.1 and 3.2) is unusual because its stability depends more on the coracoclavicular ligaments, which act as check reins, than on the local superior and inferior acromioclavicular ligaments. In fact, if these superior and inferior ligaments are damaged, there is little displacement of the joint. Within the A-C joint lies a meniscus, as in the knee, but this meniscus commonly becomes worn, and by the age of 30 is often only a peripheral tag. The A-C joint allows movement between the scapula and clavicle, which is required to allow the scapula its 60°–70° rotation on the chest wall during a full range of arm movement.

The *scapulothoracic joint* (Fig. 3.1) is important in sportsmen because it can be the site of inflammation, and later fibrosis, due

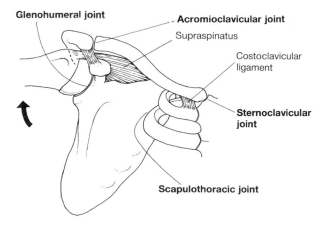

FIG. 3.1 The glenohumeral, acromioclavicular, scapulothoracic, and sternoclavicular joints are demonstrated.

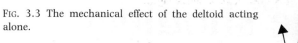

Origin of middle fibres
of deltoid from acromion

FIG. 3.3 The mechanical effect of the deltoid acting
alone.

to overuse. If this happens, adhesions develop in the layer
between the subscapularis and serratus anterior muscles and the
chest wall. These adhesions cause abnormal soft tissue tethering,
and result in a condition called 'snapping scapula'. This is normally painless, but occasionally can be a cause of pain and may
result in limitation of further sporting activity—particularly in
weight-lifters.

The *subacromial joint* (Fig. 3.2) has been ignored by
anatomists for many years. It is formed by (1) a roof, the
acromion posteriorly and the coracoacromial ligament and coracoid anteriorly, and (2) a floor, the supraspinatus tendon medially and the greater tuberosity of the humerus laterally. The
joint cavity is formed by the subacromial bursa—a sac which
contains only a thin film of fluid. The interesting feature of this
subacromial area is that if a large force is transmitted across the
subacromial joint, then pain occurs due to local soft tissue
injury. As a consequence, *this joint is responsible for the majority
of painful shoulders.*

The *sternoclavicular joint* (Fig. 3.1) lies outside the region of
the shoulder, but it makes an important contribution to movements of the shoulder girdle, and if injured can result in limitation of shoulder movement. The joint is similar in some ways to
the acromioclavicular joint. Although it does have joint ligaments passing from the sternum to the clavicle, the main stabilizing ligament of the joint is the costoclavicular ligament, which
is attached to the clavicle lateral to the joint. The joint is divided
into a medial and lateral compartment by an intra-articular
meniscus, which also acts as a stabilizing ligament. This joint
has no inherent mechanical stability, and is very dependent on
these different ligamentous structures to hold the bones in place.

The biomechanics of the shoulder complex are difficult to
grasp, but are perhaps best understood by concentrating first on
the kinetics—the study of the actual movements of the joints—
and secondly on the dynamics—the forces required to produce
these movements.

The *kinetics* of the shoulder movement are as follows. When
an arm is raised, the movement is usually divided into two
phases. The first 30° is described as the setting phase—during
this there is a variable pattern of shoulder movement, but
Poppen and Walker (1976) have noted that, for most shoulders,
movement during this phase occurs at the glenohumeral joint
while the scapula remains fairly static. From 30° onwards,
however, there is a uniform pattern of movement, with 2° of
glenohumeral movement for every 1° of scapular rotation. This
means that if the arm is raised to 90° elevation, then 60° is

glenohumeral while 30° is scapular; for 180° of elevation, 120°
is glenohumeral and 60° is scapular. For the A-C joint, studies
have shown that there is little movement if the arm is raised to
90°, but movements increase from 90° upwards, with the
maximum movement and the largest strain to the A-C joint
occurring from 140° to 180° of arm elevation (Wallace and
Johnson 1982).

The *dynamics* of shoulder movement highlight a delicately
coordinated group of muscles, all of which are required for
normal shoulder movement. If one considers the deltoid acting
alone on the dependent arm trying to raise it (see Fig. 3.3) it can
be seen that its action is to push the humeral head upwards,
forcing it to impinge on the acromion and the coracoacromial
arch through the subacromial joint. In order to prevent this, the
infraspinatus and teres minor posteriorly and the subscapularis
anteriorly tend to apply traction to the shoulder through the
greater and lesser tuberosities of the humerus, respectively,
pulling the head back down (see Fig. 3.4). This is helped further
by the tendons of the supraspinatus and the long head of biceps
which have a bowstring-type action which also pushes the
humeral head down. An excellent study (van Linge and Mulder
1963) has demonstrated that if the supraspinatus and infraspinatus muscles are put out of action by a local anaesthetic
block to the suprascapular nerve, then considerable weakness
and loss of endurance of the strength of the shoulder for
elevation occurs. This was highlighted by a reduced ability to lift
a weight to shoulder height and keep it there, although in most

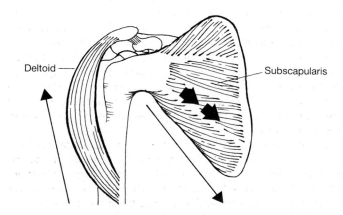

Deltoid   Subscapularis

FIG. 3.4 The mechanical effects of subscapularis, infraspinatus, teres
minor, and supraspinatus.

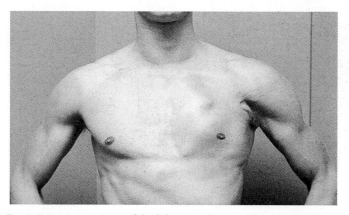

FIG. 3.5 Previous rupture of the left pectoralis major due to water-skiing is demonstrated.

cases the subjects were able to lift their arms up fully without any weights. Howell *et al.* (1986) have confirmed this finding in their studies using isokinetic dynamometry.

An integrated system (the brain and spinal cord) controls these groups of muscles, and usually does this very well, but if the coordination of muscle contraction is not good then the humeral head will be driven up through the subacromial joint, which will result in shoulder pain.

Besides the deltoid (which flexes and extends the shoulder as well as acting as an abductor), other muscles also act as prime movers of the shoulder joint. The pectoralis major is a powerful adductor, and also medially rotates the arm. The latissimus dorsi extends, medially rotates, and depresses the shoulder. The deltoid is rarely injured, despite the fact that referred pain is commonly felt over its inferior attachment. Pectoralis major occasionally is ruptured (Scott *et al.*, 1992), for instance in weight-lifting or water-skiing (Fig. 3.5). Partial rupture of the latissimus dorsi has been observed (M.A.H.), although it is uncommon.

The relationship between neck pain and shoulder dysfunction is an interesting and ill-understood phenomenon. It is common for those with neck pain from disorders of the cervical spine to suffer secondary shoulder pain—particularly the subacromial impingement-type of pain. In the authors' opinion, this occurs as a consequence of pressure on the C5 and C6 nerve roots, causing incoordination of the C5 and C6 innervated muscles (supraspinatus, infraspinatus, deltoid, and biceps), and pain is produced as a result. The opposite also occurs—shoulder pain secondarily produces neck pain because with shoulder dysfunction there tends to be increased tone in the trapezius, levator scapulae, and rhomboid muscles as well as the sternomastoid, all of which may disturb the mechanics of the cervical spine and result in neck pain. It follows that examination of the neck and of the upper limb for evidence of adverse neural tension (ANT) should always be undertaken in patients presenting with shoulder pain (Hutson, 1997)

Dyscoordination of muscle action also occurs in shoulder instability—subluxation (which is a partial dislocation) and dislocation of the joint. In these situations, muscle incoordination, either voluntary or subconscious (involuntary), may be the sole cause of the instability, and is perhaps the most common cause of multidirectional instability of the shoulder in teenagers. The forces required to produce normal shoulder movement are much larger than many realize. In a study carried out in Nottingham (Wallace 1984) the force required in either the supraspinatus or the infraspinatus to lift the arm was of the order of 30–40 kilograms, or 50 per cent of bodyweight.

Overuse syndromes of the shoulder

Problems with repetitive propulsive and explosive stress ('thrower's shoulder')

It may be seen from the foregoing account of the biomechanics of shoulder function that repetitive stress may give rise to a number of problems, of which attrition of the rotator cuff under the unyielding coracoacromial arch is a major one. The freely mobile glenohumeral joint is also at risk from the relative paucity of restraining capsular ligaments. A number of sports—for example, swimming, tennis, and those with a throwing component (for instance, baseball, American football, and cricket)—involve repetitive propulsive, and sometimes explosive, activity in the overhead position (Fig. 3.6). The size of the problem may be gauged from the estimation of Richardson *et al.* (1980) that over 40 per cent of elite swimmers, particularly those using the crawl, the butterfly, and the backstrokes, complain at one time or another of shoulder pain. Perhaps this is not surprising when one appreciates that the competitive swimmer may perform up to ten thousand overhead strokes in any one week of training. In the game of cricket, it is not unusual to find that at least one member of a team is unable to throw in a conventional overhead manner because of pain or the complaint of 'throwing the shoulder out'. A distinction should be made between throwing and bowling, as they have different biomechanical characteristics: a smoother action is required for bowling, which is less likely to cause injury. Pitchers in baseball and quarterbacks in American football also spend a considerable amount of time throwing during training as well as in matches. American sports physicians have developed a considerable insight into these problems, especially as they are advising a group of highly paid athletes. As a result of careful documentation of shoulder injuries, physicians have been instrumental in drawing up changes in the rules applied to baseball both in the junior 'Little Leagues' and in the senior games. Tennis, which is played more universally, imposes a considerable strain during the serve or overhead smash (see Fig. 1.4, p. 4). Although at first sight there may appear to be major differences between these various activities—for example, swimming as opposed to throwing—the following shoulder actions are common to all:

cocking (or recovery phase in swimming) involving abduction, external rotation, and extension;
acceleration (pull-through in swimming) involving forward flexion, internal rotation, and adduction;
follow-through (deceleration).

Each phase with its attendant problems will be described separately.

Cocking

The muscles responsible are the posterior deltoid, infraspinatus, and teres minor. In addition there is biceps brachii activity to flex the elbow. In the fully externally rotated and abducted posi-

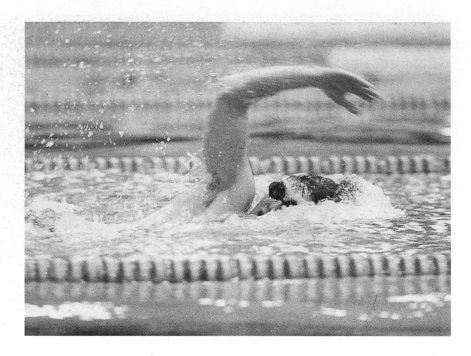

FIG. 3.6 A number of sports involve repetitive propulsive, and sometimes explosive, activity of the shoulder in the overhead position—crawl stroke swimming, baseball pitching, and cricket bowling.

tion, the subscapularis is stretched across the anterior aspect of the joint, and is active during this restraining function. In this position, the anterior capsule is stretched, and the shoulder is at risk from anterior subluxation. Such a risk applied to the underwater turn in backstroke swimming before the change of rules allowed a turn onto the front and the use of a tumble turn, as in front-crawl, on the approach to the wall. The main problems are thus related to anterior capsular strain and anterior instability, in addition to infraspinatus overactivity.

Acceleration

This is the main propulsive phase in throwing and racket overheads, and in company with follow-through accounts for the pull-through phase in swimming. The muscles involved are the anterior deltoid, pectoralis major, latissimus dorsi, subscapularis, and teres major. Attrition of the rotator cuff, principally the supraspinatus and the biceps brachii tendons, by *impingement* under the coracoacromial arch occurs in this situation, and probably accounts for the majority of those injuries that do not show much sign of early resolution. Other overuse conditions include stress fracture of the coracoid process, tendinitis of the conjoint tendon of the short head of biceps brachii and coracobrachialis, proximal epiphysitis of the humerus in youngsters, and stress fracture of the humerus. Tendinitis of the long head of the triceps, due to repeated elbow extension, occurs in swimmers and is also recognized in javelin throwers. Ringman's shoulder (insertional tendinitis of pectoralis major) is due to repeated maintenance of the iron-cross position in gymnastics. Andrews *et al.* (1985) have described superior labrum detachment in the region of the attachment of the long head of biceps. In throwers, this is presumably related to overuse of the biceps (acting through the long head) during cocking and again in the deceleration phase. Snyder *et al.* (1990) differentiated superior labral lesions into four types and labelled them SLAP (superior labrum anterior and posterior) lesions. Pain and clicking (often palpable as well as audible) on overhead activities are common complaints. Ectopic calcification may be visible on radiographs in any of the above situations.

Follow-through

The restraining action of the infraspinatus and the further activity of biceps brachii in this phase may contribute towards shoulder soreness. Posterior shoulder strain is common, and posterior subluxation (probably responsible for the arm being 'thrown out') may occur.

Impingement

Many factors may contribute to the development of impingement. A simple mechanical reason is a reduction in the subacromial gap—narrowing the subacromial space that is available for the rotator cuff. This can occur as a consequence of encroachment by inferior osteophytes from the acromioclavicular joint (Petersson and Gentz 1983), and may result in thinning of the cuff due to degenerative processes in the mature athlete (Fig. 3.7; see Fig. 10.20(a), p. 179). It has already been established that the rotator cuff is subject to attrition. The posterolateral aspect of the head of the humerus is particularly affected during the repeated combination of internal rotation, flexion, and adduction. 'Swimmer's impingement', for instance, typically occurs at the end of the recovery phase when the arm is brought into maximal internal rotation and forward elevation. Studies have shown that blanching of the cuff is a feature (Rathburn and McNab 1970), indicating that reduced vascularization plays a significant part, in combination with repeated microtrauma (Kennedy *et al.* 1978).

It is likely that a vicious circle develops: inflammatory swelling surrounding overused tendons provokes a friction effect underneath the coracoacromial arch, which gives rise to further microtrauma and further swelling. An inflammatory reaction occurs in the adjacent subacromial bursa, which initially is oedematous and invaded by inflammatory cells, and subsequently becomes fibrotic. Partial or full-thickness rotator cuff tears may develop as a result. Impingement of the humeral head occurs with a rotator cuff tear, as the head is allowed to rise up during abduction (Weiner and McNab 1970). Overuse tendinitis of the tendons of biceps brachii, subscapularis, supraspinatus,

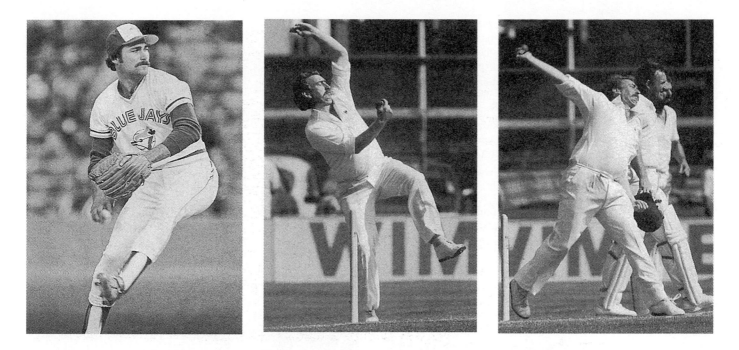

and infraspinatus may occur as a result of unaccustomed overhead exercise, giving rise to the painful arc syndrome as the affected tendon and the adjacent subacromial bursa are squeezed between the humeral head or greater tuberosity and the coracoacromial arch. Degenerative changes in the cuff may give rise to calcific deposits (Fig. 3.8), usually found in the supraspinatus tendon of the middle-aged. These give rise to acute subacromial bursitis and contribute further to subacromial impingement.

Instability

Chronic instability usually manifests itself as recurrent bouts of subluxation which follow an initial dislocation episode. Beware the 'sprained shoulder', which is often the presentation of the first acute dislocation episode. These shoulders should be treated with a broad arm-sling under the clothes for four weeks to reduce the chance of recurrence. Recurrent anterior dislocation is particularly common in younger patients (aged 18 to 30). What is rarely appreciated is that if a dislocation occurs at this age, the chance of a normal shoulder later is only 20 per cent, with 60 per cent having recurrent dislocation episodes and 20 per cent recurrent subluxation symptoms (Simonet and

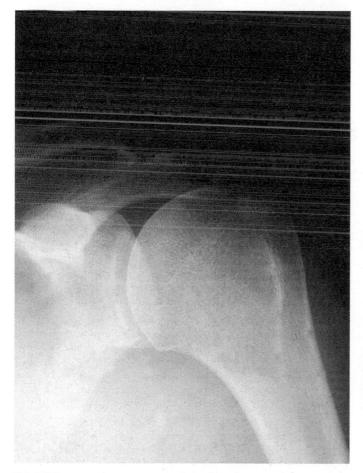

FIG. 3.7 Downward-pointing osteophytes from the A-C joint.

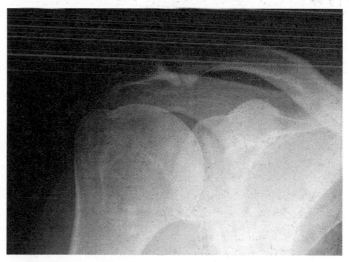

FIG. 3.8 Calcium (hydroxyapatite) deposits in the rotator cuff—usually the supraspinatus tendon. These may contribute to subacromial impingement.

Cofield 1984). A similar situation may apply to the less common posterior dislocation. Subsequent dislocations may be reduced by the patient; nevertheless, he should be referred to an orthopaedic surgeon for consideration of surgical stabilization of the shoulder. The general rule is that patients are expected to 'earn' their operations, and most orthopaedic surgeons will only operate if there have been at least three dislocation episodes. Sometimes, however, the subsequent episodes take the form of subluxation rather than dislocation. These can be very disabling, and are often associated with a sudden click in the shoulder, a popping sensation, a 'dead arm', or a pain shooting down the arm or into the hand. These episodes occasionally are followed by a few days of shoulder dysfunction.

It is important to separate recurrent traumatic subluxation or dislocation, which is usually unidirectional, from recurrent atraumatic subluxation or dislocation, which is often multi-directional. Beware of the habitual dislocator who has no history of trauma, but is able to dislocate the shoulder either anteriorly or posteriorly at will. These patients are special cases. They should not be treated by surgery, and are best referred early to an orthopaedist with a special interest in shoulders, to have reassurance and rotator cuff-strengthening exercises.

Careful attention should be paid to the history, and in particular a detailed enquiry should be made into the position of the arm at the time of the initial dislocation and also the position of the arm during subsequent episodes of subluxation or dislocation.

Assessment

The history

Full details of the history should be obtained from every patient with a shoulder problem. As in the knee, approximately 50 per cent of patients can have a diagnosis made from the history alone. The pain from conditions in the subacromial region is often felt at the anterolateral aspect of the shoulder or close to the insertion of the deltoid, and frequently it radiates to the upper arm. In the condition of capsulitis, which enters into the differential diagnosis in patients aged 45 years or over, pain comes on gradually and may radiate down the arm as far as the wrist. However, pain may come on suddenly and, if associated with a fall on to the point of the shoulder, this is strongly suggestive of a rotator cuff tear, a fracture, an A-C joint injury (see p. 48), or occasionally a gleno-humeral joint dislocation with spontaneous reduction. The pain may be accompanied by a click and be grossly disabling for a short while, suggesting instability. It may take the form of the typical overuse syndrome, in which the pain gradually becomes more severe and is felt earlier in the exercise programme, eventually totally preventing training or any exercise. Such a story is strongly suggestive of impingement. As with all cases of shoulder and arm pain, any associated or preceding neck pain should be noted. A history of paraesthesiae and numbness in a dermatomal pattern, suggesting true nerve-root irritation, should always be sought.

The examination

ALWAYS examine the neck, and include a test for neural tension, prior to examination of the shoulder.

A logical pattern of examination of the shoulder is crucial:

LOOK *then* MOVE *then* FEEL *then* INVESTIGATE FURTHER.

(1) LOOK—*observation* might reveal muscle-wasting in the region of the deltoid or in the supraspinous or infraspinous fossa.

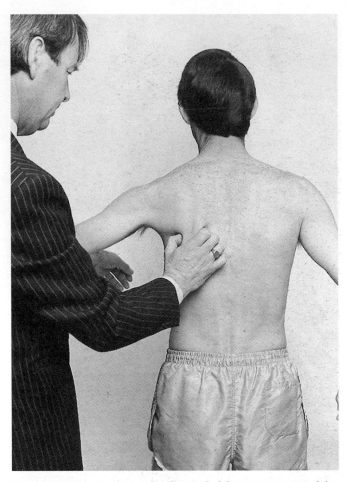

FIG. 3.9 Assessment of true glenohumeral abduction requires stabilization of the scapula.

Localized soft tissue swelling is sometimes observed over the humeral head, particularly in acute bursitis, but this is uncommon. The subacromial bursa is more commonly swollen in the presence of a full-thickness rotator cuff tear or in rheumatological conditions.

(2) Move—*active movements* are assessed first. Active abduction yields information on the presence of a painful arc (see later), and on any restriction of range of movement. Abnormal scapulo-humeral rhythm should be observed by standing behind the patient. One useful sign is to study the anterior bulge formed by the top part of the humeral head during the initiation of abduction or flexion. In the presence of a rotator cuff tear or weakness of the cuff the head will ride up at the start of movement. If the shoulder is normal, the head position does not change. Included at this stage are tests of serratus anterior function to identify winging of the scapula due to a long thoracic nerve palsy. This can occur from excessive stretching of the nerve from an indirect injury.

Passive movements are assessed next. The full range of passive shoulder movements is performed with care, so that the examiner is clear in his own mind exactly which movements or combinations of movements are being tested. Initially the patient is examined in the standing position. True glenohumeral abduction is assessed by passive abduction of the arm, using one hand supporting the elbow for leverage and the thumb and index fingers of the other examining hand to stabilize the inferior angle of the scapula

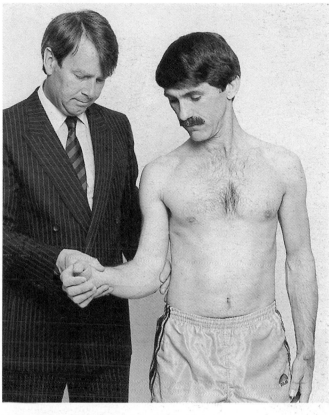

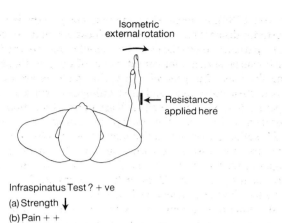

Isometric
external rotation

Resistance
applied here

Infraspinatus Test ? + ve

(a) Strength ↓

(b) Pain + +

FIG. 3.10 The elbow should be held by the examiner at a right angle prior to assessment of both the passive range of external rotation and the power of the external rotators (the infraspinatus test).

FIG. 3.11 Functional internal rotation (a) is compared with the normal side (b) by determining the number of the spinous process reached by the dorsum of the patient's hand.

(a)

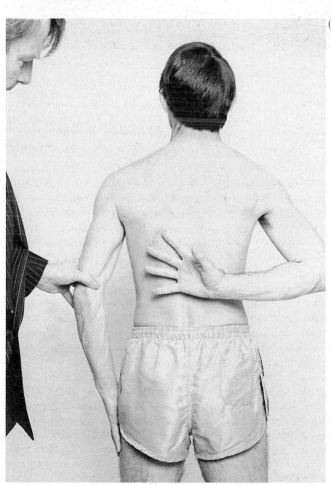

(b)

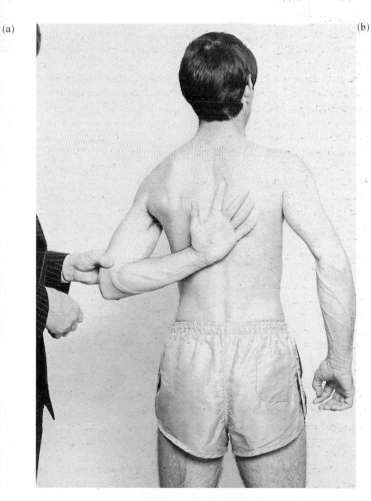

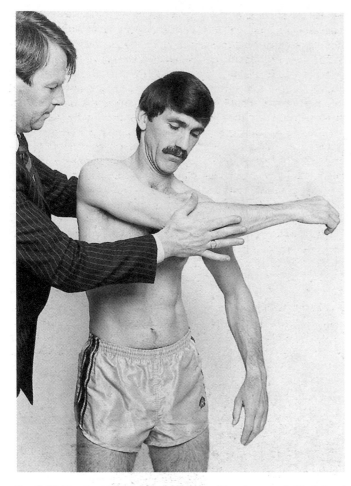

FIG. 3.12 Passive adduction is tested by pushing the arm, held at shoulder level, across the front of the chest. (This is also used as the A-C joint stress test.)

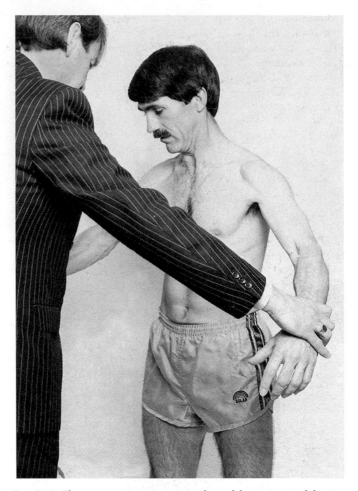

FIG. 3.13 The supraspinatus test is performed by resisting abduction with the arms in 20° abduction and 20° flexion.

(Fig. 3.9). The degree of arm abduction from the vertical is measured to the point at which the scapula starts to rotate. External rotation (Fig. 3.10) should be performed initially with the arm dependent and the elbow held at a right angle. Functional internal rotation (Fig. 3.11) is compared with the normal side by determining the number of the spinous process reached by the *dorsum* of the subject's hand at the full range of movement. There is now increasing awareness that a tight posterior capsule can give rise to impingement. It is therefore important to check full passive internal rotation in patients with impingement. Passive adduction (Fig. 3.12) is tested by pushing the arm, held at shoulder level, across the front of the chest. In all these movements, a note is made of any restriction in range and the degree of pain elicited.

Patterns to emerge

(a) *The capsular pattern.* The capsular pattern of the shoulder is greater restriction of passive external rotation than of abduction or internal rotation. At its earliest stage, external rotation alone may be restricted; subsequently all movements are restricted, so that in its most severe form there is up to 20° of fixed internal rotation. These signs denote capsulitis, either post-traumatic or adhesive ('frozen shoulder').

(b) *The non-capsular pattern.* Chronic subacromial bursitis is one cause of a restriction of passive movements in a non-capsu-

lar pattern, although the possibility of more serious pathology (for instance, metastatic deposits) in the middle-aged and elderly should always be borne in mind. A typical pattern might be significant restriction of abduction and internal rotation, coupled with well-maintained external rotation. In acute bursitis, such as that which occurs in gout, all movements are grossly restricted. In this situation, the short history (hours or days), with no history of trauma, reduces the differential diagnosis to either gout or acute calcific tendinitis.

Assessing muscle balance

Apparent gross muscle weakness may be due to either pain inhibition or to neurological deficit, and should prompt regular examination over a few months. Winging of the scapula due to weakness of the serratus anterior may be a presenting feature of neuralgic amyotrophy—a disease which is still not clearly understood. Weakness of pectoralis major may be secondary to C7 nerve-root compression, but could also be due to direct injury (see Fig. 3.5). Occasionally, minor tears of latissimus dorsi occur, giving rise to pain on resisted depression of the arm. Lesser degrees of muscle imbalance, possibly associated with loss of flexibility, may not only indicate incomplete recovery, but may also be the precursors of a more substantial injury.

Assessment of the rotator cuff—the supraspinatus, infraspinatus, and subscapularis tests

The clinical assessment of the rotator cuff is an integral part of every examination of the shoulder. Rotator cuff injury in athletes and those participating in recreational sport is very common indeed. The muscles and their relationship to the subacromial bursa are examined as follows.

(a) *The supraspinatus test* (Fig. 3.13) is carried out with the patient standing. With the elbow straight, the arm is placed in about 20° of both abduction and flexion, and the patient attempts to abduct the arm against resistance. The examiner assesses the strength of abduction, and the patient reports the amount of pain produced by this manoeuvre. The examiner then tests the opposite (normal) shoulder for comparison. If the test is painful, but there is no significant weakness, then this indicates supraspinatus tendinitis. Weakness on testing, however, indicates a rotator cuff tear. Unfortunately, if there is a lot of pain during testing, weakness due to pain inhibition occurs, and the situation should be evaluated again after carrying out an impingement injection test.

(b) *The impingement injection test* (Neer 1983) allows the doctor to establish the exact site of the painful arc syndrome. An injection of 5–10 ml of local anaesthetic (such as 0.25 per cent bupivacaine or 1 per cent lignocaine) is given into the subacromial bursa in the region of the supraspinatus tendon. After ten minutes, the patient is re-examined, and if the painful arc is improved or abolished, then the site of the pain has been established. After a supraspinatus test which is positive for pain, an impingement test should be carried out to confirm the location of the pain, and then a further supraspinatus test should be carried out.

(c) *The infraspinatus test* (Fig. 3.10) is very similar to the supraspinatus test, and is a test of resisted (isometric) external rotation of the shoulder. The infraspinatus is the only efficient external rotator of the glenohumeral joint. Pain and weakness on testing are sought; pain denotes a tendinitis and weakness indicates a tear. Infraspinatus tears are particularly common in throwing athletes, but as the infraspinatus is almost totally muscular, tears usually heal, although they may have a protracted course.

(d) The *subscapularis test* (Fig. 3.14) is similar to but the opposite of the infraspinatus test—that is, resisted (isometric) *internal* rotation is assessed. Unfortunately, this movement is produced by pectoralis major and latissimus dorsi, as well as subscapularis, and therefore this is not such a sensitive test.

(e) The *biceps test* (Fig. 3.15) is supposed to indicate biceps tendinitis. It is a test of resisted (isometric) elbow flexion, this being the activity which stresses particularly the long head of the biceps tendon. As biceps tendinitis is rare (despite comments made by other authors to the contrary), and a false-positive test is common, particularly with subscapularis tendinitis, this test is unreliable. If the test is performed with a supinated forearm (instead of in neutral forearm rotation), an unstable biceps tendon may sublux from the bicipital groove.

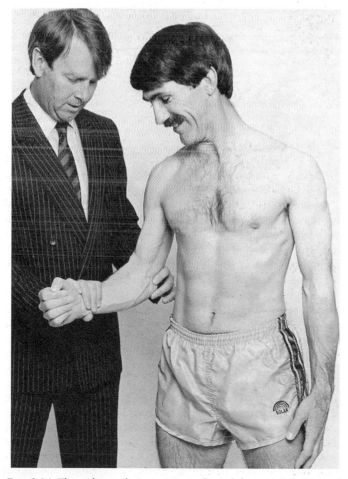

FIG. 3.14 The subscapularis test is performed by resisting internal rotation.

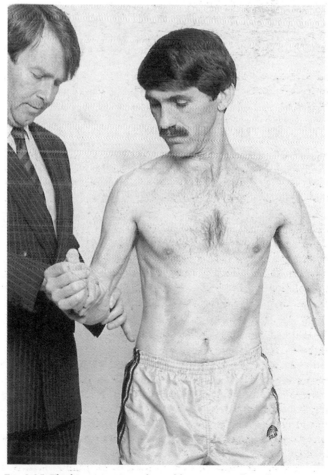

FIG. 3.15 The biceps test is performed by resisting elbow flexion.

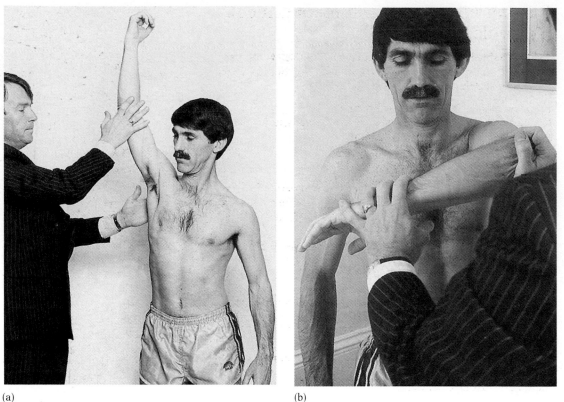

FIG. 3.16 The impingement signs: (a) full passive flexion; (b) 90° forward flexion combined with internal rotation.

(a)   (b)

(f) *Impingement signs* (Fig. 3.16) are produced by pushing the greater tuberosity upwards against the inferior aspect of the acromion—first when the arm is fully flexed, and secondly when the arm is internally rotated with 90° of forward flexion (Hawkins and Kennedy 1980; Gerber *et al.* 1985). The tests are positive when painful. Passive external rotation of the shoulder is *not* restricted; internal rotation is painful and often restricted in range. Thus the non-capsular pattern emerges.

Other special tests to identify instability or specific joint pathologies are used at this stage. Which special tests are chosen depends on the differential diagnosis indicated by the previous history and examination. It is important not to carry out every special test on every patient, as this is both uncomfortable for the patient and time-consuming for the doctor. These special tests are described later.

(3) FEEL—*palpation* should be the final part of the examination because, again, where the examiner palpates depends on his likely diagnosis from the history and examination so far. Localized tenderness of the palpable portion of the subacromial bursa immediately inferior to the anterior margin of the acromion suggests subacromial bursitis. Tenderness of the insertion of the supraspinatus tendon is most easily elicited when the arm is internally rotated behind the back, thus bringing the greater tuberosity to the fore. In this position, a defect (representing a substantive tear) in the supraspinatus tendon may be palpated by the experienced examiner.

Tenderness of the infraspinatus musculotendinous area should be detected with the patient prone, leaning on the elbow, and with the arm externally rotated 10°. Biceps tenderness (a non-specific sign) may be found in the bicipital groove. Subscapularis tenderness is felt more medially, over the anterior head of the humerus. Other anatomical sites—for instance, the coracoid process and the superior aspect of the A-C joint—may be palpated at this stage.

(4) FURTHER INVESTIGATIONS. Although most overuse syndromes of the shoulder are related to the soft tissues, radiographs can be helpful—particularly in excluding serious disorders (metabolic bone disorders and secondary tumours). Initially conventional AP and axial views are required. Two views of the shoulder are essential, and if it is not possible to abduct the arm sufficiently for a conventional axial view, then a modified axial view as described by Wallace and Hellier (1983) should be taken. Ectopic calcification, resulting from degenerative change, may be seen in the region of the supraspinatus tendon (see Fig. 3.8). However, its presence is not necessary for the diagnosis of supraspinatus tendinitis; indeed it may be quite incidental, as demonstrated by one patient with clinical adhesive capsulitis who recovered fully following intra-articular steroid injections, but still had a large calcific deposit after treatment in a shoulder which was then painless. Nevertheless, calcium may interfere mechanically with normal shoulder function. Not uncommonly, after a prolonged period lying 'dormant' within the cuff, an acute calcific tendinitis may develop suddenly. As the calcium liquefies, an acute inflammatory response develops, causing the patient severe pain resulting in disturbance of sleep and inability to move the arm. Degenerative changes within the A-C joint are common in middle-age, and again are usually of little significance. However, in weight-lifters and men doing heavy manual work, the A-C joint occasionally develops a painful osteolysis, in which loss of bone, usually on the clavicular side of the joint, may be clearly seen on X-ray (Cahill 1982; Leyshon and Kessel 1982).

Further assessment and management of shoulder injuries

As highlighted in the previous section, the history is very important. In sportsmen and sportswomen, the four common conditions which do not settle are:

(1) recurrent subluxation of the shoulder;
(2) chronic subacromial impingement syndrome (which may be secondary to recurrent subluxation);
(3) a rotator cuff tear;
(4) acromioclavicular disorders.

To this list one might add lesions of the superior labrum, including SLAP tears, which, although relatively uncommon in comparison with the afore-mentioned conditions, have assumed greater prominence in recent years.

The assessment of the shoulder by an orthopaedic specialist will involve the following questions.

(a) What is your problem?
The problem will be pain, the giving way of the shoulder in certain positions, or inability to practise the sport to as high a standard as the athlete would wish. It should be remembered that it is not uncommon for a sportsman or sportswoman to fail to achieve a high standard and then to blame an injury for this, rather than to recognize that their failure of achievement is indeed due to a lack of skill.

(b) Where is the pain?
The pain will be identified either by the finger directed at the A-C joint area or by the palm of the hand directed to the front of the shoulder region or to the deltoid muscle.

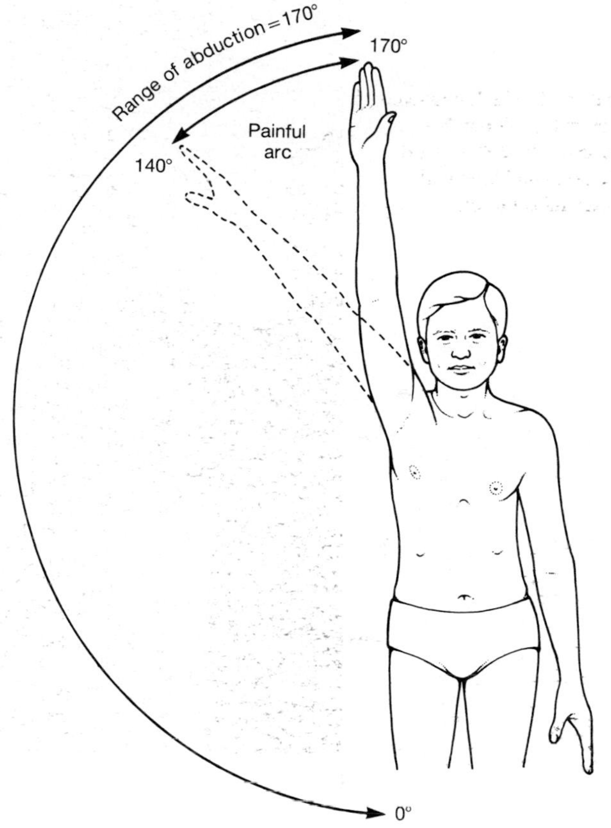

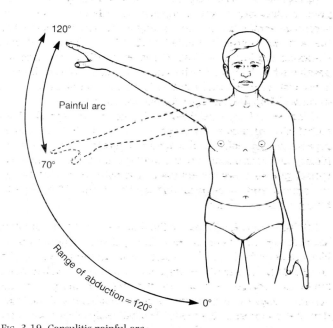

FIG. 3.18 A-C painful arc.

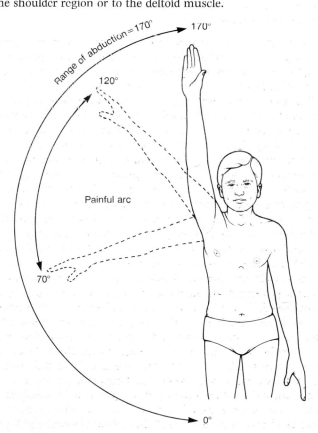

FIG. 3.17 Subacromial painful arc.

FIG. 3.19 Capsulitis painful arc.

(c) When does the pain occur—at rest? during activity? which activity?
Pain at rest normally indicates either early arthritis in the shoulder or a developing capsulitis ('frozen shoulder'), both of which are uncommon in the sportsman. Adhesive capsulitis may occur in the 45- to 60-year-old and, although not due to

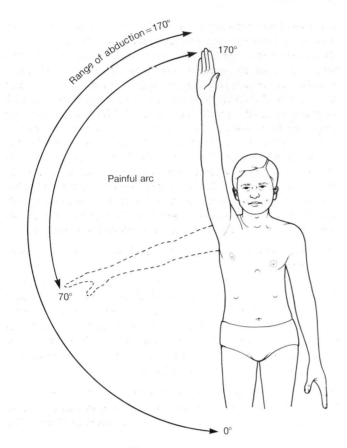

FIG. 3.20 Composite painful arc.

sport, nevertheless restricts activities, particularly racket sports. The capsular pattern of loss of movement is found on examination (Cyriax 1982). Management by intra-articular injection (see Fig. 12.9, p. 213), followed by stretching exercises (see Fig. 11.14, p. 198), has been found to be beneficial in most cases (Wallace and Echeverri 1987).

Pain on movement usually indicates a painful arc, and it is then necessary to identify which type of painful arc. There are four types: the subacromial painful arc, the A-C painful arc, the capsulitis painful arc, and the composite painful arc.

The *subacromial painful arc* (Fig. 3.17) typically produces a mid-arc pain during abduction (and less commonly during flexion) in the arc between 70° and 120° of elevation. It is accentuated by pronation of the forearm. This arc indicates pain arising from subacromial impingement. It will normally be improved or abolished by the impingement injection test.

The *A-C painful arc* (Fig. 3.18) is a painful arc at the extreme of flexion or abduction of the shoulder, occurring between 140° and 170° of elevation.

The *capsulitis painful arc* (Fig. 3.19) is a terminal painful arc which occurs in a shoulder with a restricted range of movement—that is, elevation may be reduced to 120°, and the painful arc lies between 70° and 120°.

The *composite painful arc* (Fig. 3.20) is one where there is a near-normal range of shoulder elevation, but a painful arc from 70° to the top of the range. This is a fairly common situation. It occurs in patients who have dual pathologies, such as A-C joint pain and a subacromial impingement, or subacromial impingement and an early capsulitis.

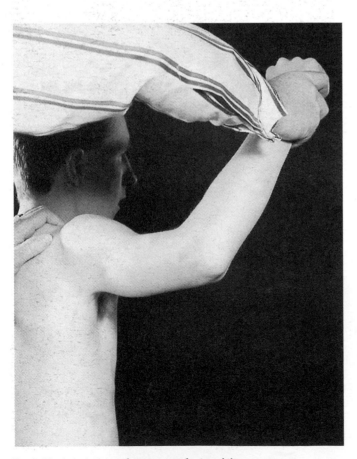

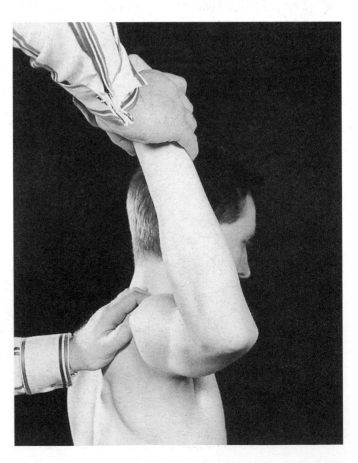

FIG. 3.21 Anterior apprehension test for instability.

AN APPARENT SUBACROMIAL IMPINGEMENT SYNDROME IN A PATIENT UNDER THE AGE OF FORTY IS A TRAP FOR THE UNWARY—this is often a sign of shoulder instability, which produces secondary impingement.

(d) Is the shoulder unstable?

The patient will sometimes clearly say, 'I feel the shoulder jump out' or 'In some positions my shoulder seems to catch'. The patient is usually right, and it is important to explore the past history for a previous episode of possible traumatic dislocation. In a patient of under 30 years, there is more than an 80 per cent likelihood of recurrent subluxation or recurrent dislocation following a reported past dislocation. A useful question to ask the patient is, 'Does your hand ever feel funny or develop pins and needles when your shoulder jumps?' If so, one can be confident that the problem is indeed an unstable shoulder.

Assessment of the shoulder for instability—anterior, posterior, and multidirectional

The doctor should assume that all patients with shoulder pain or a sensation of instability might have an unstable shoulder, and should carry out the following tests for instability, which have been well described by Gerber and Ganz (1984).

(a) Anterior apprehension test for anterior instability (Fig. 3.21)

The patient may be examined sitting, though greater patient relaxation is usually achieved when supine. The problem shoul-der is passively abducted to 90° and is then passively externally rotated by the examiner into full external rotation. The arm is then pushed into the fully stressed position, while the patient's face is studied for apprehension and the anterior shoulder muscles are examined for muscle spasm. If pain is produced in an unstable shoulder, pressure backwards on the humeral neck may relieve it (the Jobe relocation test). The normal shoulder may then be stressed in the same way, and the two sides compared to detect loss of the passive range of movement. Finally, on the problem side, the arm is lifted higher under stressed external rotation, and then lowered through a range of 140° to 60° of abduction in order to identify any part of the abduction arc which produces apprehension. There is a risk during this test of provoking an anterior dislocation if the shoulder is grossly unstable; if this is suspected, extra care should be exercized.

(b) The sulcus sign (described by Neer and Foster 1980) for inferior subluxation (Fig. 3.22)

The patient is seated with both arms hanging downwards on either side of the chair and is asked to relax. The examiner applies a downward traction on the arm by holding the wrist and distracting the arm downwards firmly but not roughly. If the shoulder is inferiorly unstable, a sulcus will appear under the acromion—between the acromion and the humeral head—which will be both visible and palpable.

(c) Posterior stress test for posterior instability (Fig. 3.23)

The patient is examined lying supine on an examination couch. The arm is brought passively into 90° elevation in flexion. For

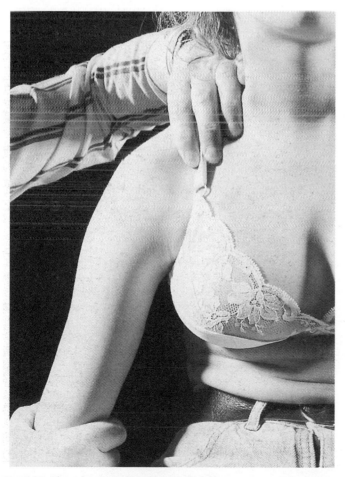
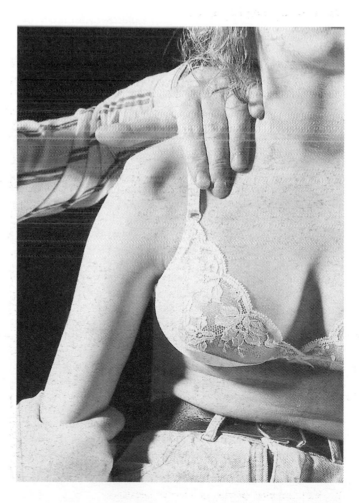

FIG. 3.22 The sulcus sign for inferior instability.

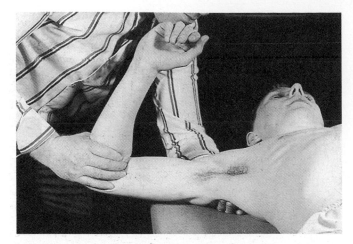 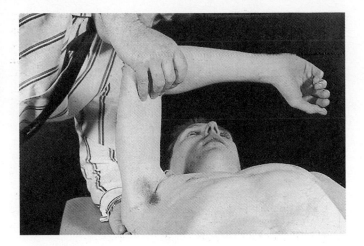

FIG. 3.23 Posterior stress test for instability.

examination of a right shoulder, the examiner's left hand is placed behind the glenohumeral joint—that is, under the shoulder blade. The humeral head is then pushed posteriorly by holding the elbow with the examiner's right hand and applying an axial loading to the humerus with the elbow at a right angle—that is, by pushing along the arm from the elbow, trying to push the humeral head backwards out of joint. If the joint is posteriorly unstable, it will sublux posteriorly, and the examiner's left hand may feel this happening. However, it may not be picked up at this stage. The shoulder is next abducted in its 90° flexed position, with the shoulder axially loaded by the examiner's right hand—that is, the examiner continues to push hard along the length of the humerus, while *abducting* the shoulder. If the shoulder was posteriorly subluxed initially, as it is *abducted* it will jump back into joint and a clunk will be felt. Again, in the grossly unstable shoulder, there is a definite risk of producing a complete posterior dislocation using this stress test.

The afore-mentioned tests are very valuable in the assessment of the problem shoulder. If one is positive the patient has a unidirectional instability, but if two or three tests are positive, then the instability is multidirectional and in general a very much more difficult condition to treat. In addition to these three standard tests, the degree of laxity, hence instability, at the glenohumeral joint may be assessed by anteror-posterior translatory movements undertaken in either the sitting or lying position. In concept, this examination is similar to the detection of increased movement in the horizontal plane at the knee and ankle following capsular/ligamentous injuries. As at the knee, the experienced clinician may have early difficulty in becoming proficient at this type of joint-play examination. A reasonably firm grasp of the acromion is required with one hand, whilst the other hand grasps the *proximal* humerus and introduces the required A+P translation. Excessive movement and/or a chick are sought.

A chick, indicative of a superior labral tear, is more likely to be present when the humeral head is loaded into the glenoid by the examiner. (This test is sometimes referred to as the 'load and shift' test.) A further test for a labral tear described by Liu *et al.* (1996) is the 'crank' test which is positive if a click is produced when the fully flexed shoulder is internally and externally rotated under axial load.

Further investigations for instability

All patients should have good quality radiographs—two AP views, one in external rotation and one in 60° internal rotation (Crawford Adams 1948). In addition, a Stryker view is valuable in picking up the Hill–Sachs (Hill and Sachs 1940) or Broca (Broca and Hartman 1890) lesion, which is a bony dent in the humeral head. The other lesion typically found in 85 per cent of anterior dislocation patients (Rowe *et al.* 1978) is the Bankart lesion—an avulsion of the capsule and glenoid labrum from the anterior inferior portion of the glenoid rim. Usually this can be picked up only on an arthrogram (preferably a double-contrast CT arthrogram) or by arthroscopy; however, straight X-rays often show infraglenoid new bone formation (Hastings and Coughlin 1981). The indication for these further investigations is only when the diagnosis of instability is not definite or where there have been recurrent episodes of trouble with the shoulder and it has not been possible to make a diagnosis. Finally, if the diagnosis is still in doubt, it may be necessary to perform an examination under anaesthetic (EUA), which should be carried out by an orthopaedic surgeon with experience of shoulder instability.

Treatment for instability—anterior, posterior, and multidirectional

Anterior instability

If the shoulder is subluxing and not frankly dislocating, it is better to achieve stability, if possible, with rotator cuff-strengthening exercises. The supraspinatus will be built up with isometric and isokinetic abduction exercises, the infraspinatus with external rotation exercises with the arm by the side, and the subscapularis with internal rotation exercises. In general, exercises should be restricted to below shoulder level, as subluxation is usually precipitated by elevation of the arm above shoulder level, and there is usually no problem with range of movement of the shoulder in these patients. The patient should be warned that some multi-gym activities do stress the shoulder and provoke rather than help anterior instability, and they should be given physiotherapy or medical guidance about which exercises are most appropriate for their instability.

If anterior instability fails to respond to non-operative treatment for more than twelve months *and* the instability is unidirectional, then surgical stabilization of the shoulder should be considered. However, it is common after shoulder stabilization operations to lose at least 20° to 30° of elevation and external rotation, and in the cases of competitive athletes such as javelin throwers, karate sportsmen, or cricket bowlers, this may end their sporting careers in these fields.

Posterior instability

This should also be treated with a conservative regime of strengthening exercise for a period of at least twelve months, again using rotator cuff-strengthening exercises, but concentrating on building up the infraspinatus and teres minor muscles posteriorly. Strengthening exercises appear to be more successful for posterior instability than for anterior instability.

If posterior instability fails to settle with conservative treatment, then surgery may be considered. Although loss of range of movement is less of a problem with posterior stabilization operations, recurrence of the subluxation is not uncommon, and the patient should be warned before surgery that the surgeon cannot guarantee long-term success from this type of operation—perhaps a success rate of only 60 per cent.

Multidirectional instability

Patients who have instability in more than one direction provide a major treatment problem. Athletes—particularly swimmers and gymnasts—often have to retire early from their sporting careers if they develop this problem. Generalized joint laxity may exist, so that examination of the wrists, thumbs, elbows, and knees should be made to detect hyperextensibility (see Fig. 1.12, p. 11). The treatment is a conservative regime of strengthening of the rotator cuff muscles, with up to two years of physiotherapy and avoidance of activities which provoke the subluxation episodes. Sport may have to be discontinued during the treatment period. It has been felt by some shoulder surgeons that certain multi-gym exercises (particularly those which stretch the anterior shoulder capsule, as occurs with movements of 90° abduction with 90° external rotation) have been responsible for producing this kind of instability, and it is also more common in butterfly swimmers.

If multidirectional instability continues for more than two years, and the patient wishes to accept a failure rate of 50 per cent, then surgery can be considered. Dr Neer in New York has devised an 'inferior capsular shift' operation for multidirectional instability, but, regrettably, recurrence of instability is fairly common after this procedure, and it is essential that the patient is warned about this before surgery.

Treatment for rotator cuff impingement and tears

Chronic rotator cuff impingement causes a recurrent subacromial painful arc syndrome. In the patient under 40 years of age the diagnosis of instability must first be excluded on clinical examination. Initial management is demonstrated in Fig. 12.10 (see p. 224), by an injection of the subacromial bursa (*not* the supraspinatus tendon) with a mixture of 5 ml of local anaesthetic (for instance, 1 per cent lignocaine or 0.25 per cent bupivacaine)

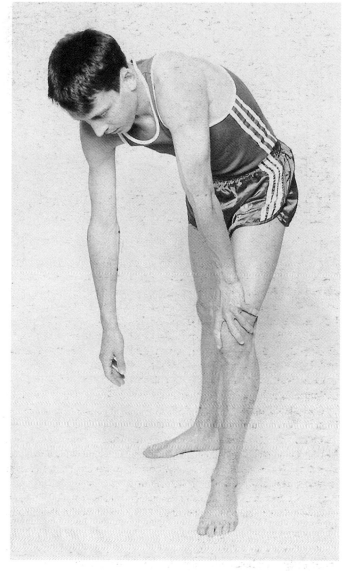

FIG. 3.24 The position of the patient is demonstrated for circumduction movements of the right shoulder under the effect of gravity (Codman exercises).

and long-acting local steroid (for instance, 1 ml–20 mg of triamcinolone hexacetonide). Up to three injections (at intervals of four weeks between injections) may be necessary. If injection treatment fails, local physiotherapy, with ice-massage, ultrasound, pulsed electromagnetic field treatment (PEMF), interferential, and particularly deep transverse frictions (Cyriax 1984) directed to an individual cuff tendon, can be very successful.

Normally tendinitis and associated subacromial bursitis resolve following subacromial injections and the use of localized physiotherapeutic anti-inflammatory modalities. Occasionally insertional tendinitis (usually of the supraspinatus) proves to be refractory.

In this situation, the insertion of the supraspinatus may be injected with low-dose steroid—such as 10 mg of triamcinolone hexacetonide (M.A.H.) (see Fig. 12.11, p. 225). If symptomatic calcific tendinitis is present, 'dry' needling may be successful, though an additional injection of steroid and local anaesthetic for the associated inflammatory reaction is a more logical approach. Rarely, the insertions of infraspinatus and subscapularis into the

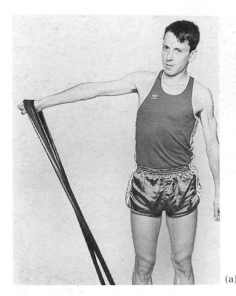 (a)

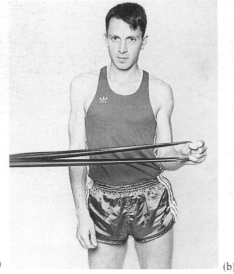 (b)

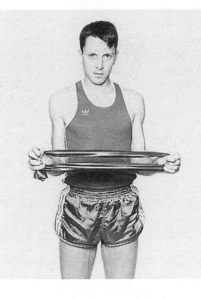 (c)

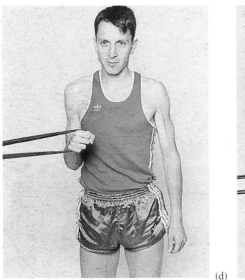 (d)

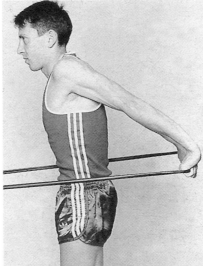 (e)

FIG. 3.25 Strengthening exercises for the shoulder muscles may be performed with Cliniband (as shown) or surgical tubing: (a) abductors; (b) and (c) external rotators; (d) internal rotators; (e) extensors.

greater and lesser tuberosities respectively require injection (see Figs 12.12 and 12.13, pp. 225 and 226). The infraspinatus lesion frequently lies at the musculotendinous junction, when it should be treated as a muscle tear. In all cases in which enthesopathies are injected, it is particularly important to follow up with strengthening exercises. Biceps tendinitis is relatively uncommon; occasionally an injection around the tendon in the bicipital groove is helpful if physiotherapy is unsuccessful (see Fig. 12.14, p. 226).

Flexibility exercises

Aggressive stretching exercises must not be used in the inflammatory phase, as they may contribute to persistence of the condition. In the presence of painful restriction of shoulder movements, the only flexibility exercises performed by the patient are Codman exercises (Fig. 3.24), which allow gravity to distract the glenohumeral joint. The therapist may utilize Maitland's passive exercises under gentle arm traction (Maitland 1986).

Once subacromial bursitis has resolved (or surgical stabilization has been achieved), graded stretching exercises with a stick or cane are encouraged on a home physiotherapy regimen (see Fig. 11.14, p. 208). Particular attention is paid to those movements which are relatively restricted: loss of passive external rotation, for instance, tends to occur in racket players and swimmers as a result of the overdevelopment of the medial rotators. Flexibility exercises should be considered later for prophylaxis.

Strengthening exercises

Isometric contraction within the painless range may be commenced as soon as there is sufficient healing of the cuff tendons to allow this to be performed painlessly. In due course exercises with surgical tubing or 'Cliniband' are instituted (Fig. 3.25), and followed if possible by isokinetic exercises. Attention is paid to the full complement of muscle groups responsible for internal and external rotation, flexion, extension, abduction, and adduction. Once it has been determined that strength in all groups

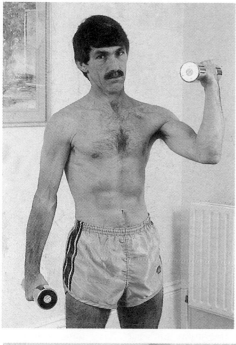

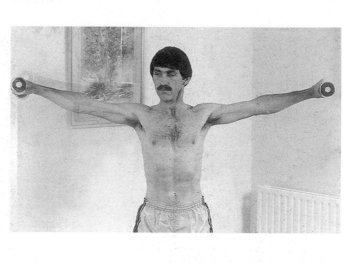

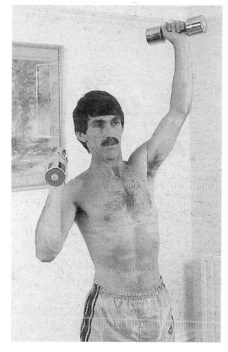

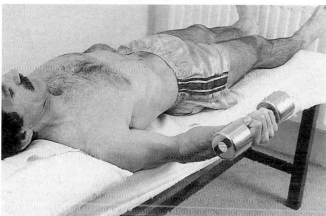

FIG. 3.26 Isotonic exercises using hand-held weights are demonstrated.

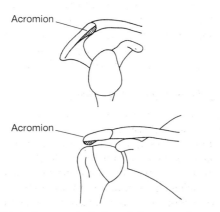

Acromion

Acromion

FIG. 3.27 Neer's anterior acromioplasty and decompression.

has improved to equal that of the normal side, isotonic contractions using hand-held weights and other available equipment may be started under the guidance of the therapist (Fig. 3.26). However, it is important that an inappropriate level of stress is not imposed on the shoulder too early in that position in which impingement or subluxation has been noted to occur.

Sports techniques

The mechanics of shoulder function, as applied to the specific sport, should be assessed to determine whether alterations of technique are possible to reduce stress. In swimming, impingement syndromes may be alleviated by measures such as raising the arm higher during the recovery phase, reducing extension of the arm by elevating the elbow at hand entry, and improving body-roll during the pull phase. Similar attention to biomechanical detail is often necessary in throwing and in racket sports, a situation which demands close cooperation with the coach. Tennis servers, for instance, learn to rotate the side of the body towards the net as the racket arm is raised above the horizontal:

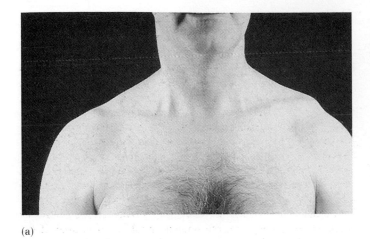

(a)

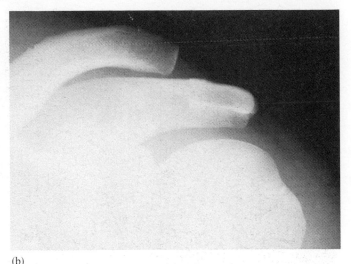

(b)

FIG. 3.28 A grade III A-C joint injury: (a) Clinical—a step may be seen and palpated, (b) X-ray—confirms A-C joint dislocation.

failure to achieve correct body rotation forces the arm to be raised lateral to the functional arc of elevation, thereby risking a recurrence of symptoms. Adjustments may be made by baseball pitchers who learn to throw 'three-quarters side-arm' rather than full overhead.

Surgery

If the problem remains chronic and lasts for longer than nine months to one year, and temporary benefit has been achieved with injection treatment, then a subacromial decompression operation may be considered. The operation described by Neer in 1972 and shown in Fig. 3.27 is preferred to that described by Watson (1978), which in the experience of one of the present authors has less good results (W.A.W.). McShane *et al.* (1978) have shown that 40 per cent of patients have residual symptoms after this procedure, which are reduced if a powered burr is used for the surgery instead of an osteotome. Post-operative physiotherapy is important, and the athlete can expect to return to sport from twelve to sixteen weeks after surgery. An improvement can be expected in 80 per cent of patients treated surgically, although only about 30 per cent will consider their shoulder completely cured. Since 1984, arthroscopic subacromial decompression operations, using a high-speed burr to remove the anterior and inferior acromion and coracoacromial ligament, have become increasingly popular in the USA (Ellman 1985). The recovery time using the arthroscopic technique is much shorter, and return to sport can be in as little as four to six weeks. However, this treatment has not yet been fully evaluated.

The most common cause of a chronic subacromial painful arc is a partial- or full-thickness rotator cuff tear. The diagnosis can often, but not always, be made with an arthrogram, but more recently arthroscopy of the shoulder has been found to be quite reliable in establishing the correct diagnosis (Bunker 1989). Full-thickness tears are categorized according to size, with small tears having a maximum dimension of 3 cm, medium tears 3 to 5 cm, and larger tears greater than 5 cm. In athletes, chronic tears are much more common in the supraspinatus tendon, and it is rare to find a large tear. Fortunately, both partial-thickness and full-thickness tears under 5 cm in maximum dimension can usually be repaired satisfactorily at the time of a subacromial decompression operation. Partial-thickness rotator cuff tears are

best treated by opening the cuff fully and carrying out a formal repair as for a full-thickness tear. The repair is carried out with interrupted non-absorbable sutures, with the repair technique varied according to the findings at operation. Again, post-operative physiotherapy is important, but recovery will take longer, with a return to sport delayed until sixteen to thirty weeks after surgery, depending on the size of the tear. Although the author (W.A.W.) has returned top-class sportsmen to their sport after surgical repair of rotator cuff tears, the outcome is not fully predictable and cannot be guaranteed.

The acromioclavicular joint

Assessment

Acute injury to the A-C joint usually results from a fall on to the point of the shoulder. It is particularly common in rugby football, and is often mistakenly diagnosed by the inexperienced traumatologist as a glenohumeral joint injury. A grade 1 injury involves a sprain of the superior A-C ligament. Further injury results in a subluxation (grade II) or a dislocation (grade III), in which the coracoclavicular ligaments are torn. On inspection, a step may be seen and palpated in grade III injuries (Fig. 3.28), but this may be missed during the first few days because of the local soft tissue swelling.

A-C joint pain is located at the point of the shoulder directly over the joint. It is aggravated by forced *adduction* of the shoulder with the arm in 90° of flexion (Fig. 3.12). However, this test may also cause pain in a patient with a supraspinatus tendinitis. An additional useful test is resisted isometric *ad*duction of the shoulder with the arm hanging close to the side (Fig. 3.29), which will aggravate pain in a patient who has pain arising from the A-C joint. In acute injuries a diagnosis of an A-C joint sprain, with subluxation or dislocation, should be explored with stress radio-graphs (Bannister *et al.* 1984). The site of the pain can be confirmed by a local anaesthetic diagnostic test—1 to 2 ml of local anaesthetic is injected into the A-C joint and 1 ml infiltrated into the superior A-C ligament (see Fig. 12.15, p. 227). If after five to ten minutes this improves or abolishes the pain on carrying out the above diagnostic tests, the diagnosis is established.

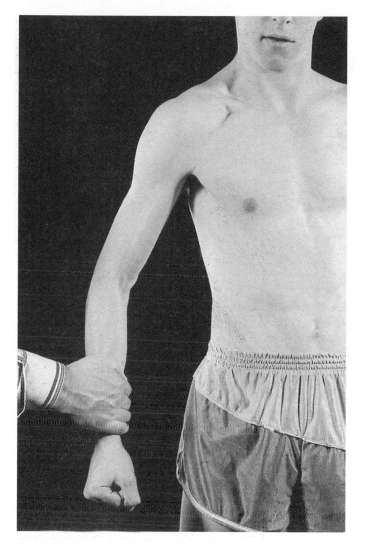

FIG. 3.29 Resisted adduction provokes A-C joint pain.

Treatment

The outcome from A-C joint injuries has been clearly high-lighted by a randomized prospective study carried out by Bannister *et al.* (1984). In general, a conservative expectant policy should be adopted, with early physiotherapy and muscle strengthening exercises. Local pain will resolve over a period of six to eight weeks, and a return to sport may follow at around the same time. For recurrent chronic A-C joint pain, osteoarthritis of the A-C joint is the most likely cause. This is best treated with one to three injections of local steroid (10 mg of triamcinolone hexacetonide) at two to three months intervals (see Fig. 12.15, p. 227). Local physiotherapy with ultrasound and 'mobilization' treatment of the joint can be very beneficial if injection treatment fails. Only a small proportion of patients fail to respond to such treatment and, if symptoms continue for longer than nine to twelve months, surgery (resection of the lateral 1 cm of the clavicle) can be considered. This is a very successful operation, with 90 per cent of patients satisfied (Taylor and Tooke 1977), but it often leaves the shoulder with a slight weakness for heavy manual tasks.

The scapulothoracic joint

Assessment

This joint is examined by positioning the patient erect and asking him to lift the arm, first in flexion and then in abduction, into full elevation. The scapula should slide smoothly over the posterior chest wall. If the scapula jerks, this indicates a disorder of the scapulothoracic joint, a glenohumeral joint disorder such as subluxation, or a subacromial joint disorder such as impingement or a supraspinatus tendinitis. If, in addition to jerking, the scapula makes a snapping sound, this indicates a problem in the scapulothoracic joint area. Crepitus may be palpated alongside the medial border of the scapula in the less severe case ('scapulothoracic bursitis'). If the snapping is pain free, it should be ignored completely and the patient should be reassured. If the snapping is painful, treatment should be considered.

Treatment

'Scapulothoracic bursitis' may be treated with local steroid injections and a short period of rest. However, a painful snapping scapula can be very disabling in an athlete, and can be responsible for prolonged disability. The first-line treatment is rest, and avoidance of aggravating the pain and snapping. This treatment is not popular with a sportsman, but should be carried on for at least four to six months. However, if the problem recurs on returning to sport and the athlete feels that the symptoms are excessively restrictive, then surgery may be offered. The results of surgical release of the plane between the subscapularis and serratus anterior and the chest wall (a subscapular mobilization) have been found to be promising (Foy and Wallace, personal communication).

The sternoclavicular joint

Assessment

The sternoclavicular joint can give rise to pain either from degenerative change (osteoarthritis) or from instability. The common situation is in the late teens when a girl athlete develops pain and an intermittent anterior displacement (or subluxation) of the medial end of the clavicle during elevation of the arm. The initial provoking injury is not usually a major one. A careful assessment of all joints is indicated because this condition may be associated with a generalized joint laxity. In particular it is vital to examine the other sternoclavicular joint very carefully, because usually it is also found to be abnormal. On examination the affected joint will be found to be slightly tender, and will displace obviously on full elevation of the arm (Fig. 3.30). The joint may also produce a palpable click on displacement. Radiographs are rarely helpful.

Treatment

For instability of the joint, non-surgical local treatment with ultrasound or PEMF therapy may result in a reduction of the tenderness. Surgical treatment should only be considered as a last resort, as most patients with this problem do learn to live and cope with it (although that may involve giving up sport). Surgery to the sternoclavicular joint area is dangerous, and deaths have occurred even in the best surgical hands. The

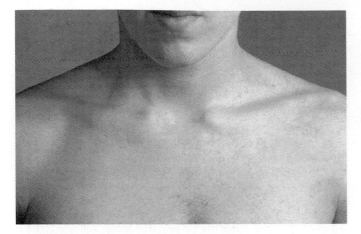

FIG. 3.30 An anterior sternoclavicular joint subluxation.

author (W.A.W.) has attempted to stabilize six joints surgically, with four relative successes; however, if the joint has been successfully stabilized there is usually a loss of up to 40° of arm elevation, and this may in itself limit the patients' capacity to carry out their chosen sport. Osteoarthritis of the sternoclavicular joint is uncommon, but when it occurs and causes persistent symptoms, surgical resection of the medial 1 cm of the clavicle can be very successful.

Don't forget the neck

The neck and the shoulder are closely related, and the relationship between neck pain and shoulder pain is complex. If smooth coordinated movements of the shoulder are lost owing to shoulder pathology, then an increased muscular strain is placed on the neck, particularly by the trapezius, sternomastoid, and levator scapulae muscles. This commonly causes secondary neck pain. A reduction of spasm with massage or relaxation therapy will help this. It is also worth trying cervical mobilization or traction, even when the problems are obviously primarily in the shoulder.

As indicated at the beginning of this chapter, the authors believe that one reason why shoulder pain is so common is because of adverse neural tension in the upper limb, often primary C5 nerve-root irritation resulting in secondary C5 muscle incoordination and weakness, and pain in the subacromial joint. Therefore, it is necessary to perform a full assessment of the cervical spine (see Chapter 5) and direct treatment, if indicated, to the neck as well as to the shoulder in patients with shoulder disability. It is also important to recognize the corollary—it is often possible to relieve neck pain, even if the neck is the primary problem, by treating a disordered shoulder.

Summary of examination procedures

(1) LOOK
Observation
- of deformity—dislocation of A-C or glenohumeral joints
                —fracture
- of swelling—acute bursitis
- of muscle wasting

(2) MOVE
(a) Active movements:
- flexion—range of movement/painful arc
- abduction—range of movement/painful arc

(b) Passive movements:
- flexion
- abduction—both combined and glenohumeral
- flexion and adduction
- rotation—internal and external

(3) FEEL
Palpation for tenderness
- A-C joint
- subacromial
- rotator cuff insertions (± defect)

(4) SPECIAL TESTS
(a) Rotator cuff (resisted contraction)
- supraspinatus test = abduction
- infraspinatus = external rotation
- subscapularis test = internal rotation
- biceps test = elbow flexion at 90°

(b) Impingement
- signs
- injection test

(c) Instability
- anterior—apprehension test
- inferior—sulcus sign
- posterior—stress test
- AP translation

(d)
- superior labral defect tests

References

Andrews, J. R., Carson, W. G., and McLeod, W. D. (1985). Glenoid labrum tears related to the long head of biceps. *Am. J. Sports Med.*, **13**, 337–41.

Bannister, G. C., Stableforth, P. G., Wallace, W. A., and Hutson, M. A. (1984). A prospective study of the treatment of acromio-clavicular dislocation. *J. Bone Jt. Surg.*, **66B**, 279.

Broca, A. and Hartman, H. (1890). Contribution à l'étude des luxations de l'épaule. *Bull. Soc. Anat. Paris*, **5me Série, 4**, 312.

Bunker, T. (1989). Shoulder arthroscopy. *Ann. R. Coll. Surg.*, **71**, 213–17.

Cahill, B. R. (1982). Osteolysis of the distal part of the clavicle in male athletes. *J. Bone Jt. Surg.*, **64A**, 1053–8.

Crawford Adams, J. C. (1948). Recurrent dislocation of the shoulder. *J. Bone Jt. Surg.*, **30B**, 26–38.

Cyriax, J. (1982). *Textbook of orthopaedic medicine*, Vol. 1 (8th edn). Ballière Tindall, London.

Cyriax, J. and Russell, G. (1984). *Textbook of orthopaedic medicine*, Vol. 2 (11th edn). Baillière Tindall, London.

Ellman, H. (1985). Arthroscopic subacromial decompression: a preliminary report. *Orthop. Trans.*, **9** (1), 43.

Gerber, C. and Ganz, R. (1984). Clinical assessment of instability of the shoulder—with special reference to anterior and posterior drawer tests. *J. Bone Jt. Surg.*, **66B**, 551–6.

Gerber, C., Terrier, F., and Ganz, R. (1985). The role of the coracoid in the chronic impingement syndrome. *J. Bone Jt. Surg.*, **67B**, 703–8.

Hastings, D. E. and Coughlin, L. P. (1981). Recurrent subluxation of the glenohumeral joint. *Am. J. Sports Med.*, **9**, 352–5.

Hawkins, R. J. and Kennedy, J. C. (1980). Impingement syndrome in athletes. *Am. J. Sports Med.*, **8**, 151–8.

Hill, H. A. and Sachs, M. D. (1940). The grooved defect of the humeral head. A frequently unrecognised complication of dislocation of the shoulder joint. *Radiology*, **35**, 690–700.

Howell, S. M., Imobersteg, A. M., Seger, D. H., and Marone, P. J. (1986). Clarification of the role of the supraspinatus muscle in shoulder function. *J. Bone Jt. Surg.*, **68A**, 398–404.

Hutson, M. A. (1997). *Work related upper limb disorders*. Butterworth-Heinemann, Oxford.

Kennedy, J. C., Hawkins, R., and Krissof, W. B. (1978). Orthopaedic manifestations of swimming. *Am. J. Sports Med.*, **6**, 309–22.

Leyshon, A. and Kessel, L. (1982). Post-traumatic osteolysis of the distal clavicle. In *Shoulder surgery* (ed. I. Bayley and L. Kessel), pp. 183–7. Springer-Verlag, Berlin.

Liu, S. H., Henry, M. H., Nuccion, S. *et al.* (1996). Diagnosis of glenoid labral tears: a comparison between magnetic resonance imaging and clinical examinations. *Am. J. Sports Med.*, **24**, (2) 149–54.

McShane, R. B., Leinberry, C. F., and Fenlin, J. M. (1978). Conservative open anterior acromioplasty. *Clin. Orthop.*, **223**, 137–44.

Maitland, G. D. (1986). *Vertebral manipulation* (5th edn). Butterworths, London.

Neer, C. S. (1972). Anterior acromioplasty for the chronic impingement syndrome in the shoulder. *J. Bone Jt. Surg.*, **54A**, 41–50.

Neer, C. S. (1983). Impingement lesions, *Clin. Orthop.*, **173**, 70–7.

Neer, C. S. and Foster, C. R. (1980). Inferior capsular shift for involuntary inferior and multi-directional instability of the shoulder. *J. Bone Jt. Surg.*, **62A**, 897–908.

Petersson, C. J. and Gentz, C. F. (1983). Ruptures of the supraspinatus tendon. The significance of distally pointing acromio-clavicular osteophytes. *Clin. Orthop.*, **174**, 143–8.

Poppen, N. K. and Walker, P. S. (1976). Normal and abnormal motion of the shoulder, *J. Bone Jt. Surg.*, **58A**, 195–201.

Rathbun, J. B. and MacNab, I. (1970). The microvascular pattern of the rotator cuff. *J. Bone Jt. Surg.*, **52B**, 540–53.

Richardson, A. B. Jobe, F. W., and Collins, H. R. (1980). The shoulder in competitive swimming. *Am. J. Sports Med.*, **8**, 159–63.

Rowe, C. R., Patel, D., and Southmayd, W. W. (1978). The Bankart procedure—a long-term end result study. *J. Bone Jt. Surg.*, **60A**, 1–16.

Scott B., Barton, M. A. J., and Wallace, W. A. (1992). Diagnosis and assessment of pectoralis major rupture by dynamometry. *J. Bone Jt. Surg.*, **74B**, 111–13.

Simonet, W. T. and Cofield, R.H. (1984). Prognosis in anterior shoulder dislocation. *Am. J. Sports Med.*, **12**, 19–24.

Snyder S. J., Karzel, R. P., Del Pizzo, W. *et al.* (1990). SLAP lesions of the shoulder. *Arthroscopy*, **6**, 274–9.

Taylor, G. M. and Tooke, M. (1977). Degenerative of the acromio-clavicular joint as a cause of shoulder pain. *J. Bone Jt. Surg.*, **59B**, 507.

van Linge, B. and Mulder, J. D. (1963). Function of the supraspinatus muscle and its relation to the supraspinatus syndrome. *J. Bone Jt. Surg.*, **45B**, 750–54.

Wallace, W. A. (1984). Evaluation of the forces, ICR and the neutral point during abduction of the shoulder. *Transactions of the 30th Annual Meeting of the Orthopaedic Research Society*, **9**, 5.

Wallace, W. A. and Echeverri, A. (1987). Intra-articular distension with local anaesthetic, steroid and air in the treatment of capsulitis of the shoulder. In *The shoulder* (ed. N. Takagishi), pp. 204–8. Professional Postgraduate Services, Tokyo.

Wallace, W. A. and Hellier, M. (1983). Improving radiographs of the injured shoulder. *Radiography*, **49**, 229–33.

Wallace, W. A. and Johnson, F. (1982). A biochemical appraisal of the acromioclavicular joint. In *Shoulder surgery* (eds I. Bayley and L. Kessel), pp. 179–82. Springer-Verlag. Berlin.

Watson, M. (1978). The refractory painful arc syndrome. *J. Bone Jt. Surg.*, **60B**, 544–6.

Weiner, D. S. and McNab, I. (1970). Superior migration of the humeral head: a radiological aid in the diagnosis of tears of the rotator cuff. *J. Bone Jt. Surg.*, **52B**, 524–7.

4 Injuries to the upper limb

M. A. HUTSON AND N. J. BARTON

Overuse injuries

M. A. HUTSON

It is a natural consequence of most sports and recreational activities that loss of balance may result in a fall onto the outstretched hand and thus incur the risks of *trauma* to the elbow or wrist. An ensuing dislocation or fracture is of the same type as that sustained in most other circumstances, although any subsequent loss of flexibility (for example, loss of extension at the elbow) may result in grave problems for the athlete. For an understanding of the major joint injuries or fractures at and above the wrist, however, the reader should refer to suitable texts on orthopaedic surgery. The team doctor or general practitioner may be called upon to advise on hand injuries, for in certain sports such as cricket there is a commonly held view that 'getting on with the game', using strapping and early mobilization, is better than the enforced rest that otherwise may be prescribed upon the diagnosis of a fracture. To clarify this situation, hand and wrist injuries are included in the second part of this chapter, 'Injuries to the hand and wrist'. *Overuse* injuries are common, especially in the forearm, and are covered in some depth. They arise particularly in racket sports and, in common with impingement problems at the shoulder, in those sports that involve throwing.

Applied anatomy/biomechanics

The function of the elbow is principally to allow the hand to be positioned for maximal efficiency; it is aided by the joints between radius and ulna. The *humero-ulnar* joint is inherently stable, being of the uniaxial hinge type. In extension, there is a natural carrying angle of 10°–15° of valgus, greater in women than men. This is obliterated when the forearm is pronated or when the elbow is flexed. The *radiohumeral* joint is a shallow ball-and-socket joint, with the head of the radius being protected by the annular ligament; it is involved in the transmission of forces across the elbow, rather than in contributing towards stability. Since most stresses to the elbow are in the form of axial compression and medial tension, the medial ligament is strong. It has several components which produce tautness in both flexion and extension. Rotation of the forearm (into pronation and supination) is allowed at the superior and inferior *radio-ulnar* joints, which are pivotal in type. Injury to the distal radius may involve the inferior radio-ulnar joint and thus affect rotation. Displaced fractures of the distal third of the radial shaft are

invariably associated with disruption of the inferior radio-ulnar joint (Galeazzi fracture-dislocation); although uncommon, they usually occur in the young adult. Angulated fractures of the proximal ulna are accompanied by a dislocation of the superior radio-ulnar joint (Monteggia fracture-dislocation). Thus it is important to examine (and X-ray) the elbow and wrist in the presence of a fracture of the radius or ulna, so that disruptions of the radio-ulnar joints may be diagnosed and treated.

The biceps brachii (Fig. 4.1) and triceps muscles are primarily responsible for flexion and extension at the elbow (as well as contributing towards flexion and extension at the shoulder). In addition, as a result of its distal attachment to the radius, the biceps is a powerful supinator of the forearm. Overall, supination is more powerful than pronation: hence the clockwise direction of the screwdriving mechanism. If greater power is required, the forearm may be locked and the rotator muscles of the shoulder recruited. Wrist and hand movements involved in the process of gripping are controlled by the extensors and radial deviators of the wrist arising from the lateral epicondyle of the humerus, and the flexors and ulnar deviators arising from the medial epi-

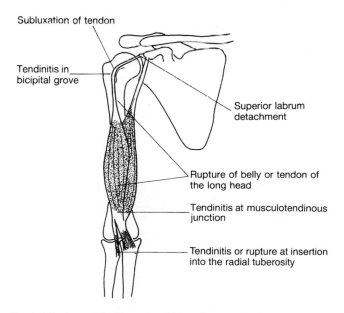

FIG. 4.1 Lesions of the biceps brachii are demonstrated.

condyle. The pronator teres also arises from the medial epicondyle—a fact which is of some significance in determining the cause of chronic medial elbow pain.

In throwing (see Chapter 3), the elbow is flexed to approximately 45° during the cocking phase, and forcibly extended towards the end of acceleration and in follow-through. The forearm is pronated, and the wrist flexed, in follow-through. Such propulsive efforts involving elbow extension may be seen in cricket, racket overheads and backhand, baseball pitching, swimming, discus and javelin throwing, and shot putting (Fig. 4.2). In these circumstances, injury may occur as a result of the olecranon being forced into the olecranon fossa and the application of valgus stress during acceleration.

Acute injury to the elbow

Injuries to the elbow usually result from a fall onto the outstretched hand with the elbow locked into extension. Should the elbow be flexed, protection may be afforded by the shock absorption of the relevant muscle groups. In a child, epiphyseal fracture and avulsion fracture of the medial epicondyle may occur. In the adult, posterior dislocation of the elbow is a potentially serious injury; it may be complicated by vascular impairment, which, if it persists after reduction, needs very urgent surgical intervention. Subsequent loss of extension is likely. In children, the common supracondylar fracture also threatens the vascular supply and, if mismanaged, may give rise to Volkmann's ischaemic contracture. If involved in rehabilitation, the physician is advised to treat the elbow with the utmost respect, as any attempt to be aggressive

towards the recovery of elbow extension may be counterproductive and lead to myositis ossificans. In the early stage, flexion exercises only should be countenanced.

In the child, the elbow may be 'pulled out' when the head of the radius is avulsed from its restraining annular ligament: further advice should be sought. Fracture around the elbow should always be referred to an orthopaedic surgeon, as fixation may be required. However, the undisplaced olecranon fracture due to forced stretching of the contracting triceps may be managed by a few weeks in a sling. Similarly, a fracture of the radial head requires no more than support for a couple of weeks, though the period required to regain a full range of movement is often frustratingly protracted.

A *haemarthrosis* may result from a relatively inconsequential undisplaced fracture. It may be recognized by the restriction in active and passive elbow movements in the capsular pattern (relatively greater restriction of flexion than extension) and by a boggy swelling which can be seen and felt either side of the olecranon process. X-rays usually show the 'fat pad' sign (Fig. 10.6, p. 182). Aspiration relieves pain—a posterolateral approach between the head of the radius and the humerus is desirable (Fig. 12.17, p. 228). Subsequently, elbow extension tends to lag behind during recovery.

Overuse injury—elbow and forearm

Impingement syndromes

Repeated high-velocity elbow extension in throwers may provoke hypertrophy of the olecranon process as a result of impingement on the humerus in the olecranon fossa (Fig. 4.3). Symptoms include pain on throwing and impairment of throwing efficiency, as the capacity to extend the elbow fully is insidiously lost. Forced passive extension of the elbow is painful. Initially an appraisal of the throwing technique is necessary, and liaison with the patient's coach is desirable. In the established case, surgery is required to trim the posteromedial aspect of the olecranon (Wilson *et al.* 1983); recurrence of hypertrophic impingement may occur nevertheless. Stress fracture of the olecranon has been described from the same cause, and would be expected to resolve uneventfully following a suitable period of rest.

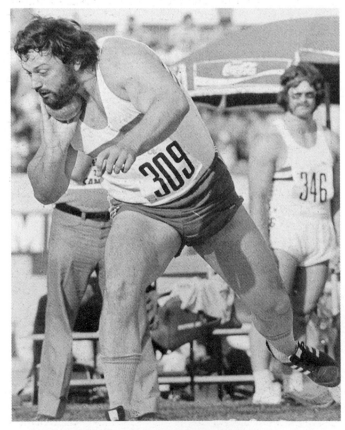

FIG. 4.2 Forceful elbow extension occurs in shot-putting.

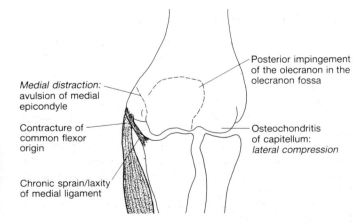

FIG. 4.3 'Thrower's elbow'. Repetitive throwing or pitching may give rise to elbow problems. These include posterior impingement of the olecranon in the olecranon fossa, valgus stress to the medial structures of the elbow joint, and compression injuries to the radiohumeral joint.

Medial joint injuries

Overload in throwing (for instance, discus throwing and baseball pitching) imposes repeated valgus stress upon the medial joint structures, principally the medial collateral ligament and common flexor origin, and compressive stress to the radio-humeral joint (Fig. 4.3). The medial collateral ligament undergoes repeated micro-tears, culminating in ectopic calcification and bony spur formation. Rupture may eventually occur. In the child and adolescent, 'Little Leaguer's elbow' (in baseball pitchers) is a descriptive label for recurrent medial joint pain, the causes of which include traction avulsion of the medial epicondyle. Baseball pitching is clearly a common source of elbow pain in the USA, and has been well documented (Slocum 1978); the combination of olecranon hypertrophy, chronic medial ligamentous strain, and contracture of the common flexors at their origin from the medial epicondyle leads to fixed flexion contracture in the elbows of 50 per cent of professional baseball pitchers (King *et al.* 1969). In the less established case, active and passive extension of the elbow are comfortable; the imposition of valgus stress with the elbow flexed to 30° provokes pain, and laxity may also be present. Isometric contractions are usually painless. Injections of small doses of steroid (for example, 10 mg of triamcinolone hexacetonide) assist in the resolution of the symptoms, though recurrences are common unless biomechanical stress is reduced by an appropriate alteration of technique.

Medial epicondylitis (golfer's elbow)

Although less common than lateral epicondylitis, this is nevertheless a troublesome condition that is often difficult to eradicate. It is an enthesitis of the common flexor/pronator origin from the medial epicondyle. Localized discomfort that may radiate to the flexor aspect of the forearm is the principal complaint. Although isometric contraction of the wrist or finger flexors may be uncomfortable, it is predominantly the pronator teres that is affected, thus reflecting the aetiology of the condition. Over-pronation of the forearm may be seen in a tennis player with a technically faulty topspin forehand, or in a golfer with an overdominant right hand. Short-term improvement may be gained by steroid injections and other anti-inflammatory measures. Correction of abnormal biomechanics is essential for a long-term cure.

Lateral epicondylitis (tennis elbow)

This is an extremely common condition, which arises from overload in industrial and domestic situations as well as in sport. The middle-aged male in particular is at risk from indulgence in occasional DIY activities, including repetitive screwdriving and bricklaying. In the sporting context, racket sports—for example, tennis, badminton, and squash—are the likely causes. Essentially it is an enthesitis, involving the common extensor origin from the lateral epicondyle, and is associated with repeated grasping. Pain or discomfort is felt over the lateral aspect of the elbow, frequently radiating either proximally or (more commonly) distally to the extensor aspect of the forearm. Grasping is painful—even simply holding a tea-cup. The aetiological factors include:

(1) overload—related to the sheer frequency of shots played;
(2) incorrect technique, particularly on the backhand;
(3) too small a racket handle;
(4) recent change of racket—particularly from one construction to another;
(5) too tight a grip between shots;
(6) muscle imbalance/loss of flexibility.

On examination, passive elbow movements are usually painless, though in the acute case extension is painful and may be slightly restricted. Passive stretching of the musculotendinous structures arising from the lateral epicondyle by the combination of elbow extension, pronation of the forearm, and palmar flexion of the wrist may be painful. The typical pattern on isometric contraction is pain on testing one or more of the wrist extensors, radial deviators, and finger extensors. Of these, the wrist extensors (extensors carpi radialis longus and brevis) are primarily affected. Tenderness is localized to the common extensor origin from the lateral epicondyle.

Initial management should be in the form of a short period of rest from sport, combined with ice and ultrasound. Subsequent treatment includes friction massage (for example, thrice a week for eight weeks) in addition to ice and ultrasound. This may be followed by Mills' manoeuvre, in which the examiner fully pronates the forearm, flexes the wrist, and then forcibly extends the affected elbow (Cyriax 1982). Regrettably, however, patients may develop a traumatic synovitis of the elbow joint if the procedure is over-vigorous. By far the most rapidly effective treatment is steroid injection. If accurately placed, one injection of 10 mg of triamcinolone will suffice in 90 per cent of cases, and two injections, ten days apart, in most of the remaining 10 per cent (Fig. 12.16, p. 228). However, it is necessary to identify any appropriate aetiological factors, often by referral to a coach. The player should be restrained from playing for several weeks, during which suitable stretching and strengthening exercises are considered. If imbalance is detected, the flexors of the wrist may be strengthened. Regular stretching of the wrist extensors is imperative. An epicondylitis clasp may be prescribed in refractory cases.

Despite all this, recurrence is sufficiently common for the sufferer to be sceptical of a 'cure' being achieved. For recurrent lesions, steroid injections tend to give relief for shorter periods, so that some cases appear refractory to all conservative methods. Cyriax has stated that, if left untreated, tennis elbow resolves spontaneously over a year or fifteen months, though few sportsmen have this patience. Alternatively, a muscle slide operation may be performed, although the results are by no means uniformly successful. At best, an attempt may be made at surgery to exclude nerve entrapment masquerading as tennis elbow (see the section on nerve entrapment).

Atypical tennis elbow

A significant minority of patients who complain of lateral elbow pain suffer from problems of neural origin. The cause of ANT (adverse neural tension) may be multifactorial, most commonly arising in the neck but not infrequently in the distal limb as a peripheral nerve entrapment. Compression of the posterior interosseous nerve (PIN) in sportsmen usually results from repetitive forceful supination, as in topspin tennis serves. Tenderness is usually felt over the anterior aspect of the radial head rather than at the lateral epicondyle. Additionally, in established lesions, tenderness on palpation of the supinator muscle combined with weakness/discomfort on resisted supination of the forearm is apparent. In PIN entrapment, tenderness is always more marked in the proximal forearm than at the lateral epicondyle.

Adverse neural tension, masquerading as tennis elbow, is a particularly common problem in the general population, no less so in sports enthusiasts. Relatively widespread discomfort in the upper limb is encountered, although it may be maximal at the lateral elbow. The diagnosis is made by the presence of diffuse muscle hyperalgesia throughout the upper limb, affecting muscle groups such as the proximal scapular fixators, pectoralis major, both the common extensor and flexor muscles in the forearm, and the interossei between thumb and forefinger. Tests for neural tension are positive. Muscle hypertonus and hyperalgesia between the cervical spine and the shoulder invariably is present.

The features that suggest that lateral (or medial) elbow pain is due to a condition other than enthesitis are widespread hyperalgesia in the upper limb, bilateral symptoms, concomitant lateral and medial elbow pain, failure to respond to local steroid injections, and the presence of distal paraesthesiae and/or numbness (Hutson 1997).

Muscle lesions

Repetitive stress may give rise to minor tears occurring in muscle bellies around the elbow. Presenting as a variety of tennis elbow, the lesion occurs in one of the extensor muscle bellies some centimetres distal to the lateral epicondyle. Similarly, on the medial aspect of the antecubital fossa, the pronator teres may be tender 2–3 cm from the medial epicondyle, as a variety of golfer's elbow. Lesions of brachioradialis may occur, and insertional lesions of biceps brachii are perhaps slightly more common (Fig. 4.1). Occasionally, the distal biceps tendon is ruptured in the middle-aged. Early surgical reconstruction should be considered; otherwise, loss of power of supination as well as elbow flexion usually results in significant loss of function. Identification should be made by tissue tension tests (pain on resisted contraction of the respective muscles) and confirmed by palpation. Most minor muscle lesions respond to a course of deep friction massage.

Osteochondritis dissecans

In common with osteochondritis at the ankle and knee, the aetiology continues to be debated, though it seems logical that repeated impingement between the articular surfaces of the radial head and the capitellum is a likely cause. Thus it is common in those sports requiring throwing or pitching (Fig. 4.2; see also Fig. 3.6, pp. 40–1), in which forceful elbow extension is combined with lateral compression in valgus overload, such as baseball (Little Leaguer's elbow). Repeated weightbearing stress resulting in injury to the radiohumeral joint also occurs frequently in gymnasts (Fig. 4.4).

It is a lesion of the articular cartilage and subchondral bone, only occurring on convex articular surfaces, suggesting a traumatic aetiology. The lesion occurs most commonly in the capitellum in the 11–14-year old girl. It is probable that the condition is the same as that described by Panner (1929) and subsequently termed osteochondrosis (Singer and Roy 1984).

In the early case, discomfort is experienced on use, but rest may prevent the occurrence of fragmentation. In the established case, loose bodies form, and give rise to temporary locking of the joint and repeated effusions. If an effusion occurs, both passive flexion and extension of the elbow are restricted; otherwise examination is essentially normal. X-rays reveal typical features. If ignored, the condition progresses to osteoarthritis in later life.

Osteoarthritis (OA) of the elbow

This may be the long-term result of a fracture, or possibly the result of a long period of stress—for instance, in baseball pitchers, weight-lifters, or gymnasts. In common with OA at other joints,

Fig. 4.4 Repeated weightbearing stress resulting in injury to the radiohumeral joint occurs in gymnasts.

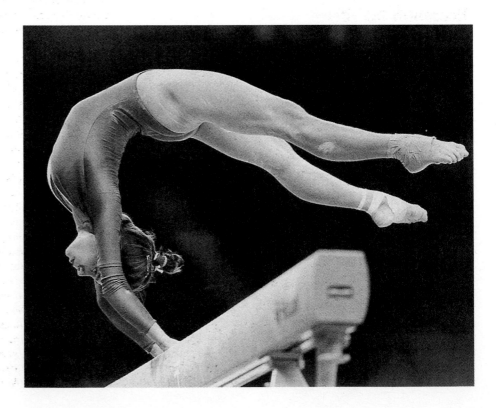

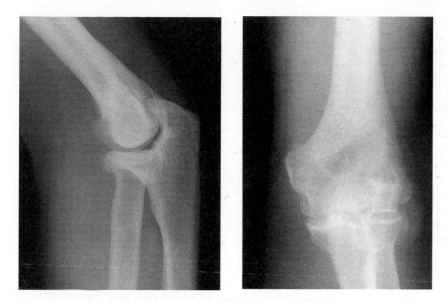

Fig. 4.5 Osteoarthritis of the elbow joint due to weight-lifting.

the onset is often insidious, being recognized by the patient when a bout of pain reveals the accompanying restriction of movements in the capsular pattern. Whether due to a loose body or micro-fracture, pain is often accompanied by an effusion that may be expected to resolve gradually. As the condition progresses, however, pain may be anticipated when the elbow is stressed, a situation that is incompatible with sports which require a throwing or racket arm. The findings are restriction of movements in the capsular pattern, that is, in the proportion of 30° loss of flexion to 20° of extension. Tissue tension tests are negative. X-ray confirms the typical features of OA (Fig. 4.5). In the absence of degenerative changes in the elbow joint, a restricted range of movements may be due to synovitis secondary to chondral damage.

Olecranon bursitis

A serous or haemorrhagic bursitis may develop as a result of repeated friction or contusion, respectively. The initial complaints are of pain and swelling; tenderness and the presence of 'seedlings' within the bursa may be noted. If accompanied by redness, there may be a significant acute inflammatory reaction which requires treatment by local anti-inflammatory measures. The presence of infection should be excluded, if necessary by microscopy and culture of the aspirate, and antibiotics prescribed if indicated. A localized steroid injection is indicated (in the non-infected case) if the acute reaction settles yet the swelling persists.

Tenosynovitis of the forearm

This condition is well recognized by the occupational medical officer and union official in a number of industries, where it is colloquially known as 'teno'. In the workplace, home, or sports arena, it is an overuse injury to those tendons that pass through the forearm and cross the wrist to be inserted into the hand. As 'intersection syndrome', it presents as a crepitating swelling of the tendon sheaths of extensor pollicis brevis and abductor pollicis longus in the forearm some 4–6 cm proximal to the wrist where they cross over the tendons of the extensor carpi radialis. Often, however, these florid features are absent and the discomfort, unaccompanied by swelling, is to be found over the radial aspect

of the wrist. At this anatomical level, it was once known as 'styloiditis radii' but is now usually referred to as 'de Quervain's tenovaginitis' or 'tenosynovitis' (see Fig. 12.18, p. 229). Although common practice, it is fallacious to label all wrist and distal radius discomfort as tenosynovitis; in the absence of gross signs, differentiation should be made from chronic dorsal wrist ligament sprain (in which localized tenderness of the relevant ligament should be sought). Stress injury to the distal radial epiphysis should be suspected in young gymnasts. In the industrial setting, many patients and unions regard 'teno' as an occupational injury, and commonly sue the employer. Thus it is particularly important not to diagnose a repetitive strain injury (RSI) without good evidence.

Rowers and weight-lifters are frequently affected by intersection syndrome. Golfers and racket sportsmen are prone to de Quervain's tenovaginitis. Dog-handlers are another vulnerable group. Whatever the cause, gripping and activities involving use of the forearm and thumb become excruciatingly painful.

Tenosynovitis may occur in any of the dorsal compartments of the wrist. Extensor digitorum tenosynovitis, often associated with considerable soft tissue swelling over the dorsum of the wrist, is rarely caused by overuse. It is usually a feature of rheumatoid arthritis. Tenosynovitis affecting the thumb extensors is a particularly common condition. The second most common tendinopathy at the dorsum of the wrist caused by overuse is extensor carpi ulnaris (ECU) tendinitis. Professional golfers are at risk. Discomfort is felt over the ulnar margin of the wrist. Tenderness may be exquisite. Passive radial deviation of the wrist with a fully pronated forearm is a reliable examination finding. ECU tendinitis has to be differentiated from a sprain of the ulnar collateral ligament of the wrist in which there is no pain on resisted muscle contraction (Hutson 1997).

On the volar aspect of the wrist, overuse injury occurs in both the flexor carpi ulnaris and flexor carpi radialis tendons. Calcific deposits may form, when the condition presents as an acute inflammatory reaction with redness and swelling (Fig. 1.10, p. 9).

Identification is made by careful examination. Although there is usually a full range of active and passive movements in the forearm and wrist, passive ulnar deviation of the wrist with the thumb forcibly opposed across the palm (Finkelstein's test) is usually painful in de Quervain's disease. Pain on resisted contraction of the respective contractile structures is to be expected, but is often absent; discomfort on stretching is a more reliable feature. In the acute case, crepitation, resulting from a synovial reaction in the sheath, may be felt. Pin-point tenderness must be elicited in the less florid case.

A short period of rest from sport is required while treatment using the normal anti-inflammatory options, including ice, ultrasound, and non-steroidal anti-inflammatory drugs (NSAIDs) is applied. Steroid injections are rapidly curative if there is tendon sheath swelling (Fig. 12.18, p. 229). Injections should be made into the sheath—that is, parallel to the tendon using the bent needle approach demonstrated in Fig. 12.24(a) (p. 231), and in no circumstances should intratendinous injections be given. A critical analysis and, if appropriate, a subsequent adjustment of sporting technique may be undertaken. In discus throwing, for instance, de Quervain's disease may be due to overemphasis of the power snap at the wrist. A graded reintroduction into sporting activity is then required. Surgical decompression may be required, and is usually successful, in relapsing cases.

In the hand, stenosing tenovaginitis of the flexor tendons may occur at the level of the metacarpophalangeal (MCP) joints, giving rise to a triggering effect—hence the term trigger finger (or thumb). A tender nodule is palpable on careful examination. Resolution may be expected after one steroid injection to the sheath; surgery is required in resistant cases.

Nerve entrapment

Direct trauma to a nerve causes paralysis. Compression (in a tunnel) of the median, ulnar, or radial nerves or their branches results in entrapment neuropathy, giving rise to pain and/or paraesthesiae in the forearm, hand, and digits.

The *median nerve* may be compressed occasionally in the proximal forearm by overactivity of the pronator teres (when it is sometimes referred to as the pronator syndrome). Since pronation is a component of the follow-through of a throw, repetitive throwing may cause nerve compression and give rise to forearm discomfort with or without sensory symptoms. Weight-lifters are also at risk, as a result of hypertrophy of the forearm muscles. Forceful isometric forearm pronation with the elbow at 90° may provoke discomfort during examination (Cabrera and McCue 1986). More commonly, the median nerve is compressed at the wrist, giving rise to the *carpal tunnel syndrome*. In the sports context, it is postulated (and disputed!) that this may be secondary to repeated wrist flexion and extension, or tight gripping, which clearly may be associated with any number of sports. In men, it may be due to an osteoarthritic wrist following old injury. Painful paraesthesiae in the radial three and a half digits, and discomfort in the wrist and forearm are typical features. Patients are woken at night, and obtain relief by shaking or using the hand in some way. The condition should be suspected, and a provisional diagnosis made, on the symptomatology: in early cases, objective sensory signs may not be detectable and motor weakness may not be evident. Only in late untreated cases will thenar atrophy and weakness of abduction and opposition of the thumb become obvious. Tinel's sign or Phalen's test may be positive. Diagnosis is confirmed by nerve conduction studies or by the therapeutic response to the injection of 5 mg (0.5 ml) of triamcinolone and 0.5 ml of lignocaine into the carpal tunnel (Fig. 4.6 (a); see also Fig. 12.19, p. 229). When

the compression is due to sport, surgical decompression is rarely necessary.

The *ulnar nerve* may also be compressed at the elbow or wrist. In its canal posterior to the medial epicondyle it is superficially positioned, and at risk from direct trauma; more insidiously, it may be compressed by osteophytic encroachment. Deadness in the ulnar one and a half fingers, with additional extension to the dorsal aspect of the ulnar border of the hand (distinguishing it from distal compression), are noted. If nerve compression is unremitting, decompressive or transposition surgery should be carried out *before* motor weakness becomes evident. Should a patient present at a later stage, weakness of the small muscles of the hand supplied by the ulnar nerve—for instance, the thumb adductor, the interossei, and the hypothenar muscles—may be detected. At the wrist, the nerve is at risk in the canal of Guyon between the pisiform and hamate bones (Fig. 4.6). Direct trauma may result in contusion, though in the case of cyclists, repeated pressure from handlebars is the cause ('handlebar neuropathy'). A similar situation may arise in golf and racket sports. A sensory branch is given off in this region: entrapment syndromes may be motor and/or sensory, depending upon the exact site of compression. In the case of chronic compression, suitable padding may eliminate the symptoms. Gradual resolution is usually to be expected in distal entrapment neuropathy if the source of external compression is identified and remedied.

The *radial nerve* may be injured by fractures of the humerus. More commonly, in the proximal forearm, radial nerve entrapment may arise as a result of localized direct trauma or, particularly in sports people, by overuse of the adjacent muscle groups. Entrapment of the PIN (posterior interosseous nerve) by the supinator or by the extensor carpi radialis brevis muscle has been recorded (Kopell and Thompson 1963). Resisted extension of the middle finger with the elbow extended (thereby tightening the origin of extensor carpi radialis brevis) is stated to be invariably painful (Roles and Maudsley 1972). Patients complain of weakness of grip which should therefore be assessed on clinical examination. There is no sensory loss as the PIN is purely a motor nerve. Myofascial tenderness (sometimes referred to as a trigger point) may be detected in the supinator muscle or in the common extensor muscles in the proximal forearm.

Other neuropathies have been described (Cabrera and McCue 1986). Compression of the anterior interosseous nerve in the forearm gives rise to weakness of 'pinch' between the tips of the thumb and the index finger. Repetitive digital compression may cause paresthesiae and numbness—for example, compression injury of the ulnar digital nerve of the thumb in ten-pin bowlers.

Overuse injury—the wrist

Stress fracture of the distal radial epiphysis

This occurs principally in gymnasts, and is considered by Read (1981) to result from compression loading during rotation, for instance in the Tsukahara vault. The complaint is usually of dorsal wrist pain. Examination reveals localized tenderness and slight swelling, but no articular or tissue tension signs. Radiographic changes (Fig. 4.7) include widening of the distal radial epiphysis, cystic changes, beaking of the distal or proximal

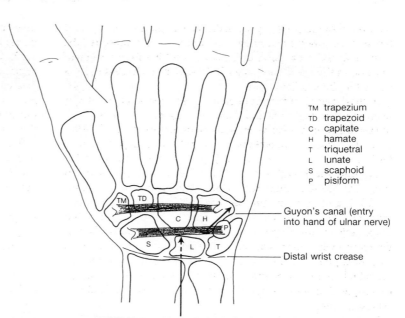

FIG. 4.6 (a) The ulnar nerve is at risk, for instance in cyclists, in the canal of Guyon. 'Handlebar neuropathy' may ensue. The site of injection of the carpal tunnel for median nerve entrapment is also demonstrated. (b) Various handlebar grip positions are shown by these cyclists. Padded gloves help prevent 'handlebar neuropathy'; the use of upright or aero bars may also be helpful.

TM trapezium
TD trapezoid
C capitate
H hamate
T triquetral
L lunate
S scaphoid
P pisiform

Guyon's canal (entry into hand of ulnar nerve)

Distal wrist crease

Injection at the level of the distal palmar crease, angled at 30° to the skin, to reach the carpal tunnel

(a)

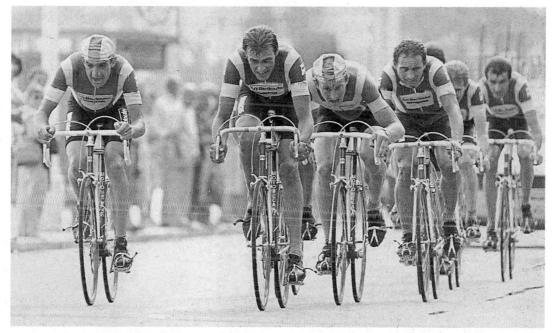

(b)

aspect of the epiphysis, and haziness within the growth plate area (Roy *et al.* 1985). Stress changes at the epiphysis due to incorrect water entry when diving have been noted by the author in adolescents who complain of dorsal wrist pain while high diving. Abstinence from provocative stress for up to three months is normally sufficient for symptoms to resolve.

Ganglia

These occur over the dorsal aspect of wrists and feet, and occasionally elsewhere—for instance, over the flexor aspect of the wrist. If asymptomatic, which is often the case, they should be left. If painful during activity—for example, during racket sports or golf—aspiration with a 20 G needle (anything less is ineffec-

tive) may release the typically viscous fluid. If recurrent, surgical referral is indicated. It should not be assumed that any wrist pain is due to the ganglion, and other causes should be considered and excluded.

Chronic ligament sprains of the wrist

These occasionally occur, and should be differentiated from tenosynovitis by the pattern of discomfort felt on passively stretching the ligament (for example, the dorsal wrist ligament or ulnar collateral ligament) and the absence of pain on isometric contraction. Transverse friction massage is usually curative once the relevant ligament has been located by fingertip palpation.

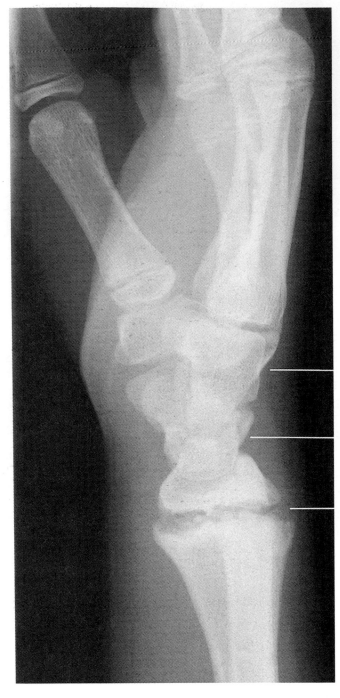

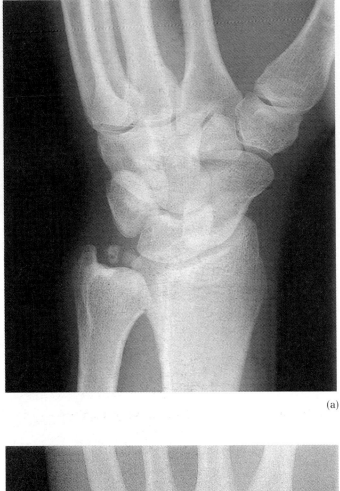

(a)

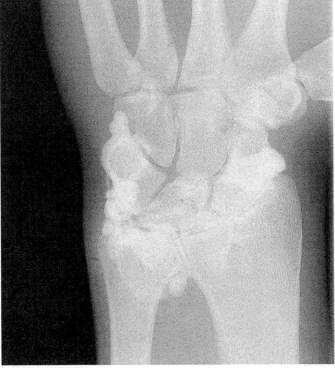

(b)

FIG. 4.7 Stress fracture of the distal radial epiphysis, due to compression loading during rotation, occurs in gymnasts. In this patient, the injury resulted from incorrect water entry in high diving.

Degenerative conditions

Osteoarthritis of the wrist is usually secondary to an old injury, such as an ununited scaphoid fracture. It causes a chronic ache that is aggravated by exercise. A restricted range of palmarflexion and dorsiflexion is found. Disturbance of the inferior radio-ulnar joint (for example, following a Colles' fracture) may give rise to permanent loss of rotation. A chronic sprain of the ulnar collateral ligament (which may also result from Colles'

FIG. 4.8 (a) and (b) An arthrogram of the wrist joint reveals leakage of dye through a disrupted triangular cartilage. The additional presence of loose bodies in this patient gave rise to considerable disability.

fracture) should respond to friction massage or steroid injection. Disruption of the triangular cartilage that forms the ulnar border of the proximal articular surface of the wrist joint results in recurrent pain and clicking on repeated wrist movements. There are few signs on examination: an arthrogram of the wrist reveals dispersal of dye into the proximal radio-ulnar space (Fig. 4.8).

Summary of examination procedures

For elbow, forearm, and wrist

Inspection
: Malalignment or deformity—for instance, cubitus valgus
  Effusion of elbow joint
  Swelling—for instance, olecranon bursitis, ganglia
  Muscle wasting—for example, thenar eminence

Active movements
: Elbow flexion and extension
  Forearm pronation and supination
  Wrist flexion and dorsiflexion

Passive movements
: Elbow flexion and extension (note 'end-feel')
  Forearm pronation and supination
  Wrist palmarflexion, dorsiflexion, ulnar deviation, and radial deviation

Stress tests
: Valgus/varus stress to the elbow in 30° flexion
  Finkelstein's test: thumb opposition with ulnar deviation of wrist

Resisted movements (tissue tension tests)
: Resisted elbow flexion in neutral, then in supination (to differentiate biceps from brachioradialis)
  Resisted elbow extension
  Resisted pronation and supination
  Resisted wrist palmarflexion and dorsiflexion, ulnar deviation, and radial deviation
  Resisted thumb movements—abduction, adduction, flexion, extension, opposition
  Resisted finger movements—flexion and extension (plus adduction and abduction if neuropathy suspected)
  Functional tests—pinch and grip

Additional tests
: Tinel's sign (reproduction of paraesthesiae on pressure over a nerve, such as the median nerve in the carpal tunnel, plus sensory examination if required)
  Phalen's test (reproduction of the sensory symptoms of median nerve compression by maintaining full palmarflexion of the wrist—usually performed by pushing the dorsal surfaces of the hands together—for one minute)

Palpation
: Localized tenderness
  Crepitus (tenosynovitis)
  Nodules (rheumatoid, stenosing tenovaginitis)
  Warmth (bursitis)

For examination of the thumb and digits add:
  active and passive flexion, extension, abduction and adduction at MCP, PIP, and DIP joints,
  abduction/adduction stress tests at MCP and IP joints in 30° flexion
  resisted flexion/extension at IP joints
  specific 'fingertip' tenderness

Injuries to the hand and wrist

N. J. BARTON

Almost any type of hand injury could occur during sport—for example, the hand might be pierced by a flying javelin or crushed by the collapse of a heavy stand, but in practice sports injuries to the hand and wrist are almost always closed injuries, usually to bone or joint. Therefore, the rest of this chapter will be restricted to these kinds of injury, which, of course, are by no means unique to sport but are part of the common coinage of hand injuries.

These injuries are often minor, but sometimes not as minor as they may seem at first sight. What is required is the ability to make an accurate diagnosis, and to detect those which need serious treatment.

Causes of injury

A ball

The commonest cause is that the hand is struck by a ball which is either hard, like a cricket or hockey ball (Belliappa and Barton 1991), or heavy, like a football (Curtin and Kay 1976).

In most cases, the ball knocks the finger or hand back into extension, breaking a bone or dislocating a joint, but more damage is done when the ball strikes the end of the finger, compressing it longitudinally so that the concave base of one bone is split upon the convex anvil of its proximal partner and the joint surface is disrupted.

In games in which the ball is hit with an implement, it may strike the player's hand instead as he holds the implement. There is then an element of crushing, with skin damage, but this is usually not serious, and fractures tend to be comminuted but undisplaced and stable. Occasionally, this mechanism may produce the damaging end-on blow to the fingertip.

The ground

In those games where players run around, they may fall onto an outstretched hand and sustain any of the injuries which this can produce, from a fractured finger to a dislocated shoulder. Such injuries are, of course, especially common when the nature of the sport is to move on a slippery surface, as in skating or skiing. They are likely to be worse if the sportsman is travelling at speed (for example, in skiing and cycle, motorcycle, or car racing) or falls from a height, as in jumping sports, gymnastics, riding (especially over jumps), mountaineering, or—the extreme cases—hang-gliding or flying.

The boundary of the playing area

In games such as squash or fives, which are played in small courts surrounded by a wall, the players sometimes run into the wall. This can result in injuries similar to those caused by falling on the outstretched hand, but the impact may be on the back of the hand or wrist, causing a contusion or a forcible flexion injury. In games played on a large field, the player may run into a fence surrounding the ground, and, since his finger or hand may go in between the rails or wires, this can produce more complicated injuries.

An opponent

Clearly this is most likely to occur in sports whose aim is to injure the opponent, especially boxing; the fracture of the neck of the fifth metacarpal is sometimes known as 'the boxer's fracture'. Bennett's fracture–subluxation of the base of the first metacarpal has also been described as 'an injury which owes its origin to the disparity between an individual's pugnacity and his pugilistic technique' (Blum 1941). Unfortunately, it is not unknown for similar blows to be exchanged in anger between players of other games, or in the semi-secrecy of the rugby football scrum. In the latter situation, the finger may also be pulled, wrenched, or twisted backwards or sideways to detach it from the ball, and similar injuries may occur in wrestling.

A special type of injury occurs in rugby football, where a player trying to tackle another succeeds only in catching his grasping fingers in the opponent's clothing, and the opposing extension force can rupture the tendon of the flexor digitorum profundus, usually to the ring finger.

A sporting implement

The player may be hit accidentally (or on purpose) by an opponent's racquet, stick, club, bat, etc. However, the damage may be done by his own implement, especially if it suddenly strikes a hard object in mid-swing, as when a golfer's club hits the ground. The upper end of the handle is driven forcibly against the front of the wrist, and this is actually the commonest cause of a rare but important injury—fracture of the hook of the hamate.

Sporting guns may, of course, also cause hand injuries, though it is more common for the victim to shoot himself in the foot while climbing over a fence.

Assessment of acute injuries to the hand and wrist

The first step in this process is to obtain a detailed history, as the mechanism of the damage often suggests the precise nature of the injury.

Clinical examination follows the usual pattern for orthopaedic assessment of an acute injury in which a fracture is a possibility: look, feel, move. Bruising, swelling, and deformity are looked for. In sportsmen seen immediately after the accident, bruising and swelling may not yet have appeared, but careful palpation with the tip of one finger to localize tenderness as precisely as possible is a most valuable—often *the* most valuable—part of the examination.

In palpating the wrist, it is particularly important that care is taken in the region of the anatomical snuff box. It is *normal* to be tender there because of pressure on the terminal sensory part of the radial nerve. Therefore, tenderness must always be assessed by comparison with the opposite wrist. Additionally, although the scaphoid is the most common carpal bone to be fractured, it is not the only one: any of the carpal bones may be fractured, and all are palpable clinically except the trapezoid. Moreover, the injury may be a fracture of the distal end of the radius or ulna, or the base of a metacarpal. Therefore, palpation should start with the distal radius, and progress around the wrist at that level. Subsequent levels of examination are the proximal row of the carpus, the distal row of the carpus, and the bases of the metacarpals. It should not be forgotten that the injury may be to a joint, not a bone: this is especially important because, if that is the case, it will probably not be revealed on the X-ray, and the localization of the tenderness may be the only positive finding. As palpation proceeds along the metacarpals to the digits, it is equally important that tenderness is localized precisely.

The patient is asked to put the part through a full active range of movement. If he can manage a *full* range, there is probably no serious joint injury. If one is suspected, it is necessary also to examine for abnormal movements (for example, sideways laxity of finger-joints), but it is probably wise, and certainly kind, to defer this until after an X-ray in case there is a fracture.

X-rays are usually necessary, but they are no substitute for clinical examination. X-rays may not reveal a joint injury, and will not reveal a fracture unless they are taken at the correct projection and angles to show that particular type of fracture. If X-rays of the wrist are requested, ordinary postero-anterior (PA) and lateral views are taken, which often do not reveal a scaphoid fracture, for which scaphoid views are needed. In the same way, fractures of the hook of the hamate will be visible only on special views taken for that purpose. *Therefore, clinical examination is necessary, not only in its own right* because of the information which only it can yield, *but to enable the examiner to order the appropriate X-ray views* without which the diagnosis will not be made.

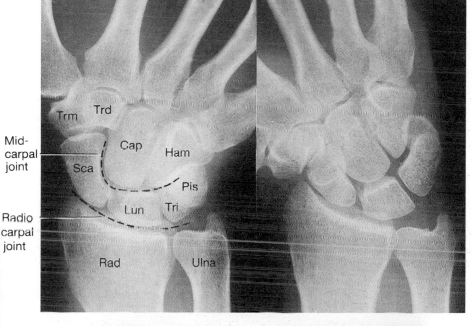

FIG. 4.9 PA views of the wrist in ulnar (left) and radial (right) deviation. In radial deviation, the scaphoid flexes and is therefore seen more end-on: a better view is obtained in ulnar deviation. Therefore, if 'scaphoid views' are requested, they will be taken with the wrist in this position. The shallow bowl of the radiocarpal joint and the deeper cup of the mid carpal joint are seen in both positions.

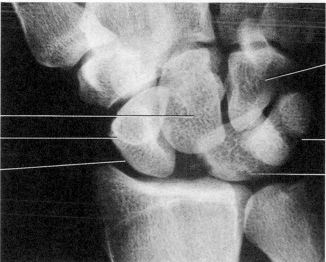

FIG. 4.10 The smooth C-shape of the mid-carpal joint is not present, indicating a dislocation: in this case, a dislocation of the lunate, which instead of being four-sided, looks five-sided. There is not always a gap between the dislocated lunate and the scaphoid; if present, it indicates an injury to the scapholunate ligament which may be isolated (see Fig. 4.16) or part of a dislocation.

It is necessary to study the X-rays carefully—something which does not always happen, as the examining doctor may not be familiar with the anatomy seen from certain angles, for example the lateral view. For this reason, important injuries such as dislocation of the lunate or of the carpo-metacarpal joints are more often overlooked than diagnosed.

On the PA view of the wrist, one must look at each bone in turn: radius, ulna, scaphoid, lunate, triquetrum, pisiform, trapezium ('articulates with the thumb'), trapezoid, capitate, hamate, and each of the five metacarpals. In addition, one should always and specifically look for the C-shape of the mid-carpal joint (Fig. 4.9); if it is not there, or is discontinuous, then something is badly wrong with the wrist (Fig. 4.10). The radiocarpal joint forms a second but shallower C.

On the lateral view of the wrist (Fig. 4.11), one can identify the radius with the proximal pole of the lunate fitting into it (a third C), the capitate fitting into the distal pole of the lunate (a fourth), and the superimposed second to fifth metacarpals, which should be in line with the capitate. At an angle of about 45° to these, one can also see the scaphoid, with its proximal pole overlapping the lunate and its distal pole and tuberosity projecting anteriorly, overlapping the pisiform. Figure 4.12 shows an abnormal lateral view.

In the fingers, one must not diagnose as a fracture the nutrient artery, the overlapping skin edge of the web between the fingers, an epiphyseal line, or the pseudo-epiphysis sometimes seen at the distal end of the first metacarpal.

Having studied the X-rays, it is usually wise to examine the patient again. Any doubtful features on the X-ray will be assessed in relation to the clinical findings: if it is not tender, it is probably not a recent injury. If there are no fractures, then the joints should be tested for lateral stability to detect injury to the collateral ligaments. It is especially important to do this after reducing a dislocation.

Fractures around the wrist

Fractures of the distal radius and ulna

Colles' fractures, though most common in elderly people, also occur in athletes, in whom they are more serious. The athlete will make greater demands upon the wrist and therefore expect a higher standard of result; in addition, the bone is stronger, requiring a more violent force to break it, so that the injury is inherently worse. Treatment will be along orthodox lines (Charnley 1961; Burke 1988) but with a greater readiness, if the fracture slips, to remanipulate or resort to other methods such as external fixation.

Smith's fractures, in which the distal end of the radius displaces forwards instead of backwards, are often unstable and frequently require internal fixation. (Smith was Colles' pupil and successor, and it was he who carried out the post-mortem examination on Colles' body.)

Fractures of the scaphoid

Almost everything that is taught about scaphoid fractures rests upon sand rather than rock. Texts are full of dogmatic statements which are passed on to medical students, but the truth is that it is not really known what the answers are to any of the

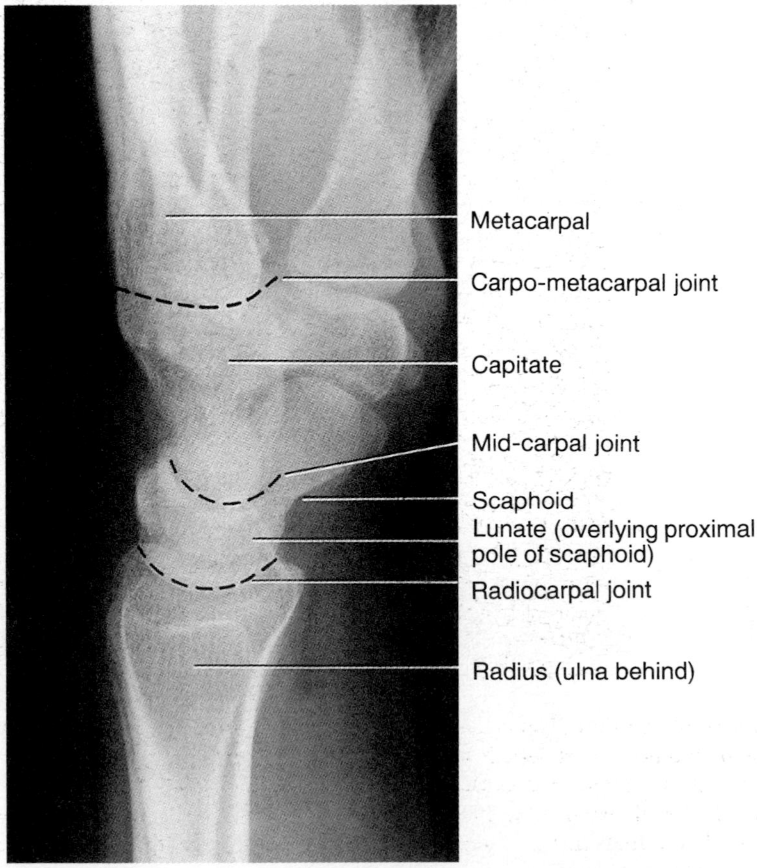

FIG. 4.11 Lateral view of a normal wrist: the proximal convex curve of the lunate ('moon-shaped') fits into the concavity of the distal radius and the convex head of the capitate fits into the distal concavity of the lunate: two more Cs. These three bones should be in line with each other and with the bases of the finger metacarpals.

Metacarpal

Carpo-metacarpal joint

Capitate

Mid-carpal joint

Scaphoid

Lunate (overlying proximal pole of scaphoid)

Radiocarpal joint

Radius (ulna behind)

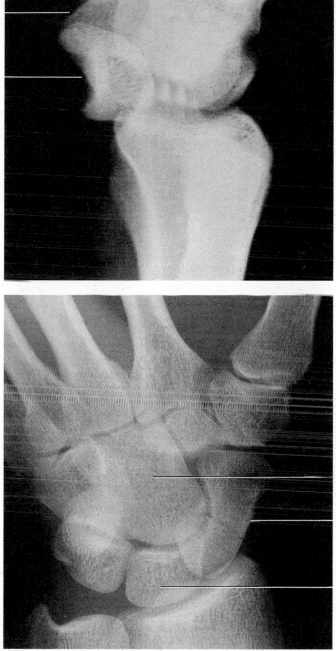

Trapezium –

Scaphoid –

Lunate –
(rotated
forwards
through 90°)

Capitate

Fig. 4.12 Abnormal lateral view: anterior dislocation of the lunate which is rotated through 90°. Its proximal convex curve is not contained within the radius and its distal concavity does not contain the head of the capitate.

Fig. 4.13 Fracture of the waist of the scaphoid. Often the fracture is less obvious than this.

Capitate

Scaphoid

Lunate

important questions, such as how to diagnose them, how to treat them, and how to tell whether they are united (Barton 1992).

What is known is that they are fairly common, that they usually result from a dorsiflexion injury, that they are often missed, and that they are subject to non-union, especially if they are not treated.

Clinical signs, apart from tenderness and some pain on movement, are conspicuous by their absence, and indeed the triviality of the symptoms is the reason why many patients dismiss the injury as a sprain, and do not seek medical advice at all—only to turn up some time later with an un-united fracture of the scaphoid.

X-rays are essential (Fig. 4.13). A sprained wrist should never be diagnosed unless at least one set of adequate X-ray films has been taken. One of the myths is that fractures of the scaphoid often 'do not show up' on the original films, and only become visible a few weeks later after resorption of the bone ends adjoining the fracture. In fact, Leslie and Dickson (1981) found that the fracture was visible on the first X-rays in 98 per cent of cases. In 75 per cent it could be seen on the PA film, and in 77 per cent on the semi-pronated view; in only six out of 222 patients was it not visible on one of these two films taken at the first attendance.

Nevertheless, it remains the usual practice for a patient with a suspected scaphoid fracture to be treated in plaster for two weeks and then have further X-rays out of plaster, despite the fact that this hardly ever results in a fractured scaphoid being discovered later. The main reason for this practice is fear of medico-legal problems and of being considered negligent; but it seems reasonable as a symptomatic method of treatment, even if, at the end of the day, no fracture is shown and the retrospective diagnosis of a sprain is made. The real advantage of repeating the x-rays is simply that more films are taken (often, by chance, at a slightly different angle) and studied.

The variety of methods of conservative treatment is amazing, varying both in the extent of the plaster and the position of immobilization. The traditional method in Britain, now sanctified by description as a 'scaphoid plaster', is in a below-elbow plaster extending to the interphalangeal joint of the thumb, with the wrist slightly extended. There is no convincing evidence that this is any better than the type of cast used for Colles' fractures, in which the thumb is left free; it has been shown to make no difference (Clay et al. 1991).

The real difficulty, though this is not mentioned in any of the textbooks or even in most of the papers in specialist journals, is in deciding for how long the plaster should be kept on or, to put it another way, when the fracture is united. The bone is too short to test by angular stress, as one would in the tibia. Tenderness is very subjective. The assumption is that the decision can be made on radiological grounds, despite the fact that on X-rays taken after eight or even twelve weeks of immobilization it is often—even usually—very difficult to decide whether the fracture is united or not. Dias et al. (1988) have shown that a group of eight expert consultants (four orthopaedic surgeons and four radiologists) frequently disagreed with each other as to whether the fracture was united, and, more significantly still, when they were shown the same films again some time later, often disagreed with what they themselves had said the first time! Thus all the papers which say that such-and-such a treatment led to union in X weeks must be taken with a large pinch of salt.

The author's current practice is to immobilize all fractures of the waist of scaphoid in a Colles' plaster for eight weeks and then assess them clinically and radiologically. If union is doubtful on either ground, they are given a further month in plaster; at the end of that time, no further films are taken, as they will be left free of the plaster anyway. Most will progress to union. Those who develop non-union but have no symptoms do not need an operation. Those who have symptomatic non-union need a bone-grafting operation, though even this is not invariably successful (Green 1985; Barton 1997).

Thus the need to diagnose and treat these fractures in the first place is emphasized. Even if the sportsman has an important contest pending, it is not worth taking a chance by failing to immobilize a scaphoid waist fracture adequately and for long enough; the risk of lasting disability from non-union is too high.

Currently, there is a wave of enthusiasm for early internal fixation of scaphoid fractures, especially in sportsmen. A limited surgical approach, with or without the use of an arthroscope, is employed and the wrist is not immobilized afterwards. Although this makes it *possible* to resume sport earlier, I do not consider it wise: the threads on the screw may provide an adequate hold to

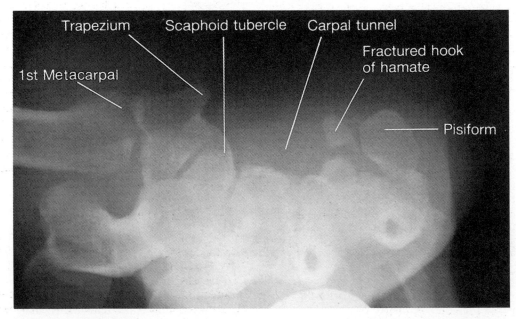

FIG. 4.14 Carpal tunnel view of the wrist of an international cricketer showing, on the right, pisiform and fractured hook of hamate and, on the left, first metacarpal (almost end-on), trapezium, and scaphoid tuberosity. The trough in the centre is the carpal tunnel.

allow unresisted movement but, if the patient resumes his sport early and falls again, the screw could cut out and a very difficult situation would result. Better safe than sorry.

In contrast, fractures of the scaphoid tuberosity are seldom a problem, and need only four weeks in plaster.

Other carpal fractures

The most common is a flake of bone pulled off the back of the triquetrum by the distal attachment of the capsule of the wrist joint. It is visible only on a lateral X-ray, where it may look as though it has come from the lunate. This is essentially a ligamentous injury, and four weeks in plaster is adequate treatment.

Uncommon, but interesting because it is almost exclusively a sports injury, is the *fracture of the hook of the hamate*. It occurs when a golf club, tennis racket, cricket bat, or similar implement hits something in mid-swing and the force is transmitted through the end of the handle to the base of the palm over the hook of the hamate. This lies about 1 cm distal and radial to the pisiform, where it can be felt by deep palpation. Stark *et al.* (1977) reported twenty patients (four tennis players, seven golfers, and nine baseball players) all with old un-united fractures of the hook of the hamate. If a golf club hits the ground instead of the ball, the impact is particularly severe and such an injury is more likely. It was always the upper hand which was injured. The correct diagnosis had been made in only two cases; the others had been treated by rest, physiotherapy, and steroid injections without benefit.

There are two reasons why this injury is usually overlooked. The first is that doctors are not aware of it. A history such as that above, with tenderness localized to the hook of the hamate, suggests the diagnosis. Pain on flexing the ring or little fingers (whose flexor tendons pass alongside the hook) or paraesthesiae in those fingers (whose sensory nerves pass over the hook) strengthen the suspicion. The second reason is that ordinary X-rays of the wrist are unlikely to show the fracture. As previously explained, the history and examination enable one to order the correct X-rays to demonstrate the fracture. In the patient whose X-ray is shown as Fig. 4.14, only two films were requested: this view through the carpal tunnel, and an oblique view, which also showed the fracture. If pain prevents the patient from dorsiflexing the wrist enough to obtain a satisfactory carpal tunnel view showing all the hook, it can be demonstrated by CT scan.

Non-union is treated by excision of the hook of the hamate. Great care is required, as it is quite deep, and there are sensory nerves superficial, a motor nerve distal, and tendons radial to the hook. The results are excellent, and professional sportsmen can quickly return to full activity. These fractures are so rarely diagnosed as fresh injuries that there is no guidance in the literature on treatment. It would appear that the attachment of the flexor retinaculum to the hook would tend to separate it, and that it might not heal even after a period in plaster. In the cricketer shown in Fig.4.14, the fractured hook was excised by the author, following which the patient resumed first-class cricket in six weeks.

Joint injuries of the wrist

A variety of *dislocations and fracture-dislocations* can occur involving the carpus. All are rare; the least uncommon are the following.

(a) An anterior dislocation of the lunate (Figs 4.10 and 4.12) which, since it has displaced into the carpal tunnel, may cause acute compression of the median nerve although, surprisingly, dislocation of the lunate is very seldom followed by avascular necrosis of that bone (Kienböck's disease).

(b) Perilunar dislocation (Fig. 4.15), where the lunate remains in its proper relationship with the radius, but everything distal to and around it is dislocated dorsally. It is thought that this is the first stage of the injury described above, after which the carpus moves anteriorly again, pushing the lunate forwards out of place.

(c) Trans-scaphoid perilunar dislocation, which is similar, except that the scaphoid fractures across its waist and its distal pole displaces with the rest of the carpus, while the proximal pole and lunate remain in the correct position. The dislocation is usually dorsal.

These are serious injuries. If PA and lateral X-rays are taken and studied carefully, they should not be missed, but it still happens. An experienced orthopaedic surgeon should carry out the reduction as soon as possible. Even if a trans-scaphoid perilunar dislocation is reduced satisfactorily, the scaphoid fracture should be treated by open reduction and internal fixation: the former because there may be torn ligament interposed between the two halves of the scaphoid (Wilton 1987), which would prevent union, and the latter because this is an unstable injury and this too means that there is a strong chance of non-union.

One would also expect carpal instability after these dislocations, which must involve considerable ligamentous damage, but in practice the wrist usually becomes rather stiff instead (Panting *et al.* 1984).

Helal (1978) has described a condition that he calls *racquet player's pisiform*. The pathology is of chondromalacia of the articular cartilage between the pisiform and triquetral bones. He wrote that 'the probable mechanism is a torsional stress upon the capsule of the piso-triquetral joint by the sharp and powerful pronation–supination movements at the wrist which occur when wielding a racquet, the racquet acting as an additional lever upon the wrist. I believe that it is only those sports in which stroke play is mainly from the wrist which give rise to the syndrome: although in tennis a heavier racquet is used, the stroke is made from the shoulder'. Three squash players and one badminton player were cured by excision of the pisiform. A similar condition is said to have been seen in a golfer.

Moving distally, *dislocations and fracture-dislocations of the carpometacarpal joints* are missed far too often (Henderson and Arafa 1987). Clinically, the displacement is obscured by the soft tissue swelling. Radiologically it is discernible, provided that lateral views are taken and that the observer checks that the distal row of the carpus and the superimposed second to fifth metacarpals are in line.

Carpal instability

It is now clear that it is possible to tear ligaments around the carpus in such a way that, although the bones do not actually dislocate on each other, their relationship is altered. The most common pattern is that the lunate tilts so that its distal surface is pointing somewhat dorsally (dorsal intercalated segment instability); this extension of the lunate is accompanied by flexion of the scaphoid. The opposite pattern (volar intercalated segment instability), in which the lunate tilts in a palmar or volar direction, is less common. In extreme cases, the ligaments between the scaphoid

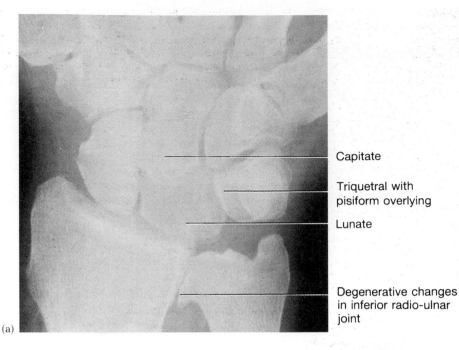

(a)

Capitate

Triquetral with
pisiform overlying

Lunate

Degenerative changes
in inferior radio-ulnar
joint

FIG. 4.15 (a) PA and (b) lateral
views of perilunar dislocation of
wrist. Note the loss of the smooth
curve of the mid-carpal joint on
PA; the adjoining surfaces of the
lunate and capitate are not parallel. The patient also has a dorsal
radial fracture and degenerative
changes in the inferior radio-ulnar
joint.

(b)

Scaphoid

Lunate

Capitate

Triquetral

Dorsal
radial
fracture

and lunate are completely disrupted, so that a gap appears between these bones, a radiological finding known as the Terry-Thomas sign from its resemblance to the gap between that actor's front teeth (Fig. 4.16). Since the instability may not be present all the time, X-rays may fail to demonstrate it. A series of films with the wrists in various positions is recommended; alternatively, the wrist may be screened whilst the patient attempts the movement that provoked pain or clicking. Both the radiologist and the physician or surgeon should be present. It is very helpful if the examination is recorded on videotape so that it can be studied repeatedly.

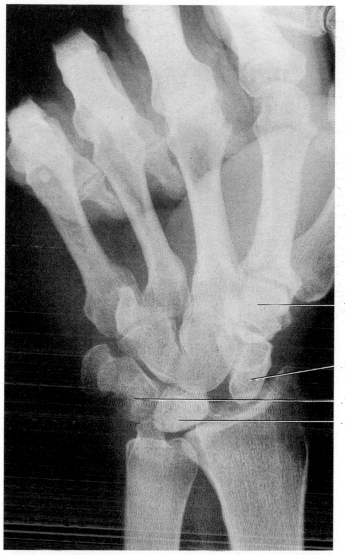

Trapezium

Scaphoid
(flexed with ring sign)

Triquetral

Lunate

FIG. 4.16 AP film with the patient gripping. This is the film most likely to show, as it does here, a gap between the scaphoid and lunate bones (Terry-Thomas sign). The other wrist must always be X-rayed for comparison. A unilateral gap indicates a ligamentous injury. The scaphoid, no longer attached to the lunate, moves into a flexed position in which the cortical outline of its tuberosity appears as a ring.

Jones (1988), in an important paper entitled 'Beware the sprained wrist', reviewed the findings in a consecutive series of 100 wrist injuries in which, in addition to the conventional X-rays, an extra AP view was taken with the patient clenching his fist tightly (Fig. 4.16); this is one of the views most likely to demonstrate carpal instability. Only those patients with obvious fractures of the distal radius were excluded; all others had this extra view taken. In 76 patients, the films were considered normal: four had fractures of the scaphoid, three of the trapezium, and fourteen of the distal radius. However, the most important finding was that nineteen patients had a gap of more than 2 mm between the scaphoid and lunate; of these, it was found that in fourteen this finding was bilateral, and therefore presumably not caused by the injury, leaving five (that is, 5 per cent) thought to have had a significant injury to the scapho-lunate ligament complex, with clinical and radiographic evidence of instability. Evidently, this type of injury is not so uncommon if one looks for it properly.

The treatment of these instability patterns in the carpus is still a problem; on the whole, ligamentous reconstructions have not proved to be very successful, but limited or partial arthrodesis (for example between the scaphoid, trapezium and trape-

zoid) is also disappointing. For further information on this complex subject, the reader is referred to the papers by Taleisnik (1988) and Larsen et al. (1995) and the books edited by Lichtman (1988) and by Barton and Mulligan (1999).

What is clear, however, is that there are patients complaining of pain in the wrist in whom ordinary examination and X-rays reveal no abnormality, but who have a genuine if intermittent instability. This is comparable to the knee, where thirty years ago the instability patterns were not understood, and the patients were either dismissed as hypochondriacs or just had to put up with it (or had their menisci removed). Unfortunately, even effective treatment of wrist instability may not succeed in allowing the patient to resume top-class sport.

Lastly on the topic of ligamentous injuries to the carpus, it must be admitted that a wrist sprain probably can occur, and this may be the pathology in those patients in whom a fracture of the scaphoid is suspected but never confirmed. The old adage 'sprained wrist does not exist' is not quite true, but it remains true that this is a diagnosis which can be made only after thorough clinical and radiological investigation and only in retrospect, by which time treatment is unnecessary as a true (acute) sprain settles quickly with rest. Persisting symptoms indicate the possibility of a more serious injury, perhaps one of the forms of carpal instability mentioned above.

Fractures of the hand

These are exceedingly common, and sport is a common cause. It is probably the *most* common cause of the end-on blows which result in severe damage to joints.

The essential principles of treatment of hand fractures are the same as for anywhere in the body, and comprise the three Rs of fracture treatment: reduction, retention, and rehabilitation. In the hand, however, the principles are applied in a rather different way (Barton 1984). The first step, of course, is to define the nature of the fracture; this requires an X-ray. In the femur, a subcapital fracture is not treated in the same way as a shaft fracture, and in the phalanges and metacarpals there are many different types of fracture, each needing different management.

Reduction

Frequently the fracture is undisplaced or minimally displaced: this does not need to be reduced. However, a displaced fracture of the shaft of the proximal phalanx will leave a step in the floor of the tunnel in which the flexor tendon runs, and this is not acceptable. Rotational deformity *must* be corrected, and therefore the finger must be examined specifically to look for this; the fingers of both hands should be studied end-on (Fig. 4.17). Usually, despite the fracture, the patient can be persuaded to flex the finger to some extent, which renders the deformity more obvious (Fig. 4.18); unless corrected, the finger will remain rotated permanently, making it almost useless. Spiral fractures, caused by a rotational force, are particularly likely to have rotational deformity.

Retention

Experience is required to determine which fractures are unstable and therefore need external or internal splintage. Figures 4.19

and 4.20, modified from London's book, give some guidance. Stable fractures should be treated by strapping the injured finger to an intact neighbour, giving some support and protection while allowing movement, with the normal finger acting as a dynamic splint (Fig. 4.21). The strapping must be applied in such a way as to *permit*, not prevent, movement. Any fracture which needs reduction also needs retention to ensure that reduction is maintained; this may be by external splintage or by internal fixation.

The hand tends to stiffen with the metacarpophalangeal (MCP) joints extended and the interphalangeal (IP) joints flexed. Therefore, it must always be immobilized in the opposite position, with the MCP joints flexed and the IP joints extended (Fig. 4.22). This is often called the Edinburgh position because it was popularized by Professor J. I. P. James of Edinburgh (James 1970); he calls it the safe position. Whatever its name, nothing is more important in the treatment of hand injuries, whether minor or major, than to ensure that the hand is immobilized correctly to minimize the chance of permanent loss of movement. There are virtually no circumstances in which the interphalangeal joints should be immobilized in a flexed position.

External splintage of a single fractured finger may be achieved satisfactorily by a padded aluminium splint, such as one made by Zimmer; this must be put on correctly (Fig. 4.23), so that the finger is immobilized in the safe position and the fingertip can be inspected end-on to check that there is no malrotation. If more than one finger is fractured, anterior and posterior plaster slabs in the safe position provide the most effective immobilization. A fractured thumb which requires immobilization may be treated in a plaster cast extending almost to the tip of the thumb but leaving the fingers free.

Many fractures of the hand do not need to be immobilized, though clearly the digit should, if possible, be protected from further injury until the fracture has healed. This is determined *clinically*. Radiological union takes a long time, and one does not need to wait for it; in fact, once the position of the fracture is satisfactory, it is seldom necessary to take any more X-rays.

A very small proportion of hand fractures, not more than 5 per cent, need operative treatment. The *indications* are as follows:

FIG. 4.17 Looking at the fingers end-on to detect rotational deformity. The ring finger is pronated in relation to the other fingers. This is best seen by looking at the line of the finger-nail.

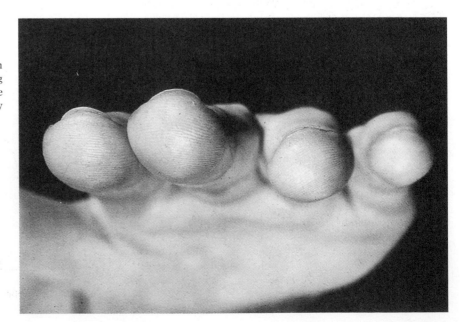

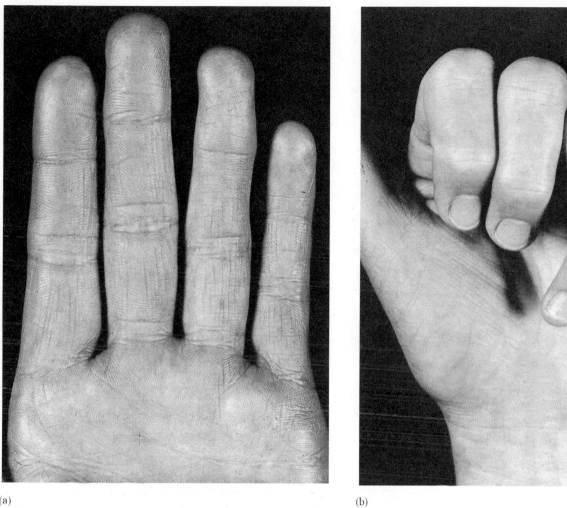

(a)

(b)

FIG. 4.18 (a) In extension, the finger looks fairly normal; (b) in flexion, rotation deformity becomes obvious.

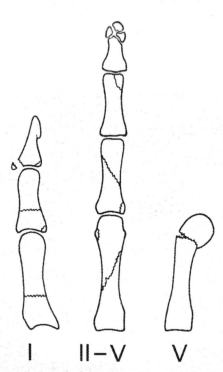

I   II–V   V

Fig. 4.19 Stable fractures, which do not need immobilization.

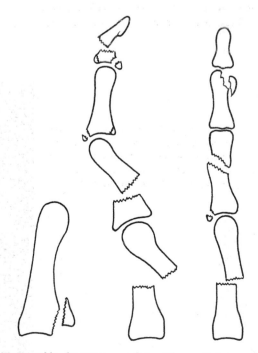

Fig. 4.20 Unstable fractures, needing either splintage or internal fixation.

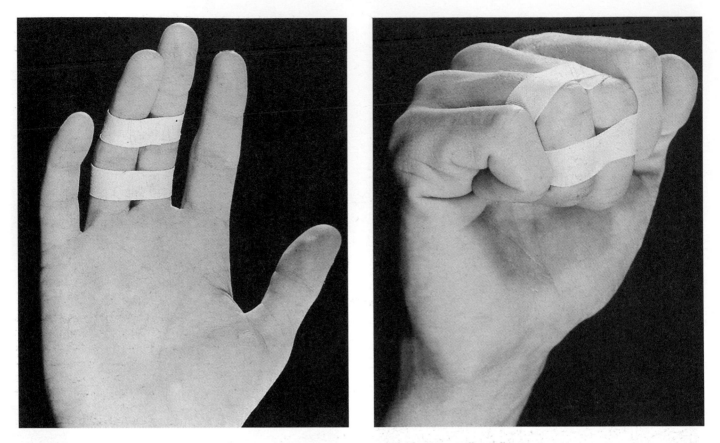

FIG. 4.21 The injured finger has been strapped to a neighbouring intact one in such a way as to allow full movement.

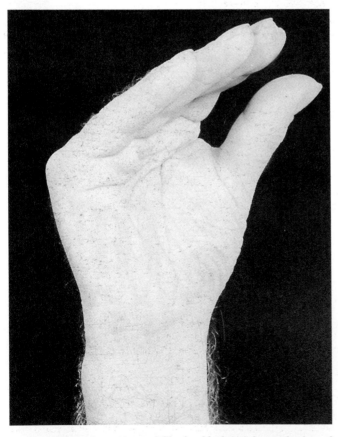

FIG. 4.22 The safe position, which should always be used when the hand has to be immobilized. It is not meant as a permanent position, but is the one from which it is easiest to regain a full range of movements.

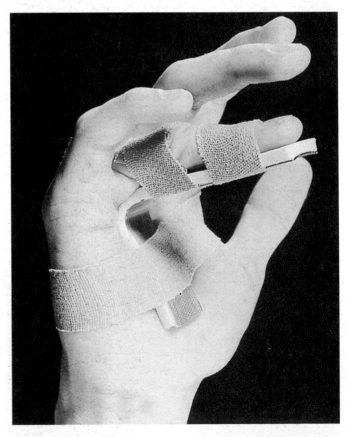

FIG. 4.23 Finger splinted in the safe position on an aluminium splint. The splint is bent to 90° at the transverse palmar creases, which overlie the MCP joint (not the crease at the base of the finger, which is halfway down the proximal phalanx). The splint should not cross the wrist joint.

(1) fractures of the shafts of the phalanges in which good reduction cannot be achieved by closed means;

(2) fractures involving joints in which there is either a large fragment carrying a lot of the joint surface or a small fragment associated with subluxation of the joint;

(3) multiple fractures within the hand.

The important early management decision is to identify the minority that must be treated by splintage or surgery from the majority, where simple strapping to a neighbouring finger is adequate treatment. Failure to do this is likely to result in permanent disability; little delay can be tolerated, as the fracture will begin to unite in the wrong position within a few days.

Rehabilitation

This is the most important part of treatment. In other parts of the body it must wait until the fracture has united, but in the hand it should start straight away. In sportsmen, this is usually no problem; on the contrary, the difficulty is to persuade patients with more serious fractures that it is in their interest as sportsmen to accept a period of immobilization in order to achieve a satisfactory long-term result.

(a)

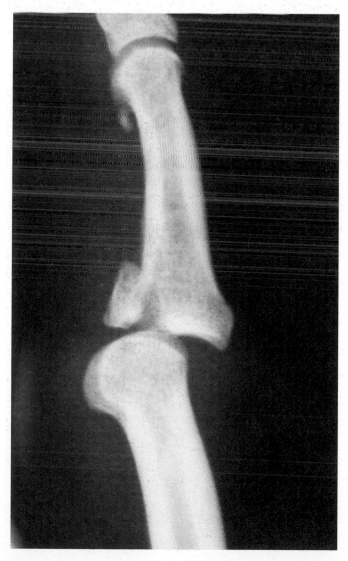

In stable fractures, active mobilization within the protective strapping is encouraged. The point when sport can safely be resumed is when tenderness has diminished to an acceptable level. Fractures which have been splinted or operated on may need physiotherapy to help the patient regain a full range of movement. Active exercises should be practised *with the hand empty:* squeezing a ball or bit of putty should be forbidden (though some well-meaning person will probably suggest it), because this promotes redisplacement of the fracture and prevents full flexion. What is required is a full range of movement, so that the finger does not stick out and become injured again; once a full range is regained, power quickly follows.

A detailed account of the management of each type of fracture of the metacarpal and phalanx is given elsewhere (Barton 1982), and so only brief comments follow on the most common or important types.

Fractures of the phalanges

Fingertip fractures

If the skin has burst or the nail is broken, the fracture is compound and must be treated as such. After careful cleansing, the nail may be replaced as a dressing (Henderson 1984). If the fracture is closed and there is a subungual haematoma, it should be released to relieve pain and speed resolution. A paper-clip may be opened up so that one end can be heated until it is red-hot and applied to the nail to burn a hole through; this is less painful than trephining and is also sterile.

The fracture itself is unimportant; it is the soft tissues which need treating.

Fractures involving joints

The most common are tiny flake fractures, avulsed by a ligament or capsule. There is no evidence that immobilization improves the outcome and so, provided that the joint is stable,

(b)

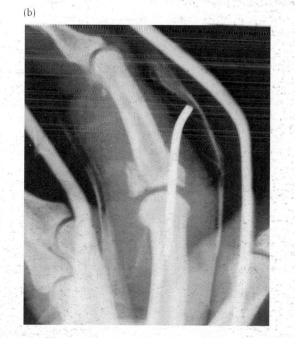

FIG. 4.24 (a) Fracture-subluxation of PIP joint in a professional cricketer injured while fielding. The fact that the base of the middle phalanx is no longer congruous with the head of the proximal phalanx is more important than the small fracture. (b) Subluxation reduced and joint held in correct alignment by transfixing Kirschner wire.

activities can be resumed as soon as pain permits, with the protection afforded by strapping the finger to its neighbour (Phair *et al.* 1989)

However, if the joint is subluxed (Fig. 4.24), a very different situation exists. This is a major injury to the joint, requiring serious treatment. It occurs quite often in fielders at cricket and in Australian Rules Football. McElfresh *et al.* (1972) have described an ingenious extension block splint which allows flexion but prevents extension (which is the unstable position). The author prefers to use percutaneous Kirschner wire fixation to maintain the reduction for three weeks, and then an extension block splint for a further three weeks. In some cases, the small fragment may also need fixation.

Fractures of the base of a phalanx without subluxation usually do surprisingly well without immobilization (Steel 1988). Fractures of the head of a phalanx nearly always need internal fixation (McCue *et al.* 1970).

Epiphyseal fractures

In boys, the epiphyses in the hand remain open until the age of 15 or later, and fractures in or near the growth plate are common in injuries sustained in games. A great deal of correction may be anticipated from the processes of remodelling with growth, but it is important to correct lateral angulation near the interphalangeal joints and malrotation anywhere, because these do not correct themselves.

Fractures of shafts of phalanges

The front of the phalanx is the floor of the tunnel in which the flexor tendon glides up and down. If this is not restored to a smooth bony surface, one cannot expect the finger to work properly. The angulation, which is into extension, must be corrected, together with any displacement. A skilled manipulation can often achieve the desired perfect reduction. This is performed with the MCP joint flexed to stabilize the proximal fragment: the MCP joint is kept in the flexed position with the IP joints extended while the finger is immobilized. If perfect reduction cannot be achieved then, in the proximal phalanx at any rate, an operation is indicated.

Comminuted fractures

These usually result from some sort of crushing injury, and the combination of many fracture-lines with skin damage means

that an operation is often contraindicated. The periosteal envelope is usually intact, so that the fracture is stable and heals surprisingly well with early mobilization. As always, any rotational deformity must be corrected.

Fractures of the metacarpals

On the whole, these cause fewer problems than fractures of the phalanges. Metacarpal fractures usually angulate into *flexion* and so, if there is any permanent loss of movement, it is loss of extension, which is less likely to result in disability. Malrotation can occur, and, when it does, is serious because there is a greater length of digit distal to the fracture and greater deformity results; however, in most cases, the deep transverse metacarpal ligaments and the interossei which connect adjoining metacarpals limit displacement of a single metacarpal fracture.

When one makes a fist and hits somebody, the impact is taken on the distal end of the metacarpal and commonly causes a fracture at that level, though the force may be transmitted down the shaft to the base of the metacarpal.

Fractures of the metacarpal heads

These are most often seen in the index and middle fingers, usually due to fighting. On the whole, they do surprisingly well, but again one cannot lump them all together. McElfresh and Dobyns (1983) have described ten different types of fracture of the metacarpal head.

Fractures of the necks of the metacarpals

These are usually the result of fist-fighting, though not in a formal manner: unhappily, this is increasingly common during sporting contests which are not intended to include fighting.

It is usually the neck of the fifth metacarpal which is broken and considerable flexion deformity of this particular fracture is acceptable and compatible with normal function afterwards, for the following reasons.

(a) Since the fracture is distal, an angulation of, say, 30° produces much less forward displacement of the metacarpal head than would the same angulation in the mid-shaft (Fig. 4.25).

(b) The joint between the hamate and the base of the metacarpal of the little finger (fifth carpo-metacarpal joint) normally allows about 30° flexion and extension, as may be observed

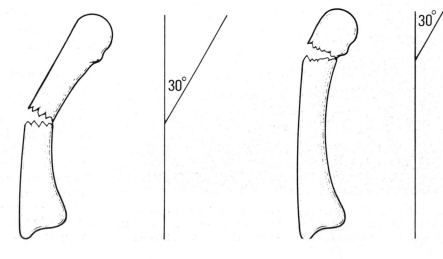

FIG. 4.25 Angulation at the neck of the metacarpal causes less deformity than angulation in the mid-shaft.

by clenching one's fist tightly when the fifth metacarpal head moves forward.

Thus any flexion deformity at the neck of the fifth metacarpal can be compensated for by extending the joint at the base of the metacarpal. This applies less in the fourth metacarpal, whose basal joint has only about 15° of movement, and not at all in the middle and index fingers, whose basal joints have virtually no movement and therefore cannot compensate for more distal deformity.

Therefore, the common fracture of the fifth metacarpal should not be overtreated. The author's practice is to treat it by a crepe bandage and early movements. The bandage reminds the patient and others that there is an injury. Often it takes some weeks to regain full active extension at the MCP joint, but hardly ever is there any permanent disability even in poorly motivated patients (Ford *et al.* 1989). The old practice of strapping the finger in flexion has been rightly abandoned; it is true that in this position one can reduce the fracture by pressure along the proximal phalanx, but it is also true that immobilization with the proximal interphalangeal (PIP) joint flexed, even for a short period, can produce a permanent flexion contracture at that joint, which is worse than the effect of the original injury.

It is said that very severe angulation (e.g. 60° or more) in fifth metacarpal neck fractures requires surgery: however, in the author's experience, surgical intervention seldom improves the result, and occasionally is very harmful.

Fractures of the shaft of the metacarpals

Often there is little or no displacement, and simple immobilization for three weeks is adequate treatment. However, it is important to make sure that there is no rotational deformity of the attached finger. Displaced or rotated fractures should be referred at once for orthopaedic assessment.

Fractures at or near the base of the first metacarpal

The most common type is a transverse fracture of the first metacarpal about 1 cm distal to the joint; the metacarpal is angulated into flexion. Since the first metacarpal normally lies in a rotated position compared with the other metacarpals, the injury results in the thumb becoming flexed across the palm— that is, extension of the thumb is restricted, and the span between the thumb and the index finger is reduced. Therefore, it is important to reduce these fractures, but they are usually easy to reduce and to hold corrected in plaster provided that the extension force is applied to the distal end of the metacarpal and not to the phalanges of the thumb, which may merely hyperextend the MCP joint.

Bennett's fracture-subluxation of the first carpo-metacarpal joint (Fig. 4.26) is a rare injury, although much has been written about it. A surprisingly good functional result may occur despite poor treatment (Cannon *et al.* 1986), but as it involves an important joint, it seems right that such an injury should be managed by an orthopaedic surgeon. It may be treated conservatively provided that a very special and careful technique of plaster application is used (Charnley 1961), but frequently percutaneous fixation with a Kirschner wire is needed (Wagner 1950). Either way, the immobilization should be maintained for six weeks; the usual three weeks is not enough, and if the joint is left free at that stage it may redisplace.

Joint injuries to the digits

Fractures into the joints have already been considered; the following account is of soft tissue injuries.

Carpo-metacarpal joints

At the bases of the second and third metacarpals, 'sprain-impaction problems are seen after flexion stress injuries resulting in volar impaction and dorsal stretch. A common example occurs when ice-hockey players crash into the wall or fend off an opponent. Compression-impaction is a serious problem in the professional boxer, whose repetitive stress to the stable longitudinal arch eventually results in cartilage damage, osteochondral fractures, and a chronically painful arthrosi.' (Dobyns 1988).

Metacarpophalangeal joints

As the *thumb* protrudes laterally from the hand at the level of the MCP joint, this joint is often injured. This is particularly common in skiing. If the ulnar collateral ligament of the MCP joint is torn (Fig. 4.27) it almost always displaces superficial to the adductor aponeurosis (Stener 1962). It cannot heal with this aponeurosis interposed between the two ends of the ligament, and operative treatment is required. Therefore, these patients must be referred to a surgeon for operation within a few days of injury. The diagnosis should be made upon the detection of bruising, the absence of fracture on X-ray, and the presence of ligamentous laxity (comparison should be made with the normal thumb).

Some experts (Abrahamsson *et al.* 1990) say that they can tell whether the ligament is displaced by clinical palpation, or failing that by ultrasound, and that if it is not displaced the

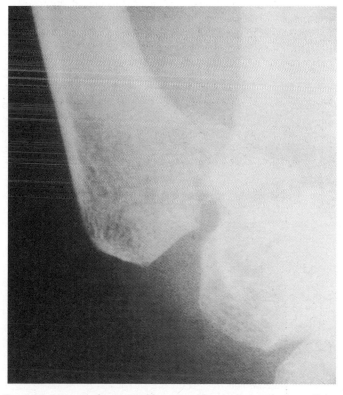

Fig. 4.26 Bennett's fracture-subluxation. The small piece broken off the base of the first metacarpal remains in place while the rest of the metacarpal, carrying most of the articular surface, subluxes laterally.

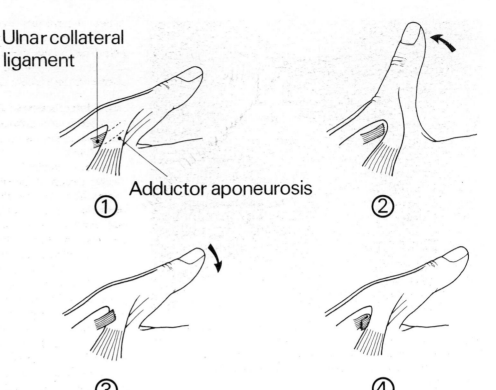

FIG. 4.27 Mechanism of the torn ulnar collateral ligament of the MCP joint of the thumb: (1) normal anatomy; (2) radial abduction injury to the thumb tears the distal end of the collateral ligament; (3) when the thumb returns to its normal position, the adductor aponeurosis comes to lie deep to the torn ligament or even (4) is folded back. Operative replacement and repair are needed.

injury can be treated conservatively. Most of us find this distinction difficult. I have always done stress X-rays and explored all those cases in which they were abnormal: only once in 25 years did I not find the ligament displaced, so I recommend early surgical repair in all cases.

The radial collateral ligament is torn less often, but can be surprisingly troublesome. The anatomy is different on that side of the thumb, with little risk of soft tissue interposition, and conservative treatment in a plaster cast is satisfactory except in the more severe cases.

The acute injury (skier's thumb) should be distinguished from chronic instability due to an old injury and from gamekeeper's thumb, a condition confined to gamekeepers, which is not due to a single injury but to gradual attenuation of the ligament over many years while breaking the necks of rabbits (Campbell 1955).

The MCP joints of the *fingers* are injured less often. If injury does occur, it usually takes the form of a dislocation of the second or fifth MCP joint. This is either easy or impossible to reduce by manipulation. One try is permissible. If it will not reduce, the torn volar plate is probably interposed between the joint surfaces, and this must be dealt with by open operation (Kaplan 1957). Repeated and increasingly forceful attempts to reduce the dislocation can only do harm.

Proximal interphalangeal joints

Dislocation is easy to diagnose clinically and often easy to reduce, but it is always wise to have it X-rayed because an accompanying fracture makes it a much more serious injury, requiring expert treatment (see above). The usual dorsal dislocation (that is with the distal part of the finger displaced dorsally) is easily reduced. The collateral ligaments are often intact, the base of the middle phalanx having swung round on them like a trapeze

artist on his arms, but, after reduction, one must always test the collateral ligaments by applying first radial and then ulnar angulation to the extended finger. If the ligaments are intact, it is not necessary to immobilize the finger, though it may be wise to do so as some authorities believe that complete immobilization for ten days in a splint or in plaster will allow the finger to make a complete recovery more quickly (Eaton 1971).

If a collateral ligament is not intact, then the injury passes into the next category.

Tears of the collateral ligament of the PIP joint result from sideways force—for example, trying to catch a ball or falling onto the finger. With a complete tear, the instability is usually obvious; in cases of doubt, the finger may easily be anaesthetized by digital block, and stress X-rays performed (Fig. 4.28). Opinions differ as to whether operative repair is required. Provided that the X-ray shows the joint surfaces to be exactly parallel (that is, the torn ligament is not displaced into the joint), the author's practice has been to strap the finger to an intact neighbour to prevent further lateral stress but allow flexion and extension; the results have appeared satisfactory.

Sprains are partial tears of the collateral ligament, in which lateral stress causes pain but no abnormal lateral angulation. These would appear to be the least serious joint injuries in the fingers, but in practice they are often the most troublesome. Pain may continue for six months, and swelling for a year or even more. No treatment seems to make any difference, but eventually they make a full recovery and all the patients need is reassurance.

The *boutonnière injury* (known in France as 'le button-hole') is caused by a flexion force which tears the central slip of the extensor mechanism over the back of the PIP joint (Fig. 4.29). This injury is easily overlooked because at first the patient is able to extend the PIP joint using the lateral bands of the extensor mechanism. However, there will be tenderness and pain on

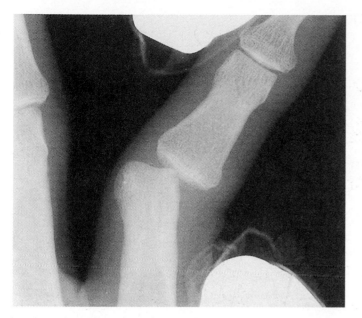

FIG. 4.28 Stress views show abnormal lateral angulation due to a torn collateral ligament of the PIP joint. The patient, a famous Antipodean fast bowler, was treated by simple strapping, and regained full stability (perhaps to the regret of the English batsmen, as later that summer he took many England wickets).

extension against resistance. Treatment is by immobilization in extension for four weeks, followed by a lively splint for another two weeks. If the injury is not diagnosed and treated, then over the next week or two the lateral bands slip forwards down the side of the joint until they can no longer extend it (Fig. 4.29(c)).

A flexion contracture quickly develops, with the joint coming through between the lateral bands like a button through its hole. This is now the boutonnière deformity and is much more difficult to treat, though lively splintage is sometimes effective. Surgery is not recommended.

Distal interphalangeal (DIP) joint

Dislocation and collateral ligament injuries at this level are uncommon, because there is such a short length of finger distal to the joint.

However, *mallet fingers* are very common, caused by forcible passive flexion of the DIP joint when the extensor apparatus is contracting. The result is an injury to the extensor tendon rather like a rupture of the Achilles tendon: it is not a transverse tear with the ends apart, but an internal shredding, with the torn ends overlapping but in a lengthened position. The result is a lag in active extension, but full active flexion (Fig. 4.30). An X-ray should be taken, as the presence of a fracture may mean that different treatment is required. If there is no fracture, a decision must be made as to whether to treat the injury or not. A minor lag (e.g. 30°) may be taken up by the extensor mechanism, and an almost normal finger results; but a more severe one will, if untreated, be permanent: however, this causes no disability. Treatment consists of continuous immobilization of the DIP joint in extension for *eight weeks*. Any splint will do, *provided it is kept on all the time and not removed for any reason, even briefly*. Stack's moulded polypropylene splint (Fig. 4.31), which comes in various sizes and is available from Pryor & Howard Ltd, Manufacturers of Orthopaedic and Surgical Appliances, Willow Lane, Mitcham, CR4 4US, is probably the most satisfactory (Warren *et al.* 1988). It should be trimmed with a scalpel if the edge is pressing on the tender dorsum of the DIP joint. If the patient is not prepared to persevere with this

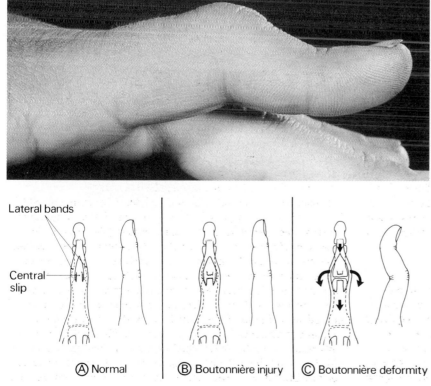

(a)

FIG. 4.29 The boutonnière injury: (a) clinical appearance; (b) pathology.

Lateral bands

Central slip

Ⓐ Normal | Ⓑ Boutonnière injury | Ⓒ Boutonnière deformity

(b)

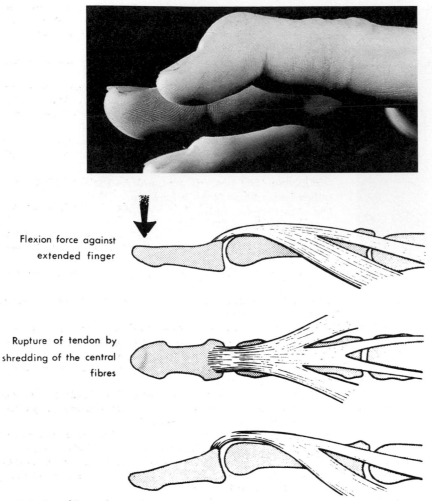

FIG. 4.30 Mallet finger injury: (a) clinical appearance; (b) pathology.

(a)

Flexion force against
extended finger

Rupture of tendon by
shredding of the central
fibres

(b)

treatment, there is no point in starting it, and he must understand that he will have to accept the minor deformity; however, function will be no problem. There is no need for surgical treatment of the acute injury, and very few indications for later surgery either.

Forcible extension of the finger can produce a corresponding, but much rarer, injury: *rupture of the flexor digitorum profundus (FDP) tendon* on the front of the finger. This is classically seen in rugby football players failing to make a tackle; they clutch despairingly at the trouser-band of the other player, whose determined departure pulls the distal end of the FDP tendon, sometimes with a fragment of bone, from the distal phalanx. It is nearly always the ring finger which is injured. This is often a more severe injury than an open cut of the flexor tendon, because the force of flexion pulls the tendon right down into the palm, ripping the vincula and filling the empty tendon sheath with blood, which will, if allowed, turn into restrictive fibrous tissue. A surgeon specializing in the hand should be given the opportunity to carry out primary repair within a day or two. If this chance has been lost, active flexion of the DIP joint can only be restored by a tendon graft—never a very predictable procedure. Provided that the patient has full active flexion of the PIP joint (by the intact flexor digitorum super-

ficialis), it may be wiser to do nothing, as lack of flexion at the distal joint seldom causes much difficulty in using the hand. If it does, a tenodesis or arthrodesis of the DIP joint in slight flexion can be offered.

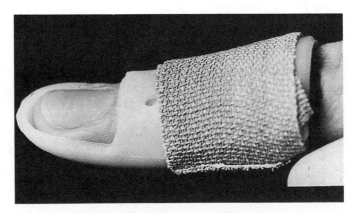

Fig. 4.31 Stack splint for mallet finger.

Conclusion

Many, but not all, sports injuries to the hand and wrist are minor and need little treatment or time off sport. Some, which may at first sight appear to be minor injuries, will cause permanent disability if not treated energetically. All must be assessed with great care including X-rays in most cases, to ensure recognition of the more serious injuries, so that they may be referred to an expert. The average casualty officer is not an expert, and the doctor in charge of the patient may be wise to arrange an urgent referral to a hand surgeon or an orthopaedic surgeon, which should take place within two or three days.

References

Abrahamsson, S.-O., Sollerman, C., Lindborg, G., Larsson, J., and Egund, N. (1990). Diagnosis of displaced ulnar collateral ligament of the metacarpophalangeal joint of the Thumb. *J. Hand Surg.*, **15A**, 457–60.

Barton, N. J. (1982). Fractures and joint injuries of the hand. In *Watson-Jones' fractures and joint injuries* (ed. J. N. Wilson), Vol. 2, pp. 739–88. Churchill-Livingstone, Edinburgh.

Barton, N. J. (1984). Fractures of the hand. *J. Bone Jt. Surg.*, **66B**, 159–67.

Barton, N. J. (1992). Twenty questions about scaphoid fractures. *J. Hand Surg.* **17B**, 289–310.

Barton, N. J. (1997). Experience with scaphoid grafting. *J. Hand Surg.* **22B**, 153–60.

Barton, N. J. and Mulligan, P. J., eds (1999). *The Upper Limb and Hand* W. B. Saunders, London.

Belliappa, P. P. and Barton, N. J. (1991). Hand injuries in cricketers. *J. Hand Surg* **16B**, 212–14.

Blum, L. (1941). The treatment of Bennett's fracture-dislocation of the first metacarpal bone. *J. Bone Jt. Surg.*, **23**, 578–80.

Burke, F. D. (1988). Colles' fractures: conservative treatment. In *Fractures of the hand and wrist* (ed. N. J. Barton), pp. 267–75. Churchill-Livingstone, Edinburgh.

Cabrera, J. M. and McCue, F. C. (1986). Nonosseous athletic injuries of the elbow, forearm, and hand. *Clin. Sports Med.*, **5**, 681–700.

Campbell, C. S. (1955). Gamekeeper's thumb. *J. Bone Jt. Surg.*, **37B**, 148–9.

Cannon, S. R., Dowd, G. S. E., Williams, D. H., and Scott, J. M. (1986). A long-term study following Bennett's fracture. *J. Hand Surg.*, **11B**, 426–31.

Charnley, J. (1961). *The closed treatment of common fractures* (3rd edn). Churchill-Livingstone, Edinburgh.

Clay, N. R., Dias, J. J., Costigan, P. S., Gregg, P. J., and Barton, N. J. (1991). Need the thumb be immobilized in scaphoid fractures? A randomized prospective trial. *J. Bone Jt. Surg.*, **73B**, 828–32.

Curtin, J. and Kay, N. M. R. (1976). Hand injuries due to soccer. *Hand*, **8**, 93–5.

Cyriax, J. (1982). *Textbook of orthopaedic medicine*, Vol. 1 (8th edn). Baillière Tindall, London.

Dias, J. J., Taylor, M., Thompson, J., Brenkel, I. J., and Gregg, P. J. (1988). Radiographic signs of union of scaphoid fractures. *J. Bone Jt. Surg.*, **70B**, 299–301.

Dobyns, J. H. (1988). Fractures and dislocations at the base of the metacarpals. In *Fractures of the hand and wrist* (ed. N. J. Barton), pp. 120–33. Churchill-Livingstone, Edinburgh.

Eaton, R. G. (1971). *Joint injuries of the hand*. Thomas, Springfield, Illinois.

Ford, D. J., Ali, M. S., and Steel, W. M. (1989). Fractures of the fifth metacarpal neck: is reduction or immobilization necessary? *J. Hand Surg.*, **14B**, 165–7.

Green, D. P. (1985). The effect of avascular necrosis on Russe bone grafting for scaphoid non-union. *J. Hand Surg.*, **10A**, 597–605.

Helal, B. (1978). Racquet player's pisiform. *Hand*, **10**, 87–90.

Henderson, H. P. (1984). The best dressing for a nail bed is the nail itself. *J. Hand Surg.*, **9B**, 197–8.

Henderson, J. J. and Arafa, M. A. M. (1987). Carpometacarpal dislocation. An easily missed diagnosis. *J. Bone Jt. Surg.*, **69B**, 212–14.

Hutson, M. A. (1997). *Work-related upper limb disorders*. Butterworth Heinemann, Oxford.

James, J. I. P. (1970). The assessment and management of the injured hand. *Hand*, **2**, 97–105.

Jones, W. A. (1988). Beware the sprained wrist. The incidence and diagnosis of scapho-lunate instability. *J. Bone Jt. Surg.*, **70B**, 293–7.

Kaplan, E. B. (1957). Dorsal dislocation of metacarpo-phalangeal joint of the index finger. *J. Bone Jt. Surg.*, **39A**, 1081–6.

King, J. W., Brelsford, H. J., and Tullos H.S. (1969). Analysis of the pitching arm of the professional baseball pitcher. *Clin. Orthop.*, **67**, 116–23.

Kopell, H. P. and Thompson, W. A. L. (1963). *Peripheral entrapment in neuropathies*. Williams & Wilkins, Baltimore, MD.

Larsen, C., Amadio, P., Gilula, L, and Hodge, J. (1995). Analysis of carpal instability. *J. Hand Surg.*, **20A**, 757–76.

Leslie, I. J. and Dickson, R. A. (1981). The fractured carpal scaphoid. Natural history and factors influencing outcome. *J. Bone Jt. Surg.*, **63B**, 225–30.

Lichtman, D. M. (1988). *The wrist and its disorders*. W. B. Saunders, Philadelphia.

London, P. S. (1967). *A practical guide to the care of the injured*. Livingstone, Edinburgh.

McCue, F. C., Honner, R., Johnson, M. C., and Giech, J. H. (1970). Athletic injuries of the proximal interphalangeal joint requiring surgical treatment. *J. Bone Jt. Surg.*, **52A**, 937–56.

McElfresh, E. C. and Dobyns, J. H. (1983). Intra-articular metacarpal head fractures. *J. Hand Surg.*, **8**, 383–93.

McElfresh, E. C., Dobyns, J. H., and O'Brien, E. T. (1972). Management of fracture-dislocation of the proximal interphalangeal joint by extension splinting. *J. Bone Jt. Surg* **54A**, 1705–11.

Panner, H. J. (1929). A peculiar affection of the capitellum humeri resembling Calve–Perthes disease of the hip. *Acta Radiol*, **10**, 234.

Panting, A. L., Lamb, D. W., Noble, J., and Haw, C. S. (1984). Dislocations of the lunate with and without fracture of the scaphoid. *J. Bone Jt. Surg.* **66B**, 391–5.

Phair, I. C., Quinton, D. N., and Allen, M. J. (1989). The conservative management of volar avulsion fractures of the P. I. P. Joint. *J. Hand Surg*, **14B**, 168–70.

Read, M. T. F. (1981). Stress fractures of the distal radius in adolescent gymnasts. *Br. J. Sports Med.*, **15**, 272–6.

Roles, N. C. and Maudsley, R. H. (1972). Radial tunnel syndrome. *J. Bone Surg* **54B**, 499–508.

Roy, S., Caine, D., and Singer, K. M. (1985). Stress changes of the distal radial epiphysis in young gymnasts. *Am. J. Sports Med.*, **13**, 301–8.

Singer, K. M. and Roy, S. P. (1984). Osteochondrosis of the humeral capitellum. *Am. J. Sports Med.*, **12**, 351–60.

Slocum, D. B. (1978). Classification of elbow injuries from baseball players. *Am. J. Sports Med.*, **6**, 62–7.

Stark, J. J., Hobe, F. W., Boyes, J. H., and Ashworth, C. R. (1977). Fracture of the hook of the hamate in athletes. *J. Bone Jt. Surg.*, **59A**, 575–82.

Steel, W. M. (1988). Articular fractures. In *Fractures of the hand and wrist* (ed. N. J. Barton), pp. 55–73. Churchill-Livingstone, Edinburgh.

Stener, B. (1962). Displacement of the ruptured ulnar collateral ligament of the metacarpo-phalangeal joint of the thumb. *J. Bone Jt. Surg.*, **44B**, 869–79.

Taleisnik, J. (1988). Carpal instability. *J. Bone Jt. Surg.*, **70A**, 1262–8.

Wagner, C. J. (1950). Method of treatment of Bennett's fracture-dislocation. *Am. J. Surg.*, **80**, 230–31.

Warren, R. A., Norris, S. H., and Ferguson, D. D. (1988). Mallet finger: a trial of two splints. *J. Hand Surg.*, **13B**, 151–3.

Wilson, F. D., Andrews, J. R., Blackburn, T. A., and McCluskey, G. (1983). Valgus extension overload in the pitching elbow. *Am. J. Sports Med.*, **11**, 83–8.

Wilton, T. J. (1987). Soft-tissue interposition as a possible cause of scaphoid non-union. *J. Hand Surg.*, **12B**, 50–51.

5 Spinal injuries

M. A. HUTSON AND F. R. I. MIDDLETON

Soft tissue injuries

M. A. HUTSON

Biomechanics/applied anatomy

The spine has a number of functions that reflect man's upright stance, his capacity to bend and lift, and his desire to indulge in sport and recreation, which demand both stability and flexibility. It may be considered to be constructed in two columns, anterior and posterior. The *anterior* column is composed of vertebral bodies, their superior and inferior margins (the end plates) and the intervening discs. Each disc has a fibrocartilaginous annulus and a gelatinous nucleus pulposus. The anterior column resists axial compression loading of the spine. Associated with this shock-absorbing function of the disc is a little intervertebral movement in all directions (Bogduk and Twomey 1987). The *posterior* column is derived from the neural arches: movement occurs at the zygo-apophyseal (facet) joints, which are diarthrodial—that is, synovial in type.

In the cervical spine, nodding movements and side flexion occur at the atlanto-occipital (C0/1) joints. At C1/2 (the atlanto-axial joint), approximately $50°$ of rotation is allowed around the odontoid peg. At the other facet joints in the neck, side flexion, rotation, and flexion/extension occur. The greatest degree of flexion/extension occurs at C5/6. Intervertebral discs are present at all levels other than C0/1 and C1/2. The intervertebral foramina are reduced to their smallest diameter on ipsilateral side flexion, rotation, and extension—a fact of clinical significance when examining for evidence of nerve-root entrapment.

The thoracic spine is inherently stable because of its kyphosis and its rib attachments. A limited range of movements (flexion, extension, rotations, and side flexions) occur at the facet joints. Most rotation/side flexion takes place between T10 and T12 and at the thoracolumbar junction. As a result, these distal joints are vulnerable to injury. The ribs articulate with the vertebral bodies at the costovertebral joints and between T1 and T10 at the costotransverse joints; both these sets of joints are synovial. Further joints are found between the ribs and the costal cartilages (costochondral joints), between ribs 1 to 7 and the sternum (sternocostal joints), and between ribs and adjacent costal cartilages (ribs 5 to 9). The 'false' ribs 8, 9, and 10 join only with the costocartilage of the ribs above, and 'floating' ribs 11 and 12 do not have a distal articulation.

In the lumbar spine, the facet joints are orientated to resist torsional and shear strain: rotation is minimal. Flexion/extension occurs maximally at the lumbosacral junction, thereby constituting a physiological pivot between trunk and legs. Trunk flexion is a combination of pelvic rotation (around the transverse axes of the hip joints) and lumbar flexion (essentially a reversal of lumbar lordosis). The smooth simultaneous movement at these different levels constitutes the dynamic *lumbar–pelvic rhythm* (Cailliet 1981). The extensor muscles of the spine are divided into three distinct groups. The erectores spinae (sacrospinales) are the longest and most superficial group, extending from the lumbosacral spines and the iliac crest inferiorly to the ribs and thoracic transverse processes superiorly. Lying underneath the erectores spinae are a second group of muscles (semispinalis, multifidus, and rotatores) which span three segments only. The third group of muscles in the lumbar spine (only) connect the spinous processes and transverse processes of adjacent vertebrae.

Intradiscal pressure studies (Nachemson and Elfstrom 1970) have identified the increased loading of the L3 disc in different postures and during different lifting techniques: both sitting and lifting with straight legs increase intradiscal pressure considerably. Farfan (1973) emphasizes the importance of torsional overload that results in injury to the facet joints and annulus. Cailliet (1981) identifies faulty posture as a major cause of 'static' back pain, and advises strengthening exercises for the abdominals and gluteals to reduce the lumbosacral angle (Fig. 5.1). Exercise-related (kinetic) problems are due to poor training and technique, inadequate flexibility, muscle imbalance, and fatigue caused by overload. In contrast, muscle-strengthening and spinal flexibility exercises improve the dissipation of forces arising from compression loads in particular, and reduce the incidence of injury.

On bending forwards and lifting, the powerful hip extensor muscles (the gluteals and to a lesser extent the hamstrings) may allow a dead lift of over three times bodyweight. In the lumbar spine, the strain is then taken by the combination of contraction of the trunk musculature (powerful, though not as powerful as the hip extensors) and the ligamentous system. The paraspinal muscles create a compressive effect on the disc and some degree of shearing force. The ligaments comprise the spinal ligaments (supraspinous, interspinous, ligamentum flavae, posterior and

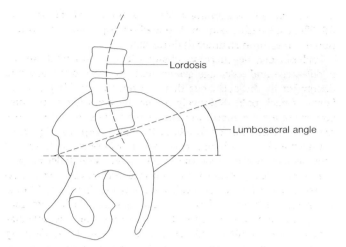

FIG. 5.1 The lumbosacral angle is made between the plane of the upper border of the sacrum and the horizontal in the standing position: it is affected by posture, and may be reduced by corrective exercises (using the abdominal and gluteal muscles).

anterior longitudinal ligaments, and facet capsules) and the lumbodorsal (or 'dorsilumbar') fascia. The abdominal muscles create extra tension in the lumbodorsal fascia, and are thus essential in the balance of external loads applied to the spine. An important function of the ligaments is to minimize the compressive and shear forces applied to the intervertebral joints.

Two important points may be emphasized. The first is the importance of a satisfactory range of extension at the hip joints. If this is absent, and fixed hip flexion develops as a result of

degenerative disease, excessive extension strain occurs at the low lumbar joints during walking and lifting. This explains the increased risk of low back problems in association with hip disorders. The second is the importance of strong abdominal musculature, which is understood by weight-lifters who often employ a tight abdominal/lumbar belt during lifting (Fig. 5.2). The abdominal muscles help increase tension within the abdominal cavity, and thus assist with transmission of lifting stress through arms, shoulders, thorax, abdomen, and pelvis. They also help to reduce shear forces posteriorly and reinforce ligamentous function as described.

With the exception of spondylolysis, which is caused almost exclusively by repetitive hyperextension, for example during back walkovers in gymnastics, the patho-anatomical changes in evidence when an athlete injures his back are the same as in the general population. In the latter group, however, inadequate musculature, particularly in the abdomen and thighs, and poor working positions are often aetiological factors. In sport, the usual causes are excessive loads applied repetitively to the spine. Inadequate or imbalanced muscle function may be seen under occasional circumstances—for example, inadequate strength in the neck muscles in adolescent rugby players or in the lumbar and abdominal muscles in the middle-aged who do not maintain regular physical conditioning. A correct technique is thus crucial when recurrent loading of any type is applied to the spine in sport. This is particularly important in weight training (as well as weight lifting), the more so as this type of training is now used in a multitude of different sports. The maintenance of the correct degree of lumbar lordosis and pelvic angle during heavy lifts requires adequate coaching. Fatigue is more of a problem in circuit training, particularly with barbells, so that the athlete may not be aware of the tendency towards hyperextension that may accompany upper body work. Faulty technique in almost all (if not all) sports may allow overload to create structural problems of any of the pathoanatomical types subsequently described.

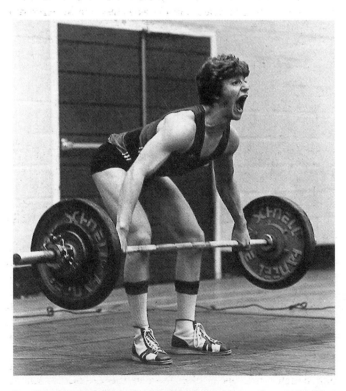

FIG. 5.2 Strong abdominal musculature is necessary for weight-lifters, who often use a tight abdominal belt (courtesy of Supersport).

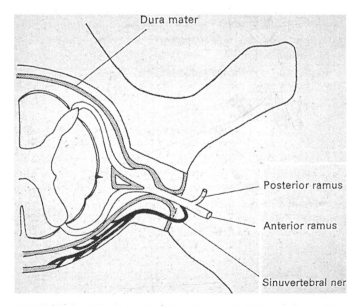

FIG. 5.3 The sinuvertebral nerve supplies the dura, the contents of the epidural space, and the posterior margin of the annulus of the disc. The articular nerves to the apophyseal joints are branches of the posterior primary rami

Pain transmission has been researched, though it continues to be debated. The articular nerves supplying the facet joints are branches of the posterior primary rami. Although the intervertebral discs were thought at one time to contain no sensory nerve endings, it is now apparent that the sinuvertebral nerves (small branches from the common spinal nerve) supply the posterior annular margins (Fig. 5.3). Accordingly, a tear of the posterior annulus is a potential source of low back pain. The sinuvertebral nerves also supply the dura and contents of the epidural space. It is probable that dural compression and irritation are responsible for the pain caused primarily by disc herniation.

A comment about 'spondylosis' is necessary: this radiological entity, present in the cervical and lumbar spines as a response to stress at the vertebral margins above and below the disc, does not cause pain, has no relationship to painful syndromes, and is not referred to again in the text.

Cervical injury

Patho-anatomy and epidemiology

In addition to fractures and fracture-dislocations, injuries to the soft tissues are naturally most common in those sports in which physical contact is part of the game. Rugby football, American football, and wrestling are three of the sports associated with a relatively high incidence of cervical spinal injury. In common with the other regions of the spine, facet strains and disc injury also occur in the absence of a history of direct trauma.

The injury that is typically found in American football and wrestling is the 'burner' or 'stinger'. This takes the form of a temporary painful loss of function in the affected arm immediately following a blow to or angulation of the neck. There are two types of causation. In one, the neck is laterally flexed away from the site of injury whilst the ipsilateral shoulder is depressed, thus stretching the brachial plexus. In the other, the neck is extended and rotated/side-flexed towards the injured side; it is likely that this mechanism irritates the nerve-root by diminishing the size of the intervertebral foramen. The feeling of electric shocks in the arm (from shoulder to fingers) is followed by numbness and partial paralysis lasting for several minutes. Complete subjective and objective recovery is often made within a few minutes, though neurological deficit occasionally persists for longer.

Neurological deficit in the arm may also result from a cervical disc prolapse, though the onset is not so acute. Radicular pain, paraesthesiae, and numbness are usually preceded by a short history of stiffness and discomfort felt in the neck. Occasionally, particularly in C7 root palsy, the pain may be felt principally in the pectoral region and axilla. Dermatomal identification is made from the distribution of paraesthesiae/numbness (confirmed by subsequent neurological examination). The most common sites of prolapse are at C5/6 and particularly C6/7. The root that emerges inferior to the vertebral body is traumatized, commonly C6 (tingling in the thumb and index finger) or C7 (tingling in index, long, and ring finger). If the C5 root is involved (due to C4/5 disc prolapse), the radicular pain is usually unaccompanied by sensory symptoms.

Segmental dysfunction in which the predominant feature is loss of movement at the facet joints is particularly common. Underlying structural pathological changes in the form of facet joint degeneration or intervertebral disc degeneration/bulging are often absent. Accordingly, MRI scanning is usually unhelpful. The osteopathic concept is one of neurophysiological (functional rather than structural) disturbance.

Undoubtedly, degenerative changes in the facet joints in the middle-aged and older age groups may give rise to stiffness and discomfort in the neck, but they are not responsible *per se* for bouts of neck pain. Relatively minor trauma, often with components of axial compression and/or torsional stress, may cause reversible segmental dysfunction. Patients complain of pain in the neck and referred pain to almost anywhere in the head and shoulders, depending upon the level of dysfunction. Referred pain from both facet syndromes and disc prolapses in the distal cervical spine to the base of the neck and the region just medial to the superomedial border of the scapula is particularly common. Tenderness may also be elicited, either in the skin and subcutaneous tissues (positive skin rolling) or within the underlying proximal scapular fixator muscles (trapezius and levator scapulae). Hyperalgesia to palpation and muscle hypertonus (the characteristic features of a 'trigger point') are particularly common. Facet joint injury also occurs in whiplash, when sudden hyperextension of the neck stresses both facet joints and connecting ligaments, and, in more severe cases the intervertebral disc and ligamentum flavum. This is most commonly seen in car accidents, when a stationary vehicle is hit from the rear, but it occurs too in field sports—particularly in 'high' tackles in rugby.

Examination

In the standing position, active movements, followed by passive movements, are performed in the six directions: flexion, extension, rotations (right and left), and side flexions (right and left). Pain and restriction of movement are noted; end-feel is noted at the extremes of passive movements. Neurological assessment in the upper limbs concentrates particularly on the examination of the motor system to detect muscle weakness due to nerve-root compression:

Shoulder shrug	C4
Shoulder abduction	C5
Shoulder external rotation	C5
Elbow flexion	C5, 6
Wrist extension	C6
Elbow extension	C7
Shoulder adduction	C7
Wrist flexion	C7
Wrist ulnar deviation	C8
Thumb abduction/extension	C8
Fingers 4/5 approximation	T1

Muscle wasting—for example, pectorals in C7 root entrapment—should be looked for.

In the presence of arm pain, a neural tension test with the patient relaxed and supine should be used. The starting position for a neural stretch of the C5 and C6 roots is depression, abduction to 90°, and extension of the ipsilateral shoulder. The forearm is supinated, the wrist is dorsiflexed, and the elbow is extended gradually from 90° of flexion. The examiner detects tension and the patient experiences neuritic symptoms. A comparison is made with the contralateral side.

The patient remains in the supine position on the examination couch, with his head cradled in the examiner's hands. Accessory passive movements known as joint-play are performed (Fig. 12.6(a), p. 220):

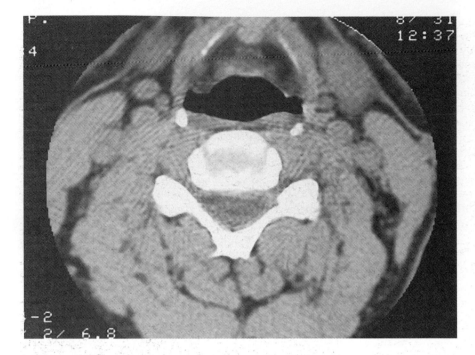

FIG. 5.4 CT scan at C4/5 revealing a disc prolapse on the left. Compression of the emerging C5 nerve-root affected the anterior deltoid, supraspinatus, and infraspinatus muscles, resulting in inability to actively abduct the arm beyond 30°.

anteroposterior glide;
lateral glide;
side bending.

These tests yield further information on the mobility at each cervical segment. Palpation of the facets for localized tenderness and muscle spasm assists in localization. Maitland's segmental vibratory techniques may also be used (Maitland 1986). Assessment of function of the neck muscles by isometric contraction may be performed at this stage, although it is unlikely to be helpful as a diagnostic procedure (as intrinsic muscle lesions are very uncommon). X-rays should be taken when there is root involvement: although of limited value, they help to exclude bony pathology, and to identify the capacity of the intervertebral foramina. Occasionally CT scans and MRI are helpful (Fig. 5.4).

Interpretation and management

The capsular pattern in the neck is limitation of all movements other than flexion. This is seen in (painless) osteoarthritis in the elderly, and ankylosing spondylitis in the young. When spondylitis is present in the neck, the lumbar spine is 'flat' on examination, and the sacroiliac joints are sclerotic on X-ray (see Fig. 6.9, p. 118).

All the soft tissue lesions subsequently described give rise to a partial articular (non-capsular) pattern, in which some movements of the neck are painful and restricted, and others are not. The only exception to this pattern occurs in the acute stage of an injury such as whiplash, burner, or torticollis caused by acute disc protrusion, when all movements may be uncomfortable and appear to be restricted. The partial articular pattern navertheless emerges before long.

The presence of persisting radicular pain in the arm, particularly when radiating below the elbow and when associated with paraesthesiae/numbness, strongly suggests *disc prolapse*. The nerve-root is affected, and the radicular pain is usually provoked by a combination of passive neck extension and ipsilateral rota-

tion. Additionally, the neural tension test may be positive. The presence of motor palsy should be sought: it has some prognostic significance. If absent, cervical traction is likely to be successful. It is not unreasonable for an experienced therapist to initiate treatment using gentle mobilization techniques to the affected segment. If the affected nerve-root is irritated rather than severely compressed, it seems probable that the accompanying oedema may be improved by passive motion (Elvey 1986). In the author's experience, traction is normally required nevertheless. If motor weakness is present, there is little prospect of improvement of symptoms by repeated distraction force, although nerve blocks may produce dramatic relief of pain. However, the patient may be reassured that spontaneous resolution is to be expected within three months: since nocturnal pain is troublesome, the patient may gain relief by sleeping with the ipsilateral hand placed behind the neck.

In *facet dysfunction*, a partial articular pattern is also found, though the restriction in mobility is not gross. Usually rotation towards the painful side is restricted. Joint-play signs are particularly useful; when combined with palpation for tenderness, they localize the level and give a guide to the type of mobilization or manipulation that is required (Fig. 12.6(b), p. 210). Mennell suggests that manipulation is merely an extension of the examining technique (Mennell 1960). Cyriax insisted on manipulation being carried out during manual traction (Cyriax and Russell 1984). Stoddard's techniques are also commended (Stoddard 1980). In general, 'mobilization' is the use of passive stretching without thrust. 'Manipulation' uses thrust at the extreme of range. A few sessions of treatment, using a technique with which the physician or therapist has become familiar, at intervals of two or three days is a reasonable regime. 'Muscle energy' techniques may also be helpful: passive stretching is facilitated by a preceding isometric contraction of the relevant muscle groups. In recovery from neck injury and for prophylaxis in those sports requiring strong neck musculature, for instance in forward play in rugby football, neck-strengthening exercises should be prescribed.

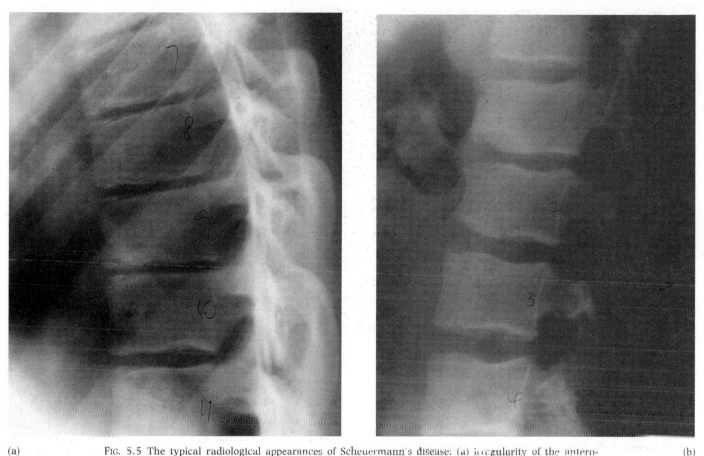

(a)

(b)

FIG. 5.5 The typical radiological appearances of Scheuermann's disease: (a) irregularity of the antero-inferior epiphyseal ring and adjacent sclerosis at D9; (b) anterior erosions at L1/2 and L2/3

Thoracic injury

Patho-anatomy and epidemiology

As a result of rotation strains, injuries occur to spinal joints, intercostal muscles, and costochondral joints. In addition, a form of osteochondritis known as Scheuermann's disease affects the distal thoracic and proximal lumbar spine in adolescents. Although the aetiology of this growth disorder is unproven, it is possible that repeated trauma is responsible for the vertebral end-plate degeneration, with subsequent propulsion of nucleus pulposus into adjacent vertebral bodies and anterior wedging (Fig. 5.5). Occurring in 14–18-year-olds, it may be a painless condition, though it often gives rise to discomfort on or after exercise. An exaggerated thoracic kyphosis is a feature. If symptomatic, exercise restriction needs to be applied for some months. At least one authority (Stoddard 1980) considers that there is an association between Scheuermann's disease and the incidence of low back pain in later life. More recently, Sward et al. (1991) have confirmed the correlation between disc degeneration and the presence of Schmorl's nodes in the thoracolumbar spine in an MRI study of elite gymnasts. Reduction in thoracic mobility and premature degenerative changes in the thoracic spine in the third and fourth decades may also restrict the capacity for certain types of exercise, such as rowing.

The exact nature of the patho-anatomical process involved in posterior thoracic 'strains' is unknown. Disc prolapses occasion-ally occur, though they are relatively uncommon. It is more likely that the facet joints or costovertebral joints are the source of problems which are clinically of two types. An acute sprain occurs as a result of rotational stress combined with either flexion or extension; pain is felt to one side of the thoracic spine, particularly in the D5–D8 range. Spontaneous resolution may be expected inside a week. A more chronic lesion presents as discomfort in a similar area, commonly with radiation unilaterally around the chest as far as the sternum, and occasionally presenting as anterior chest pain alone (thereby mimicking cardiac pain). Lesions at the thoracolumbar junction are not uncommon in the 30–45 year age-group: pain is often referred to the iliac fossa and iliac crest. Discomfort in thoracic joint lesions is felt predominantly after exercise.

Pain that is felt unilaterally around the chest and related to exercise may either be referred from the spinal joints or be a manifestation of more local pathology, such as intercostal muscle strain. The latter condition is seen typically in fast bowlers (cricket). In other sports, such as rowing and sculling, unilateral thoracic pain may be due to a stress fracture of a rib. Holden and Jackson (1985) consider that stress during weight training and serratus anterior overload are the aetiological factors. Resolution is to be expected with modification of activity. Mechanical derangement may occur at a costochondral junction in the form of a 'sprung rib'. Sudden well-localized pain is felt, and may be accompanied by clicking and swelling, which reflect repeated subluxation.

On the question of scoliosis, there may be a primary (structural) deformity in which there is a marked rotational element, or it may arise as a consequence of intense muscle spasm ('sciatic scoliosis') or a short leg. Although a mild degree of structural scoliosis of the thoracolumbar spine (such as idiopathic adolescent scoliosis) is relatively common, it has little or no relationship to sports injuries of any kind. The underlying reason for a secondary scoliosis must be found: leg-length inequality may be the cause, and may be present in the absence of back pain or sciatica. Of particular relevance is its association with overuse injury in the lower limbs.

Examination

The natural primary curvature of the thoracic spine may be exaggerated in the form of a kyphosis or, when acutely angulated, for instance when due to wedge fractures, in the form of a kyphus. Neck flexion is performed initially in the standing position: when pain is felt in the thorax, this indicates dural irritation—for example, by disc protrusion. Active posterior approximation of the scapulae by the patient tests the upper thoracic joints by traction on the dural sheath of the T1 and T2 nerve-roots. Active movements, followed by passive movements, of the thoracic spine then follow:

flexion;
extension;
rotations (right and left);
side flexions (right and left).

During flexion, a mild primary scoliosis may be detected by the presence of a 'rib hump' that is indicative of the rotational element of the deformity. A scoliosis that is present on standing, though absent on sitting, is probably due to leg-length inequality.

It is often easier to assess the passive range of rotation with the patient sitting with his fingers interlocked behind his neck. In the sitting position, isometric contraction may be tested; it is of more relevance in the thoracic region than elsewhere in the spine, as muscle injury may occur in the supporting (intercostal) muscles. Segmental (extension) pressure and skin rolling are best performed in the prone position to identify the affected level of spinal joint dysfunction. Tests for the stability of the thoracic cage include rib springing (both AP and bilateral), pain on deep inspiration, and localized tenderness or swelling (indicating the possibility of rib callus or a sprung costochondral joint).

Interpretation and management

The partial articular pattern in which two, three, or four active and passive movements hurt, though not all are restricted, denotes *thoracic joint dysfunction*. Usually at least one rotatory movement is affected. Resisted contraction is painless, and localizing signs are positive (localized segmental pressure and skin rolling). Treatment is by manipulation, which should be successful over two or three sessions (see Fig. 12.7, p. 221). Recurrent dysfunction may require management by sclerosant injections to the interspinous and (facet) capsular ligaments. The uncommon thoracic disc protrusion is characterized by pain on neck flexion and substantial restriction of forward flexion of the thoracic spine. Any suspicion of cord compression (symptoms or signs of an upper motor neuron lesion in the legs) should stimulate further investigation for the presence of disc prolapse or spinal tumour.

Although an *intercostal muscle strain* will also give rise to discomfort on certain thoracic movements (by stretching the

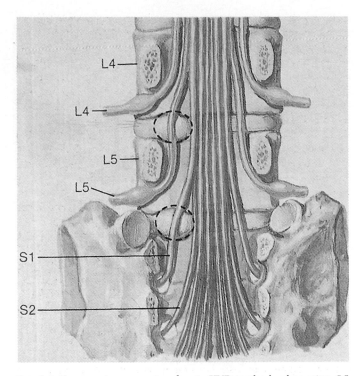

FIG. 5.6 Nerve-root compression due to HNP in the lumbar spine. L5 root entrapment results from L4/5 disc prolapse. S1 root entrapment results from L5/S1 disc prolapse.

affected muscles), there is likely, in addition, to be pain on coughing and deep breathing, and localized tenderness. Although it is difficult to resist the temptation to prescribe localized treatment, the muscle tear will nevertheless take two to three weeks to heal. The important aspect of management is the initial restriction of rotational stress, followed during rehabilitation by graded passive rotational stretching exercises in order to prevent recurrence.

A *sprung rib*, indicating at least a sprain, and more probably instability of the affected costochondral joint, may be a difficult problem to resolve. In the presence of swelling and clicking, intra-articular steroid injections may be tried: occasionally surgical excision is required.

Lumbar and sacroiliac injury

Patho-anatomy and epidemiology

Acute injury

An acute bout of pain as a consequence of a strain at a motion segment (the intervertebral disc and its accompanying facet joints) often occurs in the presence of pre-existing patho-anatomical changes in both the anterior and posterior columns. Thus degenerative changes in the disc and ligamentous laxity in the facetal supporting structures are probably coexistent in the majority of cases. However, on a clinical basis, specific syndromes are identifiable, which may be localized to the individual parts of a motion segment and demand a variety of therapeutic approaches.

As a result of a crack in the annulus of the disc, prolapse of nuclear material may take place (herniation of nucleus pulposus (HNP)). Initially, mild lumbar discomfort may be experienced, worsening overnight to give rise to the typical appearance of lumbago the following morning: low lumbar pain and stiffness accompanied by restricted flexion, and possibly by a 'pelvic tilt'. Such a protrusion is *central*—that is, posterior—and gives rise to severe low back pain (LBP), often referred to the thighs. Commonly the protrusion moves *posterolaterally*, and compression of the nerve-root ensues (Fig. 5.6). Sometimes HNP may be primarily posterolateral, in which case sciatica is not preceded by LBP. Paraesthesiae and numbness may be experienced in the dermatomal pattern: the most commonly involved of the dermatomes are L5 and S1, giving rise to posterolateral and posteriorly distributed symptoms, respectively. L4 root symptoms are felt anterolaterally in the leg, and account for approximately 5–10 per cent of cases. Disc prolapse is not confined to middle age: patients in their twenties and thirties are commonly affected. Porter and colleagues (1978) have stressed the relationship between symptomatic disc disease and the diameter of the spinal canal: patients with narrow canals are at considerable risk.

The nature of the benign 'mechanical' lesion that gives rise to acute LBP, often felt unilaterally without sciatic referral and with less pronounced articular signs, is subject to much debate. Although devotees of the Cyriax approach consider that a common cause would be a displaced tag of annular fibrocartilage (Cyriax 1982), the author's opinion is that *facet dysfunction* is a more plausible concept. Disturbed function at a motion segment is also associated with inefficient muscular stabilization. The characteristic features of somatic dysfunction are localized tenderness and skin changes, localized muscle hypertonus, and loss of intervertebral movement. The relevance of structural (patho-anatomical) changes in an acute bout of back pain when there no evidence of significant disc prolapse is conjectural. Stress (provocation) tests for the facet joints are usually painful. Rotational stress in flexion is an important aetiological factor. Repetitive hyperextension may also be incriminated. Thus backache in oarsmen has been considered to be facetal in origin (Stallard 1980). Cricket bowling may cause a number of different types of back injury, of which facet dysfunction is common. A technically correct golf swing is less likely to be associated with facet dysfunction unless overload is extreme: youngsters, in attempting to achieve extra distance on their drives, may sustain back strain by exaggerating the arched and rotated position on the backswing or follow-through.

Pain felt over the sacroiliac joint is a common symptom, and commonly ascribed (wrongly) to a lesion at this joint. It is often *referred* from a lumbar segment. However, despite the fact that normal sacroiliac joint mobility is apparently minimal (a few millimetres only on clinical measurement, by Colachis *et al.* 1963, of the inter-PSIS distance in different postures such as sitting and lying), mechanical problems do arise. Hypermobility is the underlying cause of *sacroiliac dysfunction*: pain may radiate from the sacroiliac region into the groin and posteriorly down the thigh as far as the heel.

A stress fracture of the pars interarticularis (*spondylolysis*) (Fig. 5.7) has a relatively more subacute onset. Although it was thought at one time to be present as a congenital abnormality, studies have shown that the lytic defect develops principally during childhood and adolescence (Fredrikson *et al.* 1984). The overall incidence of spondylolysis in the population is of the order of 2–6 per cent, becoming rather higher in selected groups such as female gymnasts (11 per cent in a group of average age 14 years studied by Jackson *et al.* 1976, 1981). Little (or no) backache may have been recalled on retrospective enquiry amongst such groups. Spondylolysis that develops in the teenager may give rise to exercise-dependent backache, either unilateral or

(a)

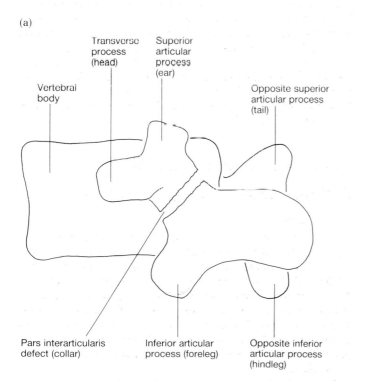

(b)

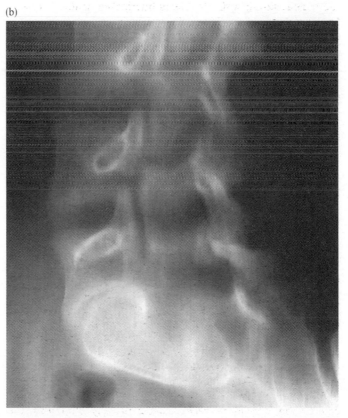

Fig. 5.7 (a) A stress fracture in the lumbar spine (spondylolysis) affects the isthmus (pars interarticularis) of the neural arch at L5, L4, or occasionally L3. A scottie dog with a collar is seen on the oblique X-ray. (b) A tomogram reveals a spondylolysis at L4

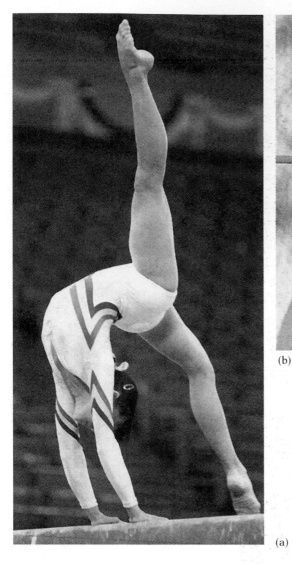

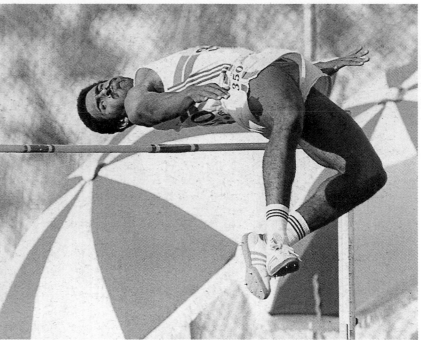

(b)

FIG. 5.8 Spondylolysis is more common in those sports in which hyper-extension of the lumbar spine is repetitive, for example (a) back walkovers in gymnastics and (b) Fosbury flop in high jumping.

(a)

bilateral. It is particularly common in children who indulge in repetitive hyperextension and rotation, as in gymnastics, circuit training, field athletics, and cricket bowling (Fig. 5.8; see also Fig. 11.5(a), p. 198). Apprentice soccer players are also at risk if they are trained too vigorously. Although the author has seen an acute spondylolysis (confirmed by bone scan) in a 26-year-old, it is most uncommon after the late teens (Elliott *et al.* 1988). The identical biomechanical stresses may give rise to facet strain in an older age group.

Chronic or relapsing injury

As degenerative changes progressively take place in the facet joints and are associated with disc degeneration and narrowing, the likelihood of *lumbar instability* increases. Loss of disc height results in 'offsetting' of the superior and inferior articular processes, accompanied by inadequate capsular and ligamentous support in the posterior columns (Kirkaldy-Willis *et al.* 1978). Frequent bouts of lumbar pain, with apparently normal lumbar function in the intervening periods, are experienced.

If 'offsetting' and degenerative hypertrophy of the facet joints worsen, the intervertebral foramina are narrowed, and sciatica due to *lateral canal stenosis* may ensue. Although the age group (55 years and over) is at the upper range for indulgence in

vigorous sporting activity, nevertheless it is not uncommon to see patients whose symptoms arise during recreational exercise such as badminton or sailing.

Chronic ligamentous insufficiency may occur in the young athlete, when it is usually associated with hypermobility. Assessment may be made by the use of a scoring system that refers to mobility of the trunk, elbows, little fingers, thumbs, and knees (Beighton *et al.* 1973). With respect to forward flexion of the trunk, hypermobility may be primary or secondary; in the latter case, ligamentous stretching results from specific exercises required to promote flexibility in activities such as ballet and gymnastics. In either event, low backache may become increasingly troublesome, though usually it is not felt during exercise. Prolonged immobility—for example, sitting or standing for some time—is painful. Therefore, ligamentous insufficiency is often referred to as the 'cocktail party' or 'theatre-goer's' syndrome.

Ligamentous insufficiency may also be associated with progressive degenerative changes in the posterior columns. Sports such as squash, which necessitate considerable twisting and turning, may cause premature degenerative changes in the facet joints at a relatively early age—for example, in the fourth decade. Peri-articular ossification around the L4/5 or L5/S1 facet joints may develop as a reaction to stress (Fig. 5.9), and has been noted by

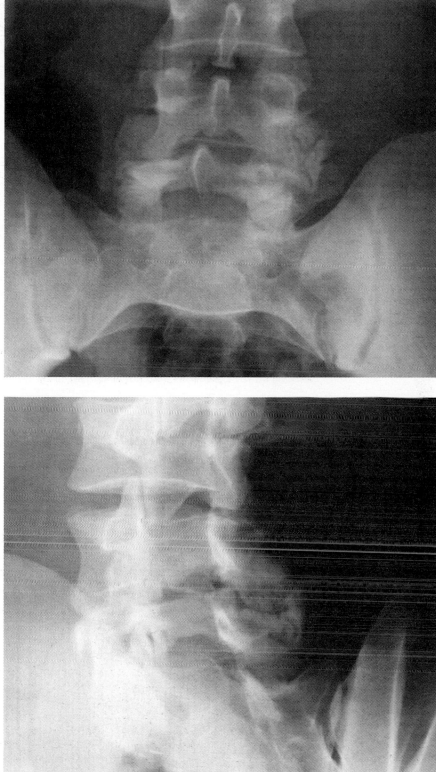

(a)

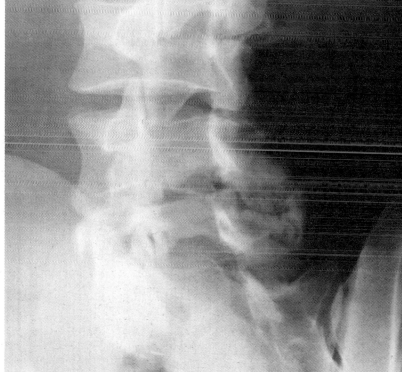

(b)

Fig. 5.9 Periarticular ossification (around the L5 posterior apophyseal joints) in this professional soccer player is a reaction to repetitive rotational stress: (a) PA X-rays, (b) oblique X-rays.

the author in relatively young sportsmen such as professional footballers. Symptoms from nerve-root entrapment as well as exercise-related LBP may result. At a later age, frank *arthrosis* of the facet joints may give rise to stiffness and discomfort, which are particularly noticeable after immobility such as prolonged sitting—the more so when provoked by injudicious exertions on

the squash court or in the garden. The 45–60-year-old is principally affected; such degenerative change is a direct consequence of the commitment to vigorous exercise over the previous decades.

Morning stiffness in the younger age group raises the possibility of *sacroiliitis* associated with one of the spondyloarthritides, such

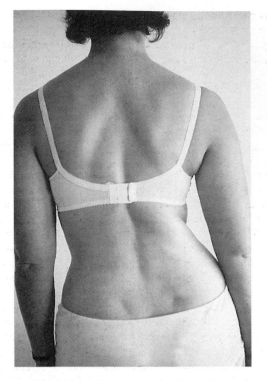

FIG. 5.10 A marked pelvic tilt is associated with a sciatic scoliosis due to a lumbar HNP.

as ankylosing spondylitis. Low backache and alternating sciatic ache, bearing little relationship to posture or exercise, are the main features. It is not unusual for the presentation to be as a sports injury, as the patient often assumes that symptoms are due to physical strain.

Although backache in the older age group may be due to more serious pathology, patients do not usually present with exercise-related pain: indeed the feature of chronic infective and malignant conditions is one of nagging persistent pain that is unrelated to posture or exercise.

Examination

Gait and posture. A patient walks, sits, and stands awkwardly when in severe pain from an acute lumbago or sciatica.

Standing. Pelvic tilt or sciatic scoliosis may be observed (Fig. 5.10). Neck flexion assesses dural irritation. Active forward flexion, extension, and lateral flexions are attempted. Range, pain, and abnormal rhythms are observed. Since the examiner may not have a record of the normal range of motion, particularly flexion, the degree of movement may be recorded with a note of whether the patient feels this is normal for him/her. Alternatively, the Schober test may be used: the distance (identified by a tape measure) between skin markers over the L1 and S1 spinous processes is recorded in the upright position and in the fully flexed position. Deviation on forward flexion is typical of an L4/5 protrusion. An arc of pain or 'hitch' on recoil

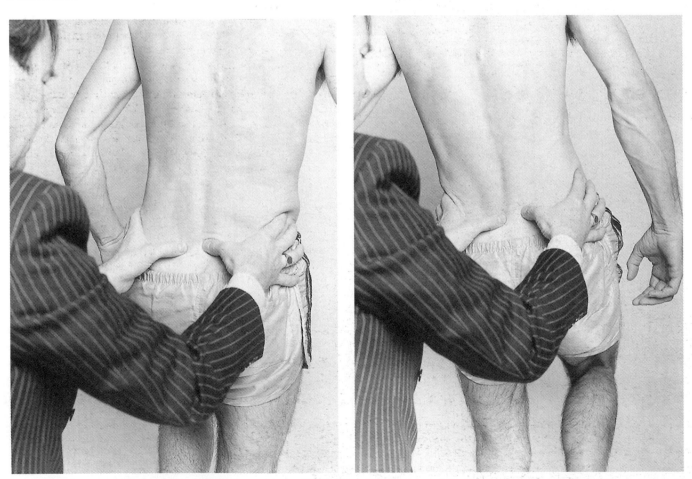

FIG. 5.11 Unilateral sacroiliac mobility may be assessed by noting the inferior movement of the PSIS (posterior superior iliac spine) when the patient flexes his ipsilateral hip in the standing position: normal (left); abnormal (right).

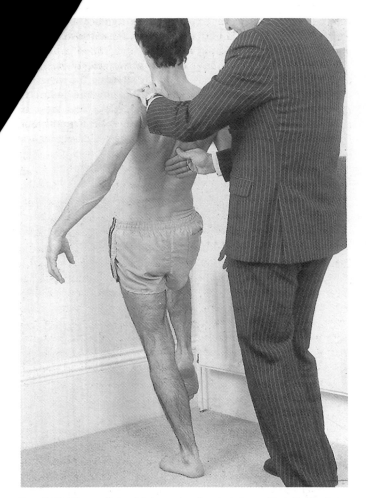

FIG. 5.12 The unilateral hyperextension test is positive (indicating a possible spondylolysis) if pain is reproduced when the patient flexes his ipsilateral hip and extends his lumbar spine.

from flexion indicates segmental instability. The lower lumbar spine may be palpated for the existence of a ledge indicating spondylolisthesis. The sacroiliac mobility test is performed by asking the patient to stand on one leg and flex the opposite hip. Inferior movement of the posterior superior iliac spine (PSIS) on the side of the flexed hip is the normal response. If the sacroiliac joint is dysfunctional, the PSIS does not descend (Fig. 5.11).

The one-legged hyperextension test may be performed if there is a suspicion of recent spondylolysis (Fig. 5.12). While standing on one leg, the spine is extended: the test is positive if pain is felt on the weightbearing side. Extension may be reinforced by rotation (as in the Fitch catch test in which the raised heel is touched by the opposite hand).

Isometric paraspinal muscle contraction may be tested (by resisting lateral flexion) and is found, even with intense muscle spasm, to be painless—primary muscle tears are most unusual. An exception is a fracture of a lumbar transverse process which, as a consequence of its muscle attachments, behaves as a muscle.

Assessment of calf power (S1/2) is made by asking the patient to stand on tip-toe on each leg in turn.

Sitting. Neural tension may be estimated by the 'slump' test: with the patient seated and the trunk flexed, the neck is gently flexed by the examiner (thereby increasing dural tension). In the presence of dural tension and irritation—for example, secondary to disc prolapse—lumbar pain is reproduced. If sciatica is predominant, the test may be modified (after Troup 1986) by extending the knee of the affected leg (Fig. 5.13). Sciatic pain is then reproduced.

Supine. The passive range of hip movements is determined. Straight leg raising (SLR) is performed for each leg individually and then together, as the lumbosacral (LS) stress test.

Experience of the normal end-feel of unilateral SLR should be gained. The usefulness of the SLR occasionally has been questioned, because there are determinants other than root compression responsible for the discomfort felt towards the end of range—for example, sacroiliac ligament strain and hamstring tightness. However, unilateral SLR does remain a most useful test, particularly when comparison with the normal side is made, and may be performed without the need for refinement.

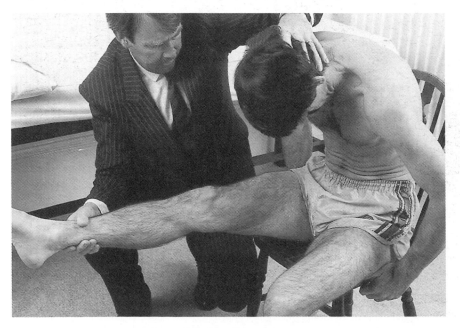

FIG. 5.13 The position of the examiner and patient on performing the slump test.

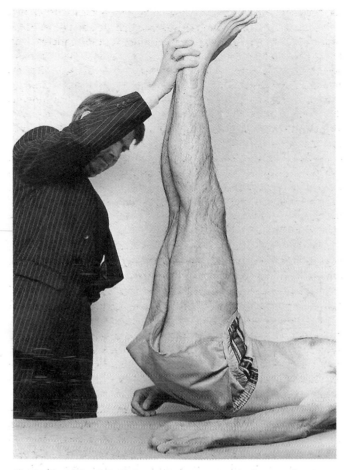

Fig. 5.14 The lumbosacral stress test is positive (indicating the presence of a lesion in either the sacroiliac or lumbosacral joints) if pain is reproduced on passive bilateral SLR.

such as the bowstring or Lasègue t
restriction is usually due to stretc'
ondary to disc herniation.

The lumbosacral (LS) stress
raising both legs simultaneously, there
and lumbosacral facet joints (Fig. 5.14).
range are indicators of dysfunction. Further
applied to the facet joints by performing passive flexion
tion/lateral flexion from a baseline position of bilateral hip
knee flexion (Fig. 5.15). Sacroiliac stress may be applied unilaterally by passive axial compression of the adducted and flexed
hip. Additional sacroiliac stress and mobility tests are described
by Grieve (1976) and Lewit (1985).

While in the supine position, neurological examination is
conducted by assessment of motor function by isometric
contraction:

Hip flexors	L2/3
Extensor hallucis longus (EHL)	L4/5
Tibialis anterior	L4
Peronei	L5

Additionally, the knee jerk (L3/4) is assessed, and the Babinski
response determined.

Prone. Once more, hip movements may be examined and
passive rotations recorded with the hip extended. The femoral
stretch test (FST) is painful with L3/4 root compression (or in a
lesion of the quadriceps muscle). Vertebral compression (performed by a downward thrust on each spinous process when
grasped between thumb and forefinger) is painful when there is
facetal dysfunction, acute or chronic. Paravertebral compression
('positive' when pain is reproduced) is helpful in localizing the
segment involved. Tenderness may be palpated over the posterior sacroiliac ligaments in chronic sacroiliac ligamentous
insufficiency. Muscle hyperalgesia—associated with muscle
hypertonus—is a relatively common but relatively poorly discriminating feature in lesions of the lower back. It is often

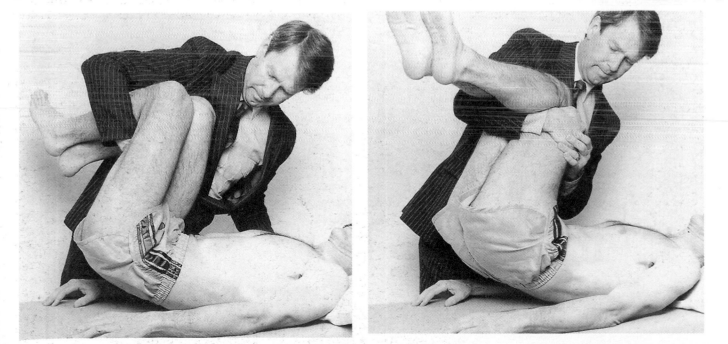

(a)   Fig. 5.15 The lumbar apophyseal joints may be stressed by passive flexion and rotation of the spine as demonstrated: (b)
(a) to the right; (b) to the left.

present in lumbar disc herniation, facet dysfunction, and sacroiliac dysfunction. Further neurological assessment is made by isometric contraction:

Glutei	S1
Hamstrings	S1
Quadriceps	L3/4
Ankle jerk	S1/2

Interpretation and management

Mechanical dysfunction gives rise to the partial (non-capsular) articular pattern, in which some movements are painful and may be restricted, whereas others are not. HNP is characterized by painful restriction of forward flexion of the lumbar spine and positive dural stretch tests (restricted SLR at the L4/5 and L5/S1 levels, restricted FST at L3/4). In the presence of a substantial protrusion at either of the two lowest intervertebral levels, particularly L4/5, both ipsilateral and contralateral SLR may be restricted, and deviation is noted on attempted trunk flexion. A pelvic tilt or sciatic scoliosis may be observed. Side flexion towards the painful side is usually restricted, and neurological signs, in a strict dermatomal distribution, are commonly found when there is sciatic root compression. Prolapse at the L3/4 level often gives rise to a reversed pattern—that is, to limitation of extension (possibly a fixed flexion posture) and less limitation of flexion. Management of a prolapsed disc is by sustained lumbar traction which is given daily as an outpatient procedure for two weeks (Fig. 5.16). In the presence of neurological signs, caudal epidural injections of 25–50 ml of 0.5 per cent procaine HCl are indicated; the addition of steroid—for example, triamcinolone hexacetonide 20 mg—is logical for reduction of the inflammatory reaction at the disc–dura interface. A positive response, manifested by improvement of both symptoms and signs, is to be expected in over 80 per cent of cases.

Investigation by X-ray conventionally is performed, although nothing is gained other than exclusion of bony pathology. If conservative management fails to control the symptoms, or improve the signs of sciatic root compression, further investigation by CT scan or particularly by MRI (Fig 10.25, p. 190) is necessary. Referral to an orthopaedic surgeon or neurosurgeon

for consideration of discectomy is indicated in the presence of a substantial HNP and unremitting sciatica. It should be noted that discectomy is an inappropriate procedure for patients with back-dominant pain (that is, in which the back pain is more severe than the sciatica). The experience of the surgeon dictates whether micro-discectomy (with the aid of an operating microscope), percutaneous micro-discectomy, or laser percutaneous discectomy will be the treatment of choice. The presence of disc sequestration or extrusion should not *per se* be considered to be an indication for surgical excision as, despite the presence of neurological signs, disc resorption may occur relatively quickly. Chemonucleolysis is an alternative approach: if suitable diagnostic criteria are satisfied (more leg pain than back pain, restricted SLR, neurological deficit, and positive imaging), a success rate of over 70 per cent is achieved, and the long-term results are as good as or better than surgery.

Lumbar segmental dysfunction is characterized by discomfort on flexion, extension, and lateral flexion away from the painful side. SLR is of full range. The LS and facet stress tests are painful. Segmental pressure is painful. The treatment of choice is vertebral manipulation (see Fig. 12.7, p. 221), which may be combined with ultrasound to the affected facet joint. If symptoms persist, infiltration of steroid and local anaesthetic along the posterior aspect of the relevant facet joints (usually L4/5 or L5/S1) is often very effective. Intra-articular facet injection under fluoroscopic screening may be performed, though it is unnecessary, in the author's experience, for therapeutic response.

In *sacroiliac dysfunction*, the articular signs on the conventional trunk mobility tests in the standing position are often unremarkable. However, the sacroiliac mobility test reveals an abnormal rhythm, and internal rotation of the hip is often uncomfortable and slightly limited (see p. 122 for further tests). Normal sacroiliac joint mobility is restored by manipulation (see Fig. 12.8, p. 221). Reassessment at the end of a week is advisable, and further manipulative procedures should be undertaken, if necessary, at weekly intervals until resolution of dysfunction is established. Recurrent dysfunction may be treated by sclerosant injections (see *Chronic ligamentous insufficiency*).

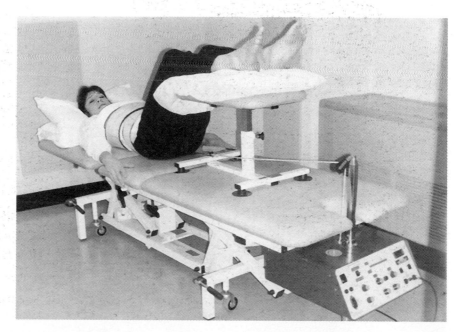

Fig. 5.16 Daily lumbar traction of 80–140 lb for 20 minutes is an effective treatment for lumbar disc prolapse without neurological signs.

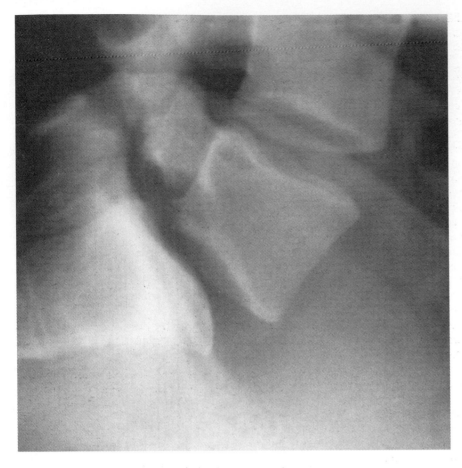

Fig. 5.17 A spondylolysis at L5 is associated with a grade I spondylolisthesis in this professional cricketer.

Minor articular signs are detected in a recent *spondylolysis*; extension is uncomfortable, and rotations variably so. Increased discomfort is felt on the one-legged hyperextension test and on the Fitch catch test. X-rays, including obliques, are necessary if there is suspicion of spondylolysis. The mere presence of a lytic defect on X-ray, however, does not indicate the vintage of the lesion: a bone scan is required to confirm a recent stress fracture. (Read (1994) has advised the use of single photon emission computed tomography (SPECT) scanning to detect very early cases.) In the presence of a positive scan, rest from sport is compulsory in any attempt to achieve satisfactory healing. Although the lysis may not necessarily be expected to heal by bony union, a sound fibrous union is required.

Three to six months' rest may be necessary, and twice that length of time is not unusual. If progress, as assessed by lessening discomfort on movement, is not in evidence after six months, it is advisable to seek an orthopaedic surgical opinion from a spinal specialist. Surgical stabilization may be required. Occasionally, spondylolisthesis develops, and requires specialist advice. Listhesis is an *early* complication after lysis, and is unlikely to develop at a later stage (Fig. 5.17). A slip of 25 per cent is considered acceptable; a 50 per cent slip increases the likelihood of incapacitating symptoms and a cosmetically undesirable posture. Surgical fusion is normally required for this degree of slip in a child.

Biomechanical assessment of sport technique may be helpful in rehabilitation (and indeed in prophylaxis). Hardcastle *et al.* (1992) analysed the delivery techniques of a group of Western Australian fast bowlers and concluded that a 'mixed' action (combining features of both side-on and front-on actions) gave rise to considerable spinal rotation and a relatively high incidence of spondylolysis.

Lumbar instability (or 'segmental instability') is characterized by recurrent bouts of acute low back pain, and is a difficult problem to influence. More often than not, the bouts appear to be provoked by relatively trivial incidents, unconnected with sport, such as reaching forward. Paradoxically, the patient comments that he is often able to indulge his back in vigorous pursuits without necessarily incurring any derangement. Acute bouts tend to last for several days, and are often helped by manipulation. The signs are usually of facet dysfunction (discomfort on flexion and/or extension, normal SLR, and pain on LS and facet stress tests), though more dominant discogenic signs may predominate (pelvic tilt, restricted flexion, and restricted SLR). X-ray is usually unhelpful, and examination between attacks is normal.

The major management problem relates to the recurrent nature of the condition. Prior to the establishment of an appropriate rehabilitative policy for an individual patient, the following biomechanical fact-file should be taken into account.

1. There is good evidence that the likelihood of recurrence is lessened by improved physical fitness (Nachemson 1984). This applies to those patients who indulge in recreational sport only, such as golf, rather than those who keep fit by more energetic means.

2. Poor muscle control and recruitment, particularly of the transversus abdominis and multifidus (the local segmental stabilisers), is associated with low back pain. Additional factors

include imbalance between segmental and global (spinal) stabilizers, and tightness of those muscles responsible for spinal motion (Mottram and Comerford 1998). An appropriate strengthening regime should be prescribed (see p. 189).

3. Although the patient may improve his dynamic stabilizers, and therefore the dorsilumbar fascial tone, by such a regime of exercises, he can do little about the capsular, lumbosacral, and sacroiliac ligaments. A course of sclerosant injections (25 per cent dextrose and 2 per cent phenol) to these ligaments should be considered. Referral to an orthopaedic physician or sports injury specialist is indicated for treatment by sclerotherapy.

In the mature athlete who is unwilling to 'hang up his boots' at an appropriate time, degenerative changes (*arthrosis*) in the facet joints are a source of low back and posterior thigh pain. The signs that accompany the typical post-exercise discomfort and stiffness are restriction of all lumbar movements (the capsular pattern), discomfort on LS and facet stress, and positive segmental pressure. Although localized steroid injections to the posterior capsular ligaments of the facet joints (or even intra-articularly under X-ray screening) give temporary relief, and sclerosant injections more prolonged relief, there is likely to be recurrence unless appropriate reduction in biomechanical stress is achieved. Despite this perfectly valid and rational approach, a lack of compliance with such guidance and the search for a 'cure' by exercise fanatics is not unusual. Participation in squash and (to a lesser extent) other racket sports is ill-advised. Swimming and cycling are usually tolerated and may therefore be prescribed, without adverse effect. Degenerative disease in the hip is a common concomitant to low back stress, and should always be considered during examination.

Chronic ligamentous insufficiency is characterized by discomfort on prolonged immobility and an absence of articular signs. Discomfort may be elicited on the sacroiliac stress test if the sacroiliac ligaments are significantly involved. Tenderness overlying the sacroiliac joints may be detected; otherwise there is little to find clinically, and all investigations are negative. Despite the absence of positive signs on examination, discomfort may be substantial. Sclerosant injections to the lumbosacral and sacroiliac ligaments are the treatment of choice, and may be repeated every few years if necessary. Ongley *et al.* (1987) have recorded improvement in chronic low back pain using the technique of sclerosant ('proliferant') injections preceded by steroid injection to the gluteus medius origin.

There remains one further condition—*unexplained sciatica* (with or without backache)—that appears to be related to exercise in the young adult. This is often associated with middle-distance or long-distance running. However, there are few, if any, signs on examination. In the older age groups, central or lateral spinal stenosis should be considered, and the spinal diameter assessed by X-ray or CT scan. This does not appear to be the cause of sciatica in the younger age group: although conjectural, the presence of dural irritation secondary to facet joint stress or previous disc herniation may be postulated. An empirical therapeutic approach by the use of epidural injections may be employed, and is often found to be successful.

Sacroiliitis gives rise to the characteristic examination findings of negative lumbar function tests (although the spine subsequently becomes progressively more stiff as spondylitis develops) and pain on sacroiliac stress tests. X-rays reveal the typical features of sclerosis of the joint margins (see Fig. 6.9, p. 108). A positive HLA B27 antigen test adds further weight to the diagnosis. Sacroiliitis is considered further in Chapter 6.

Summary of examination procedures

Cervical spine

Standing

1. Observation
   - torticollis
   - muscle wasting (in pectoral girdle)
2. Active movements
   - flexion
   - extension
   - rotation
   - side flexions
3. Passive movements
   - flexion
   - extension
   - rotations
   - side flexions
4. Resisted muscle contractions (neck)
5. Neurological—motor function in upper limbs.
6. Neural tension test
7. Trigger points—particularly proximal scapular fixators

Supine

1. Joint-play
   - A–P glide
   - lateral glide
   - side bending
2. Palpation
   - facet joints, overlying muscle tension
   - interspinous ligaments

Thoracic spine

Standing

1. Observation
   - kyphosis/kyphus
   - scoliosis
2. Neck flexion (dural stretch)
3. Active movements
   - flexion
   - extension
   - rotations
   - side flexions
4. Deep inspiration/rib cage compression

Sitting

1. Passive movements
   - rotations
   - side flexions
2. Resisted muscle contraction—rotations
3. Palpation—rib cage/sternum

Prone

1. Palpation—interspinous ligaments
2. Segmental compression
3. Skin rolling

Lumbar spine and sacroiliac joints

Standing

1. Observation
   - posture/lordosis
   - flexion deformity
   - pelvic tilt
   - gait
2. Neck flexion (dural stretch)
3. Active movements
   - flexion (hitch, deviation)
   - extension
   - side flexions

- sacroiliac mobility
- unilateral hyperextension/Fitch catch

4. Resisted muscle contraction (lumbar)
5. Calf strength
6. Palpation—ledge

Sitting

1. Slump test
2. Sacroiliac stress/mobility

Supine

1. Hip examination
2. Sacroiliac stress

3. SLR
4. Bilateral SLR (LS stress)
5. Facet stress
6. Neurology
- muscle function
- knee jerk
- Babinski

Prone

1. FST
2. Neurology
- muscle function
- ankle jerk
3. Palpation
- segmental compression
- tenderness (interspinous ligaments, facet joints)
- trigger points (glutei)

Injuries to the spinal cord

F. R. I. MIDDLETON

Introduction

This subchapter deals primarily with injury to the spinal cord. This leash of central nervous system tissue, which runs from the brain stem in the region of the foramen magnum of the skull to just above the upper border of the second lumbar vertebra, comprises mainly pathways for nervous impulses, but also a considerable number of neurons with an uncertain amount of intrinsic processing activity. Occasionally damage to the well-protected cord occurs without evident damage to the supporting structures, but in most instances the forces involved are so great that major injuries ensue, often combining instability of the spine with other injuries to internal organs or to the limbs. Brain injury may also occur, and in any unconscious patient following injury it must be assumed that cord injury exists in addition to brain injury, and appropriate precautions must be taken. It can be appreciated that the cord is a direct continuation from the brain, and that, even in the absence of overt brain injury, an insult to the cord sufficient to disrupt its function is likely to have some effect on the brain. These effects have been measured and documented using formalized psychometric testing (Wilmot et al. 1985) and have some importance in terms of further management, particularly during the rehabilitation stage for spinal cord injury.

Spinal cord injury is one of the greatest disasters that can befall the human organism; interruption of control mechanisms to muscle groups and other essential organs results in devastating loss of function and disability. Even worse, the loss of functions of sensation and feedback from these muscles and other organs creates even greater problems in terms of maintaining the organism as a whole.

Incidence

In the UK some ten to fifteen new cases of spinal injury per million of population occur each year, that is about 800–1000 new cases annually. Despite the introduction of seat belts, the alteration of rules, the introduction of protective head-gear in sport, and improvements in the health and safety code at work, this incidence has not altered significantly over the past twenty years (Smith 1999). However, there now appears to be a greater percentage of cervical injuries (lesions involving nerve-roots T1 and above which cause tetraplegia) compared with paraplegia, and more incomplete lesions (where some residual motor or sensory function remains below the level of injury) compared with complete lesions (Bette et al. 1995). Most injuries occur at the sites of maximal potential movement in the spine—lower cervical and thoracolumbar regions. Road traffic accidents and sporting injuries (rugby, gymnastics, trampoline, diving) tend to produce cervical injuries, whereas falls and jumping from heights more commonly cause thoracolumbar lesions.

There is an increasing awareness of disabled people in wheel-chairs in our communities owing to the increasing prevalence of the condition (now some 45 000 persons across the UK). This increase in awareness is due in some part to the increasing acceptability of people with disabilities in the community and to greater access to public buildings for those who are mobility-impaired, but is due primarily to a dramatic increase in life expectancy over the past forty years. When Sir Ludwig Guttmann began his work at the Stoke Mandeville Hospital in the early 1940s, cervical cord injury resulted in virtually 100 per cent mortality within a couple of months. Patients with lower cord injuries resulting in paraplegia had a life expectancy of approximately two years (death resulting in that time from complications affecting the kidneys, bowel, or skin). A major increase in life expectancy resulted from Sir Ludwig's work devising management programmes to maintain activity (Guttmann 1954) and to minimize the development of secondary complications. Nowadays, paraplegics have a life expectancy of only some 5–8 years less than that of someone of the same age and sex, and tetraplegics some 8–15 years less (DeVivo and Stover 1995). When one considers that between a third and a half of all spinal cord injuries involve young people in the age group 16–25, it is not surprising that the prevalence is increasing. There is also about a four to one male to female ratio, presumably owing to the nature of the usual underlying causes of spinal cord injury.

Aetiology of spinal injury relating to sport

Statistical analysis over the last fifteen years in the UK has revealed that some 55 per cent of all spinal cord injuries result from road traffic accidents, either involving the occupants of vehicles or pedestrians. The introduction of seat belts has made little impact on the overall numbers occurring, though this may be due to more survivors with spinal cord injury amongst those who would previously have been killed by their head injury. Great controversy still rages about the potential benefits of increasing the range of speed limits, and also about alterations in the design and manufacture of motor vehicles.

Falls from heights or down stairs are the second most common category of injuries. Deliberate jumps have become a larger group, increasing from seven per cent of admissions to the Spinal Injuries Unit (SIU) at the Royal National Orthopaedic Hospital Trust (RNOHT) in 1989, to 12 per cent in 1996, presumably an effect of more people with major psychiatric disorders living in the community. Falling injuries are approximately equally distributed between home and place of work, and again health and safety regulations do not appear to have made any significant impact on reducing in the numbers.

Sport regularly comprises about 20 per cent of spinal cord injuries. Diving into shallow water, both into swimming pools and into the sea, is the most common cause. Equestrian sports produce a large number of injuries considering the overall numbers taking part.

The increasing interest and participation in gymnastics and trampolining (Torg and Das 1985) has been paralleled by an increase in the numbers of serious injuries sustained in those sports. Rugby football continues to produce a few dramatic injuries each year (Silver and Gill 1988). It would appear that changes in the laws of the game have led to a decrease in cord injuries over the past five years. However, injuries continue to be caused by scrums collapsing, scrum 'collisions', or the practice of 'popping' (trying to drive the opposing front row upwards). Injuries also occur by axial loading, when players' heads are driven into the ground during mauls or rucks, in 'spearing' in rugby and American football, and in multiple, unskilled, or illegal tackling (such as stiff-arm neck or head level tackling in rugby union and rugby league). The small number of tragedies each year remains an unacceptable hazard, and more needs to be done by rugby authorities (Burry and Calcinai 1988; Armour *et al.* 1997). There has been increasing awareness among the organizing bodies of many sports and among schools and young people's organizations that proper rules and regulations, attention to equipment and environment, and appropriate supervision are essential if this small, but enormously important cause of injury is to be reduced. Recent trends are encouraging: analysis of 250 consecutive admissions to the SIUnit, RNOHT Stanmore between 1983 and 1988 reveals a smaller percentage (11 per cent) resulting from sport (Table 5.1). On reviewing spinal injury in rugby in the southern hemisphere in 1998, Yeo identified an apparent trend towards reduction in incidence of neurological deficits from serious cervical spinal cord injury in both New Zealand and New South Wales (Rotem *et al.* 1998) in

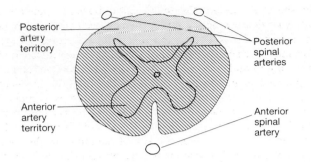

FIG. 5.18 Blood supply to the spinal cord. The anterior spinal artery is particularly vulnerable in the lower cervical and lower thoracic regions.

recent years, but no reduction in South Africa (Scher 1998). The inculcation of a responsible attitude to taking part in sporting activities will increase the pleasure resulting from the sport and will certainly help to diminish injuries.

Pathology/pathophysiology

Accurate pathophysiology of the spinal cord injury remains a poorly investigated and understood subject. Detailed definition of the anatomy of injury has become more sophisticated with the development of MRI. Measurement of cord function remains difficult and infrequently carried out. Few management decisions are made on the basis of electrophysiological testing in the acute stage. Much of what we know of spinal cord pathology results from the work of Griffiths and Kakulas (Kakulas 1988) in Perth, Australia, during the 1960s and 1970s. It is known that in injuries in which the individual survives, it is rare for the cord to be transected or cut across. The majority of injuries to the cord result from crushing of nervous tissue by surrounding bones and ligaments.

This pressure, which may be momentary or prolonged, may also cause interference with the blood supply, and it is this feature which is thought to lead to further secondary pathology (Fig 5.18). It is convenient to divide the pathology into *primary*, or that resulting directly from the force of the injury, and *secondary*, or that due to those processes which are the result of subsequent biochemical and vascular changes.

TABLE 5.1. Aetiology of spinal cord injury: cause of injury in 250 consecutive admissions to the Spinal Injuries Unit, Royal National Orthopaedic Hospital, Stanmore, 1983–88

Road traffic accident		
Driver	22%	
Passenger	12%	
Motorcycle	10%	= 50%
Bicycle	2%	
Pedestrian	4%	
Falls		
Fall from height	12%	
Fall down stairs	4%	= 27%
Fall/trip	5%	
Jump from height	6%	
Assault		2%
Heavy weight/crush		3%
Sport		
Diving	5%	
Gliding		
Skiing		
Horse riding	6%	= 11%
Jet ski		
Rugby		
Trampoline		
		7%
Other		100%

Secondary phase

The effects of altering or shutting off blood supply to major areas of tissue result in necrosis of variable amounts of the cord, proximal and distal to the site of injury. This loss of tissue may occur over a number of segments and result in significant cavitation of the cord. If there is subsequent blockage to cerebrospinal fluid flow, then further syrinx formation (classical syringomyelia) may occur and may result in further damage to the cord and loss of function if the syrinx ascends proximally. This may occur within a few months of injury, or more frequently some years later. The use of MRI has greatly increased the awareness of this condition, though the process of its development and clinical significance remain uncertain (Quencer and Bunge 1996).

In the immediate period following injury, the clinical development of neurological deficit is of some importance. It may be that there is a complete loss of function instantaneously below the site of the lesion. Not infrequently, however, patients and witnesses describe purposeful movement occurring shortly after the injury in limbs which subsequently have become paralysed. This may give some clue as to the primary or secondary nature of the injury and, particularly in the second situation, one must be guarded about eventual prognosis. The prognosis in someone who has just undergone spinal cord injury is complicated further by the presence of *spinal cord shock*. This is a condition in which there is cessation of conduction of electrical activity through the cord tissue as a result of the injury to the cord. It may last from a few seconds to several weeks or perhaps even months, and in its presence it is impossible to be certain as to the eventual outcome. Return of reflex activity in paralysed limbs and the return of tone in muscle below the level of the injury indicate the end of shock and, when this occurs, a clear indication of outcome can be given.

However, not all injuries result in total loss of function temporarily or indeed permanently after injury, and clinically lesions are said to be *complete* or *incomplete*, depending on whether there is any motor or sensory function below the level of the lesion. The definition of 'incomplete' used in the SIU, the RNOHT, Stanmore, is that given by Donovan *et al.* (1990) in the ASIA (American Spinal Injury Association) publication in which neurological status is classified. This distinction between complete and incomplete is made difficult because of the presence of spinal shock as outlined above. Nowadays, it is complicated further by the development of electrophysiology in the form of *somatosensory and motor evoked potentials*. This is an investigation in which one intentionally passes electrical current from the periphery through the spinal cord and records it through the skull over the appropriate cortical area. The reverse can also be carried out, stimulating the motor cortex through the skull and recording at the periphery. When these recordings are carried out, it is sometimes seen that, in those who have apparently clinically complete lesions, some electrical activity is capable of being transmitted along certain pathways in the cord.

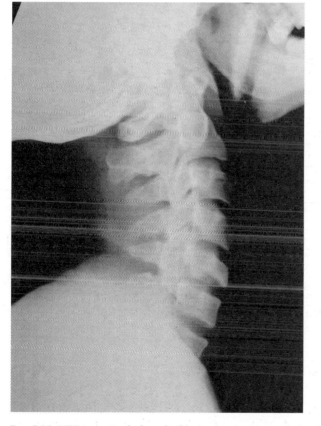

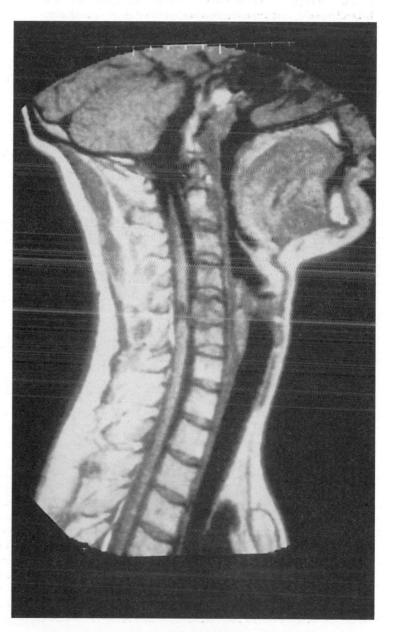

FIG. 5.19 MRI is particularly valuable in demonstrating early syrinx formation in the cord. In this patient, a crush fracture of the body of C5 (suggested by the X-ray and confirmed by the scan) is associated with cord damage (revealed by a depressed signal in the adjacent cord).

The importance of this situation is that the prognosis is markedly different when any degree of incompleteness remains.

The ability to measure what is occurring in the cord following injury is also of major importance when deciding whether or not surgical intervention should be carried out. Surgery may be carried out for several reasons; first, to stabilize the spine, thus allowing the individual to be mobilized some ten days after injury, rather than having to remain flat in bed for some three months; and secondly, to attempt to relieve pressure around the spinal cord at the site of injury, removing fragments of bone or disc, etc. from the spinal canal. Controversy has existed for many years as to whether real benefit is obtained from such interventions, and until better means of measurement are available it is likely that such arguments will continue. However, the development of MRI (Fig. 5.19) and more sophisticated computer-based somatosensory evoked potentials is leading to a capability of improved measurement. The application of such investigations to those with spinal cord injury sufficiently early after the injury remains a problem area and certainly places even greater importance on the immediate care at the injury site, the transport to Accident and Emergency facilities, and the speed with which these processes are carried out and investigations are instigated.

Immediate care at site—first aid

The first problem in first-aid management is *recognition* that a spinal cord injury has occurred. This recognition is more likely if there is a high level of suspicion and awareness of the circumstances in which such injuries may occur. Usually the injury itself has been very significant, and the immediate response must be one of saving life by maintaining vital systems—breathing and circulation. Clearly, if cardiac massage has to be carried out, the patient will have to be positioned supine. When there is an obvious misalignment of the cervical spine, that is, when there is a marked lateral flexion or rotation, the head should be brought back gently into the neutral position and a gentle traction should be maintained. This can be achieved either in the supine position, when it will be particularly necessary to pay attention to the position of the tongue if the patient is unconscious, or in full side-lying with the upper knee flexed and the head supported on the underneath arm.

The next principle which should be applied is that once the patient is in a satisfactory position and vital signs have been restored, *no further unnecessary movement should be allowed*. The patient should be kept in that position until further expert help and equipment arrive. Sandbags may be used to maintain the head position if the patient is inclined to be restless, but one person should remain at the head maintaining a neutral position at all times, if necessary by exerting gentle traction. Most ambulances and many sports centres and places of work now maintain basic equipment for removing people with spinal injury. The most commonly used are a Hines Frame for cervical injuries, or a scoop stretcher, which may be inserted beneath the patient on the ground without the need for further adjustment of position. If such a stretcher is not available, the patient will need to be lifted from the ground on to a suitable firm, well-supported, well-padded stretcher. This lifting procedure will require at least four people, with one maintaining the head in the neutral position and the others ensuring that the rest of the body remains in line throughout the procedure. One person

should act as the team leader and give instructions on the moment to lift, lower, etc.

Once the patient is in the ambulance or helicopter, his position needs to be maintained throughout the journey. Attention must continue to be paid to breathing and circulation, and because of an early specific complication of spinal cord injury, to the protection of anaesthetic skin. Accordingly, hard objects, etc. should be removed from the pockets of the individual as skin damage sufficient to cause complete ulceration subsequently may occur within ten to fifteen minutes (well within the time that it takes for an ambulance to arrive at the scene of an accident and a far shorter time than that taken by most subsequent journeys to hospital). It is tragic when a cervical cord injury is complicated by a massive pressure sore which may take several months to heal and which may well delay and dictate the course of any rehabilitation process for some considerable time.

At the site of injury, the existence of spinal cord injury is likely either to be immediately apparent or else extremely difficult to detect. The conscious patient may report the loss of movement and sensation in the legs, and simple examination will confirm this. Any further attempts at diagnosis at the site of injury are unwarranted and probably dangerous, and it is better that such actions should be reserved for the hospital Accident and Emergency department. If the patient is unconscious, then it must be assumed that injury to the spine has occurred, and the management outlined above should be strictly adhered to.

Assessment and early management

Following any significant insult to the spinal cord, a situation of conduction block of the nerve tissue is likely to be present. There will be an absence of intrinsic, electrical activity in the cord resulting in loss of afferent and efferent impulses and loss of reflexes. Once the patient is in hospital, one cannot over-emphasize the importance of proper documentation of the clinical signs on a regular basis. From a clinical point of view at this stage, when absence of movement, absence of sensation, and loss of reflexes are demonstrated, it is possible only to say that the patient is in *spinal shock*. Therefore, it is crucial that a proper and full examination of the nervous system is carried out, with particular attention to defining the neurological level of the injury and the presence or absence of reflexes, including the bulbocavernosus, the cremasteric, and the anal responses (Table 5.2). The classification of the lesion clinically into complete or incomplete will also occur at this stage, and this must be expressed from both a motor and sensory point of view. At RNOHT, Stanmore, the ASIA system of neurological examination and classification is used. Standardization of these examinations is

TABLE 5.2. Evaluation of reflexes: reflexes which should be tested routinely during the assessment of the spinal cord injured patient

Biceps	C5/6
Supinator	C6
Triceps	C7
Abdominal	T8–12
Cremasteric	L1
Knee	L3/4
Ankle	S1/2
Bulbocavernosus	S3/4
Anal	S5
Plantar	

extremely important both in terms of consistent evaluation of the patient and also for future research.

Early management strategies require the patient to be placed on a well-padded, firm supported surface and a size 12 or 14 indwelling urinary catheter inserted. The presence or absence of bowel ileus is noted, and a subsequent decision made on the need to pass a nasogastric tube. Assessment of respiration, chest injuries, and other complications should be carried out at this stage. Once these systems are under control, investigation can then proceed.

It is now well recognized that more effective resuscitation measures, with maintenance of blood pressure and oxygenation generally and specifically at the site of injury, play a highly significant role in neuroprotection of the cord. Neuroprotection implies survival of the maximum number of nerve fibres within the cord during the secondary and later phases of injury. Other measures that have been tried are high dosage steroids (NASCIS 3 1997), cord/patient cooling (Gimenez y-Ribotta and Privat 1998), a number of other drugs, for example, GM1 GK11, or decompression surgery to improve blood supply and drainage (Fehlings and Tator 1999).

Further research in this aspect of care is continuing, and it is likely that other measures, medical or surgical, will become available in the next five to ten years. Enabling even small numbers of fibres to survive may have a highly significant effect on subsequent functional outcome.

High dosage steroids, to be useful, must be given within eight hours of injury (NASCIS 3 1997), the earlier the better. They are given in all cases in the USA and increasingly in the UK.

Further investigations

X-rays of the spine and chest should be carried out to define the bony injury. In cases of thoracic and lumbar injury, a cervical spine X-ray should also be carried out to exclude cervical injury. (In ten percent of cases of damage to the spinal cord, no bony injury is demonstrated, and in a further ten per cent bony injuries occur at multiple levels.) In any unconscious patient, a lateral X-ray of the cervical spine should be carried out.

The primary decision at this stage is whether the spine is *stable* or *unstable*; instability should be assumed until further information is available. The most common injuries are due to flexion–rotation or hyperextension forces (Fig. 5.20). In the rugby scrum, hyperflexion of the neck may occur with or without rotation. A flexion injury will produce a wedge fracture of the vertebral body concerned, and may be associated with dislocation or fracture of the facetal joints. This combination is always unstable as severe ligamentous damage inevitably will be present. A 'burst' fracture of the vertebra implies an element of vertical compression in the force causing injury. This commonly arises in American football and rugby when axial loading results from the head-on tackle. Hyperextension injuries occur mostly in the cervical region, and much of the damage to the underlying cord frequently is caused by vascular compression, particularly in the elderly. Once the bony and neurological lesions have been defined and deficits demonstrated, the appropriate specialist spinal injuries unit should be contacted. The next stage of management will depend on the facilities available in the hospital concerned. CT scanning of the spine and cord may define the bony lesion and may also demonstrate material or bony fragments lying in the spinal canal. The significance of

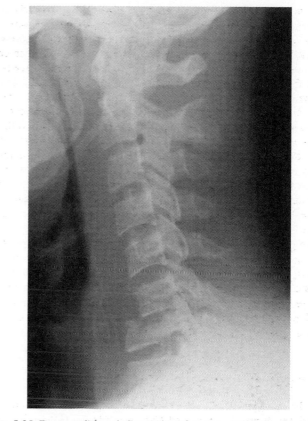

FIG. 5.20 Fracture-dislocation at C6/7 is demonstrated on the lateral X-ray of this patient who sustained a hyperextension injury.

such material, with regard to the cord injury or its potential for continuing cord injury, is difficult to evaluate, and operative decisions taken on the basis of such pictures may not produce the beneficial results expected.

From a surgical point of view, MRI scanning of the cord, with its better definition of nervous tissue, may be a better examination on which to base any future intervention (Shimada and Tokioka 1999). The development of functional MRI may be highly significant in improving clinical evaluation further. However, currently, decisions taken purely on demonstration of the anatomical situation are bound to be controversial and have been the source of much argument over the years. Residual function in the cord or potential for improvement of function may bear little relationship to the resulting anatomical structure. Difficulty in defining underlying cord function clearly at this stage after injury means that such arguments and controversy are likely to continue for some time into the future. The development of somatosensory and motor evoked potentials (SSEPs and MEPs) has given some encouragement towards a better functional definition, but this examination is extremely difficult to carry out in the environment immediately following a spinal cord injury; the recording of such minute amounts of electrical current is likely to be lost within the vast array of electrical equipment which now surrounds the acutely injured patient in the Accident and Emergency department. Also, the positioning of the patient and the necessity of not moving him make it difficult to apply good contact electrodes in the required positions. The application of skull tongs (which may well have been carried out at this stage in order to provide traction on the cervical spine in T1 lesions and above) will also inhibit electrode access to the skull over the required sensory areas. To date, no significant series of early spinal cord injury SSEP recordings have been published, almost certainly because of lack of availability of such equipment and the personnel to operate it in Accident and Emergency departments, and also because of the great difficulty in achieving adequate recordings. Therefore, few clinical surgical decisions have been taken in the early stage of spinal cord injury management on the basis of evoked potential examinations. The need for good functional measurement of cord activity to parallel the demonstration of anatomic structure remains. As a result, the surgical decision whether to decompress around the spinal cord to prevent secondary injury from compression or hypoxia remains difficult.

The decision on whether to carry out surgical internal stabilization of the spine, or to proceed with a conservative approach, is based on more clearly defined criteria. However, the decision to carry out such decompression and/or stabilization procedures is either best left to the specialist spinal cord injury unit, or carried out in conjunction with that unit as such surgical interventions will play an important role in the future management of the patient.

The ability to measure electrical function in specific pathways within the spinal cord has been demonstrated. Peri-operative monitoring, during procedures such as correction and stabilization of scoliosis, utilizing electrodes placed in the epidural space above and below the area of potential compromise, has proved reliable and sensitive.

The next stage involves the transfer of the patient to the specialist spinal unit or to the specialist unit within the district general hospital pending transfer.

Rehabilitation

This stage in the management of the majority of spinal cord injuries takes place in a spinal injury centre. The process of rehabilitation frequently is subdivided into psychological, social, and physical aspects (Mair 1972); attention to the psychological aspects in the early stages of rehabilitation is crucial. The centre should have a comprehensive team with a broad range of skills and experience appropriate to the complex task of minimizing disability, and thereby minimizing handicap for the patient. In this setting, it is likely that the team will be led by a physician or surgeon, and the members will comprise nurses, physiotherapists, occupational therapists, a social worker, a psychologist, community liaison team, special education and appropriate administration officers, and back up-support. Such a complexity of structure and expertise requires an appropriate system of ensuring that the available skills and experience are used in the most purposeful and effective way. A system of goal-planning with short-term targets within those goals can provide such a framework (Kennedy 1989), and can be a useful means of enabling the patient, his relatives, and the team to make necessary achievements. It can also provide motivation for both patient and staff in what may be an extremely difficult time in the life of the patient when such non-productive emotions as anger, denial, or depression may dominate the situation.

The use of case managers within the team to manage people with complex severe injuries is increasing. The case manager provides continuity during the acute, rehabilitation, and re-integration phases of care. He/she acts as advocate and educator, communicating with the multiplicity of agencies which may become involved in the process of social services, housing, employment, voluntary training, community nursing, etc.

Rehabilitation is essentially a learning process. During the first few months after spinal cord injury, anxiety will be high, the environment will be unfamiliar, and there may be associated high-level brain dysfunction consequent upon insult to the central nervous system. In this situation, it is inevitable that learning ability will be low. There should be an availability of psychological expertise to the patient and relatives for a significant and substantial period following the injury, certainly for at least two to three years.

Social handicap resulting from spinal cord injury may be catastrophic at worst, and is always major. As previously stated, the commonest group sustaining spinal cord injury is the age group 18–28 comprising people who are attempting to establish themselves as adults in the community independently of their parents. They are at an extremely vulnerable time in their lives, and the immense problems which spinal cord injury may present, in addition, may result in a total inability to achieve this independence without major help and support. Experience shows that relationships which are long-standing and structured are likely to continue, but those which are rather more short-lived and dependent on the ability of both parties to change together are very much less likely to survive the trauma of severe physical disability. The formation of new relationships of lasting consequence is unlikely to occur within the two years or so following injury, until the injured person has come to terms with his new identity.

With modern physical management of spinal cord injury, the period of hospitalization is becoming shorter, and although this reduces the serious danger of institutionalization, this means that the finding of suitably accessible accommodation assumes great importance. For the majority, this will involve moving from their present home or having major adaptations carried out within it.

Achieving outdoor mobility is also crucial. Re-establishing driving skills in a suitably adapted vehicle should have a high priority. The lack of employment of disabled people is one of the more depressing aspects of our society today. A recent large survey of people with spinal cord injury (Smith 1999) shows that only some 14 per cent return to gainful employment, a much lower figure than in other developed countries. Therefore, the use made by spinal cord injured people of their leisure time and their participation in sporting activities assumed great importance, as it is these activities which may well dictate their future quality of life (Creek et al. 1988). Associated with the SIU, RNOHT Stanmore, is the National Training Centre built and managed by the charity, ASPIRE. This centre is based on the integration of able-bodied and disabled through activities in sporting or vocational training. Programmes for people with spinal cord injury are provided which focus on comprehensive training and support for full re-entry and reintegration with the community at large.

Sport for the disabled has become quite highly developed in this country, led by the International Sports Centre for the Disabled at Stoke Mandeville Hospital (Fig. 5.21). The international paraplegic games have achieved considerable recognition in the primary sports of swimming, basketball, archery, and track and field, revealing extraordinary levels of quality at the higher national and international levels. Participation in sport

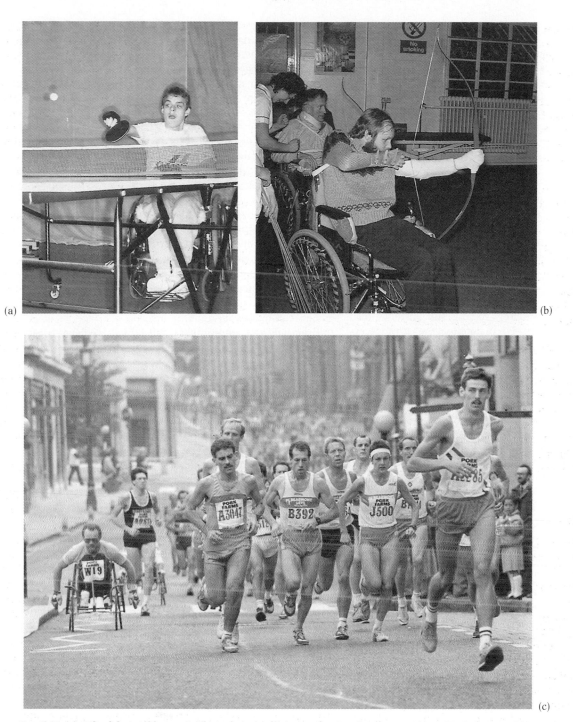

FIG. 5.21 (a) Wheelchair table-tennis, (b) archery, and (c) marathoning. Involvement in sport can be a positive beginning of reintegration into the community

can be an extraordinary confidence-builder and help along the road to adaptation for the disabled person.

Nowadays, there are developments of sporting facilities which cater for both able-bodied and disabled. Such centres can provide environments where the disabled can achieve real social integration with able-bodied people and provide for many their most useful activity in re-achieving a meaningful place in society.

The re-expression of sexuality may be achieved in such an environment, and it is therefore of paramount importance that the re-establishment of sexual function and identity have been sought and hopefully achieved during the period of rehabilitation. The majority of those with spinal cord injury are physically able, given certain compromises, to achieve satisfactory sexual physical relationships. It is likely that the majority do not, and this must reflect a great failure on the part of rehabilitation services.

Physical rehabilitation

The primary aims of physical rehabilitation are to maximize the individual's residual abilities and to prevent the development of complications. The essence of this aspect of rehabilitation is the combination of skills from physiotherapy, occupational therapy, nursing, and psychology which must be blended together in order to achieve the best possible outcome. The setting of realistic goals and appropriate targets prior to full achievement is of vital importance in maintaining purposefulness in the team and motivation for the patient. For the patient with a complete neurological lesion, the outcome objectives can be set at a relatively early stage, and some indication of the sort of time scale that it is likely to take can be given in terms of weeks. For the patient with an incomplete lesion, this is more difficult, as outcomes have to be updated frequently in terms of the changes taking place in neurological status. In this situation, it is also more difficult for individuals to maintain motivation to seek abilities of a lower level when the expectation is one of significant improvement.

In the early stages while the bony spine is still unstable, the main roles of the therapists involve maintenance of a range of movement in joints, the acquisition and maintenance of a satisfactory respiratory situation in the tetraplegic, and, as the patient comes out of spinal shock, the control of increasing spasticity.

Once the spine is stable and the phase of mobilization commences, a broader range of activities can be commenced with the goals of strengthening existing muscles, seeking and achieving mobility, achieving independence in a wheelchair, and seeking independence in the necessary activities of everyday living. When mobilization commences, the assuming of an upright posture will reveal lack of function within the autonomic nervous system, causing significant and distressing hypotension.

Sitting up after a spinal cord injury, even for quite short periods, may take several days to achieve. In most patients, this problem diminishes over a period of weeks or months, and for most ceases to be a major problem. At this stage, the physiotherapist will concentrate on the acquisition of new skills, achieving sitting balance and learning to carry out transfers from bed to wheelchair and vice versa, and will then move on to wheelchair skills. The achievement of a standing posture on a daily basis will also be sought because of its metabolic benefits primarily in keeping calcium in the bones and also in terms of kidney and bladder drainage. The continuance of maintaining a range of movement in joints, stretching muscle groups, assuming more normal postures, and achieving weightbearing while standing will all contribute to controlling spasticity, which in some patients may become an extremely important problem preventing even the simplest activities. At present, available oral drug regimes are only partially effective, and the mechanical aspects of physiotherapy or electrical stimulation provide the most hopeful means of control. The earlier that these regimens are instituted, the more likely satisfactory control will be attained. The development of intrathecal delivery systems for Baclofen (Campbell *et al.* 1995) now offers a further and potentially highly successful treatment for spasticity. As yet, this management is only available in certain specialist centres where its development is being monitored carefully as the system is not without hazards. There is an increasing use of *Botulinum* toxin injection in selected muscles or groups of muscles (Jankovic and Brin 1991).

During this phase of rehabilitation, there will be a gradual development of new skills and the re-acquisition of old abilities. It is essential that these abilities are translated from demonstration of muscle strength and range of movement in the physiotherapy department to carrying out necessary tasks in everyday living in the real world. The role of the occupational therapist becomes paramount, as does that of nurses with whom patients spend the majority of their day. The achievement of independence in everyday living skills can be approached in a logical manner, with attempts being made initially to re-achieve basic activities by utilizing the patient's remaining motor and sensory abilities. If this is not possible, the therapist will attempt to teach the patient new ways of achieving the required skill. It may be necessary to introduce splints and aids with which the individual may then achieve an independent result. The alteration of a patient's environment in order to achieve independence with the use of simple measures such as provision of ramps and the regulation of the heights of working surfaces, alongside the use of modern technology in the shape of the development of computer-based environmental controls, has become one of the major roles of occupational therapy.

If altering the environment still fails to achieve satisfactory independence then it becomes necessary to introduce attendants trained in the support situation.

In very high-level tetraplegics who require continuing ventilatory support and in those who have cognitive deficits associated with brain damage, long-term hospitalization may remain the only option. Increasingly, people who require ventilatory support are being re-established back in the community with complex nurse-led packages of care (Bach 1991). Fortunately, this is a relatively rare situation.

Although the re-achievement of independence probably remains the apparent goal of those who have sustained spinal cord injury, it is extremely important to balance the compromises necessary for such independence with some cognizance of quality of life. Frequent human contact and reassurance are important elements in providing a meaningful and satisfactory quality of life.

Education and prevention of complications

Until the 1950s, and the successful development of the Stoke Mandeville National Spinal Injuries Centre by Sir Ludwig Guttmann, the development of serious complications following spinal cord injury was inevitable, as was progression to a fatal outcome usually within a couple of years. The most frequent and devastating of these complications were massive decubitus ulceration and the combination of infection and increase in pressure within the bladder, leading to hydronephrosis and destruction of the kidneys. The presence of an indwelling urethral catheter implies a permanent route for bacteria to the bladder from the atmosphere, and a constant pressure upon the urethral mucosa causing changes in that complex structure which may result in perianal ulceration. The presence of such a foreign body in the bladder, associated with infection and an increased calcium availability consequent upon absence of bony stress, frequently led to stone formation, which aggravated bladder inflammation and renal destruction. The loss of calcium from bones also frequently led to pathological fractures which further exacerbated the problems of skin ulceration. These complications of injury to the spinal cord should now be looked on as preventable in the vast majority of patients, and modern spinal injury units exist to prevent such complications. They have been helped in this regard by the development of investigations such as video cystourethrography, which enable the clinician to have a clear picture of the anatomy and functioning of the neurogenic bladder. The use of intermittent catheterization programmes helps to maintain a more normal bladder function—an important aspect as the availability of electronic implantable bladder-controllers increased (Brindley *et al.* 1986).

Although a number of complications are preventable, a number of others remain which are not dependent upon the patient's education or discipline in managing his/her various systems. One of the causes of mortality in the first year of tetraplegia is autonomic dysreflexia, a condition where massive, and potentially fatal, hypertension can occur rapidly consequent upon stimulation of the unopposed sympathetic nervous system (McGuire and Kumar 1986). Such stimulation arises most frequently from a distended bladder, but may result from severe constipation or indeed a severely inflamed ingrowing toenail, all of which are common situations in the tetraplegic patient. The simple manoeuvres of sitting the patient up and passing a urinary catheter in this situation may be life saving.

Complications of late bony instability leading to kyphosis or scoliosis may require surgical intervention to prevent unacceptable skeletal compromise. Such bony instability in adults is relatively rare (Bedbrook and Edibam 1973); however, it is the rule in children, leading to serious deformity.

There are three major complications which occur from within the damaged cord itself: central pain, spasticity, and ascending disabilities associated with syrinx formation (dilatation of the central canal). The development of severe persistent *central pain* may be one of the most destructive aspects of spinal cord injury; fortunately, it remains relatively rare, but less severe degrees of pain are common and distressing. Such severe central pain responds poorly to the more commonly used analgesics, yet the use of a more powerful opiate analgesia is to be avoided except in an extreme case. Therefore, the first treatment of choice, for most patients, is transcutaneous nerve stimulation, which can be remarkably successful in more than 60 per cent of cases. This may be supplemented with the use of various forms of acupuncture, or nerve- or ganglion-blocking techniques. It should be remembered that central pain of this type tends to diminish over months, and its impact on the individual is greatly dependent upon mood state and on general activity.

The development of *syrinx formation*, now more commonly diagnosed with the development of MRI, may require surgical intervention to relieve a pressure drainage problem. It has already been stated that the drugs available for the control of *spasticity* are disappointing in their effects and in the frequency with which they produce unacceptable side-effects. Physiotherapy techniques remain the management choice, supplemented with electrical stimulation techniques and, more recently but still rarely, the use of dorsal column stimulation or insertion of an intrathecal Baclofen pump, which delivers, at a controlled rate, antispasmodic drugs directly to the central nervous tissues involved. Despite these measures, there remain a number of spinally injured patients whose spasticity remains uncontrolled and uncontrollable, and in whom contractures and trophic problems eventually supervene. The next research developments in

spinal cord injury management are likely to take place within these fields and to result in better management of these types of complications.

Discussion

The rehabilitation process today emphasizes the importance of the multidisciplinary involvement of an adequate range of skills and the effective and efficient education of the patient, his relatives, and his carers. Measurement of success in rehabilitation is difficult, as parameters of outcome are so extraordinarily variable. However, it is likely that the success of an education programme and a rehabilitation process can be judged by the absence of development of avoidable complications. Clearly it is of enormous importance to the individual to avoid complications, but it is also of significance to the specialist spinal cord injury centres, where, if much of their work and bed capacity is taken up with the management of preventable complications, they inevitably have less time and ability to deal with those with acute injuries, and to develop and apply to patients new developments such as bladder controllers. The development of more sophisticated calipers, of computer-controlled muscle stimulation, and of implantable motor-function controllers, requires resources in terms of personnel, equipment, and facilities.

With the increasing life expectancy of those with spinal cord injuries, the likelihood of such developments becoming applicable to them is also increased.

Neuroprotection measures, particularly in the first 6–8 hours after injury, increasingly are resulting in more people who have sustained spinal cord injury subsequently living with less severe disabilities. Awareness of the availability of such measures and when they need to be applied is thus of great importance to all, whether paramedics at the roadside or trainers/therapists, etc. at sporting venues, who are likely to be involved in the immediate care of those sustaining cord injuries.

Research aimed at achieving cord regeneration in those with established cord injury has made considerable progress in the past ten years. New fibres growing across cord lesions in the experimental situation have been clearly demonstrated. Enabling such new fibres to target muscle afflictions and produce real function remains the exciting and closer goal.

References

Armour, K. S., Clatworthy, B. J., Bean, A. R.*et al.* (1997). Spinal injuries in New Zealand rugby and rugby league—a 20-year survey. *N. Z. Med. J.*, **110**, 462–5.

Bach, J. R. (1991). Alternative methods of ventilatory support in high tetraplegia. *J. Am. Paraplegia Soc.*, **14** (4), 158–74.

Bedbrook, G. M. and Edibam, R. C. (1973). The study of deformity in traumatic spinal paralysis. *Parapelgia*, **10**, 321–35.

Beighton, P., Solomon, L., and Soskolne, C. L. (1973). Articular mobility in an African population. *Ann. Rheum. Dis.*, **32**, 413–18.

Bette, K. Go., Devivo, M. J., and Richards, J. S. (1995). The epidemiology of spinal cord injury. In *Spinal cord injury: clinical outcomes from the model systems* (eds S. L. Stover, J. A. Delisa, and G. G Whiteneck). Aspen, Maryland, pp. 21–55.

Bogduk, N. and Twomey, L. T. (1987). *Clinical anatomy of the lumbar spine.* Churchill Livingstone, Melbourne.

Bracken, M. B. *et al.* (1997). Treatment of acute spinal cord injury: results of the Third National Acute Spinal Cord Injury randomised controlled trial ('NASCIS 3'). *J. Am. Med. Soc.*, **277**, (20) 1597–604.

Brindley, G. S., Polkey, C. E., Rushton, D. N., and Cardoza, L. (1986). Sacral anterior root stimulators for bladder control in paraplegics. *J. Neurol. Neurosurg. Psychiatry* **49**, 1104–14.

Burry, H. C. and Calcinai, C. J. (1988). The need to make rugby safer. *Br. Med. J.*, **296**, 149–50.

Cailliet, R. (1981). *Low back pain syndrome* (3rd edn). F. A. Davis, Philadelphia.

Campbell, S. K., Almeida, G. L., Penn, R. D., and Corcos, D. M. (1995). The effects of intrathecally administered Baclofen on function in patients with spasticity. *Phys. Ther.*, **75**, 352–62.

Colachis, S. C., Warden, R. E., Bechtol, C. O., and Strohm, B. R. (1963). Movement of the sacroiliac joint in the adult male. *Arch. Phys. Med. Rehabil.*, **44**, 490.

Creek, G., Moore, M., Oliver, M., Salisbury, V., Silver, J., and Zarb, G. (1988). *Personal and social implications of spinal cord injury—a retrospective study.* Thames Polytechnic, London.

Cyriax, J. (1982). *Textbook of orthopaedic medicine*, Vol. 1 (8th edn). Baillière Tindall, London.

Cyriax, J. and Russell, G. (1984). *Textbook of orthopaedic medicine*, Vol. 2 (11th edn). Baillière Tindall, London.

Devivo, M. J. and Stover, S. L. (1995). Long term survival and causes of death in spinal cord injury. In *Spinal cord injury: clinical outcomes from the model systems* (eds S. L. Stover, J. A. Delisa, and G. G. Whiteneck). Aspen, Maryland, pp. 289–316.

Donovan, W. H. *et al.* (1990). *Standards for neurological classification of spinal injury patients.* American Spinal Injury Association.

Elliott, S., Hutson, M. A., and Wastie, M. L. (1988). Bone scintigraphy in the assessment of spondylolysis in patients attending a sports injury clinic. *Clin. Radiol.*, **39**, 269–72.

Elvery, R. L. (1986). Treatment of arm pain associated with abnormal brachial plexus tension. *Aust. J. Physiother.*, **32** (4), 225–30.

Farfan, H. F. (1973). *Mechanical disorders of the low back.* Lea and Febiger, Philadelphia.

Fehlings, M. G. and Tator, C. H. (1999). An evidence-based review of decompressive surgery in acute spinal cord injury: rationale, indications, and timing based on experimental and clinical studies. *J. Neurosurg.*, **91 (Suppl. 1)**, 1–11.

Fitch, K. (1981). Controversial issues in sports medicine. Proceedings of the Australian Sports Sports Medicine Federation National Scientific Conference, Adelaide, Vol. 1, pp. 282–5.

Fredrikson, B., Baker, D., McHolick, W. J., Yuan, H. A., and Lubickly, J. P. (1984). The natural history of spondylolysis and spondylolisthesis. *J. Bone Jt. Surg.*, **66A**, 699–707.

Gimenez-y-Ribotta, M. and Privat, A. (1998). Biological interventions for spinal cord injury. *Curr. Opin. Neurol.*, **11** (6), 647–54.

Grieve, G. P. (1976). The sacroiliac joint. *Physiotherapy*, **62** (12), 384–400.

Guttmann, L., (1954). Statistical survey of one thousand paraplegics and initial management of traumatic paraplegia. *Proc. R. Soc. Med.*, **47**, 1099–1103.

Hardcastle, P., Annear, P., Foster, D. H., Chakera, T. M., McCormick, C., Khangure, M., and Burnett, A. (1992). Spinal abnormalities in young fast bowlers. *J. Bone Jt. Surg.*, **74B**, 421–5.

Holden, D. L. and Jackson, D. W. (1985). Stress fracture of the ribs in female rowers. *Am. J. Sports Med.*, **13**, 342–8.

Jackson, D. W., Wiltse, L. L., and Cirincione, R. J. (1976). Spondylolysis in the female gymnast. *Clin. Orthop. Relat. Res.*, **117**, 68–73.

Jackson, D. W., Wiltse, L. L., and Dungeman, R. D. (1981). Stress reactions involving the pars interarticularis in young athletes. *Am. J. Sports Med.*, **9**, 304–12.

Jankovic, J. and Brin, M. (1991). Therapeutic uses of *Botulinun* toxin. *N. Engl. J. Med.*, **324**, 1186–94.

Kakulas, A. (1988). The applied neurobiology of human spinal cord injury: a review. *Paraplegia*, **26**, 371–9.

Kennedy, P. (1989). Psychological approaches to the management of spinal cord injury. *J. Hol. Med.* **4** (4), 169–76.

Kirkaldy-Willis, W. H., Wedge, J. H., Yong-Hing, K., and Reilly, J. (1978). Pathology and pathogenesis of lumbar spondylosis and stenosis. *Spine*, **3**, 319–28.

Lewit, K. (1985). *Manipulative therapy in rehabilitation of the motor system.* Butterworth, London.

McGuire, T. J. and Kumar, V. N. (1986). Autonomic dysreflexia in the spinal cord injured. *Postgrad. Med.*, **80** (2), 81–4.

Mair, A. (1972). *Report of the subcommittee of the Standing Medical Advisory Committee, Scottish Health Services Council, on medical rehabilitation.* HMSO, Edinburgh.

Maitland, G. D. (1986). *Vertebral manipulation* (5th edn). Butterworth, London.

Mennell, J. McM. (1960). *Back pain: diagnosis and treatment using manipulative techniques.* Little, Brown, Boston.

Mottram, S. and Comerford, M. (1988). Stability dysfunction and low back pain. *J. Orthop. Med.*, **20**, (2) 13–8.

Nachemson, A. L. (1984). Prevention of chronic back pain. The orthopaedic challenge for the 80s. *Bull, Hosp. Jt. Dis. Orthop. Inst.*, **44**, 1–15.

Nachemson, A. and Elfstrom, G. (1970). Intradiscal dynamic pressure measurements in lumbar discs. *Scand J. Rehabil. Med.*, **Suppl.** 1, 1–40.

Ongley, M. J., Klein, R. G., Dorman, T. A., Eek, B. C., and Hubert, L. J. (1987). A new approach to the treatment of chronic low back pain. *Lancet*, **8551**, 143–6.

Poster, R. W., Hibbert, C. S., and Wicks, M. (1978). The spinal canal in symptomatic lumbar disc lesions. *J. Bone Jt. Surg.*, **50B**, 485–7.

Quencer, R. M. and Bunge, R. P. (1996). The injured spinal cord: imaging, histopathologic, clinical correlates, and basic science approaches to enhancing neural function after spinal cord injury. *Spine*, **21**, 2064–6.

Read, M. T. F. (1994). Single photon emission computed tomography (SPECT) scanning for adolescent back pain. A *sine qua non? Br. J. Sports Med.*, **28**(1), 56–7.

Rotem, T. R., Lawson, J. S., Wilson, S. F. *et al.* (1998). Severe cervical spinal cord injuries related to rugby union and league football in New South Wales, 1984–1996. *Med. J. Aust.*, **168**, 379–81.

Scher, A. T. (1998). Rugby injuries to the cervical spine and cervical cord—a 10-year review. *Clin. Sports Med.*, **17**, 195–206.

Shimada, K. and Tokioka, T. (1999). Sequential MR studies of spinal cord injury. *Spinal Cord*, **37**, 410–5.

Silver, J. R. (1993). Spinal injuries in sports in the UK. *Br. J. Sports Med.*, **27** (2), 115–20.

Silver, J. R. and Gill, S. (1988). Injuries of the spine sustained during rugby. *Sports Med.*, **5**, 328–34.

Smith, M. (1999). *Making the difference.* Spinal Injuries Association, 15, 95–8.

Stallard, M. C. (1980). Backache in oarsmen. *Br. J. Sports Med.*, **14**, 105–8.

Stoddard, A. (1980). *Manual of osteopathic technique* (3rd edn). Hutchinson, London.

Sward, L., Hellstrom, M., Jacobsson, B., Nyman, R., and Peterson, L. (1991). Disc degeneration and associated abnormalities of the spine in elite gymnasts: a magnetic resonance imaging study. *Spine*, **16**, 437–43.

Torg, J. S. and Das, M. (1985). Trampoline injuries. *Clin. Sports Med.*, **4** (1), 45–60.

Troup, J. D. G. (1986). Biomechanics of the lumbar spinal canal. *Clin. Biomech.*, **1** (1), 31–43.

Wilmot, C. B., Cope, D. N., Hall, K. M., and Acker, M. (1985). Occult head injury: its incidence in spinal cord injury. *Arch. Phys. Med. Rehabil.*, **66** (4), 227–31.

Yeo, J. D. (1998). Rugby and spinal injury: what can be done? *Med. J. Aust.*, **168**, 372–3.

6 Pelvic injuries

M. A. HUTSON

Introduction

Apart from compression injuries sustained in sports such as motor racing or equestrian events, most injuries to the pelvis are to the soft tissues, principally the joints, muscle attachments, and bursae. They are caused principally by overuse. Symptoms may sometimes be localized accurately by the patient (for instance, to the groin in adductor strains), though quite often they are more diffuse in nature. The association of groin pain with pain felt in the lower abdomen, in the testes, around the 'hips', and into the anteromedial thighs is common. The combination of groin pain with backache suggests a spinal cause: occasionally difficulties in diagnosis arise when groin pain from a spinal lesion exists without coexisting backache. Lesions at the thoracolumbar junction, as well as the lumbar spine and sacroiliac joints, may refer pain to both the groin and the thigh.

Clicking or 'clonking' may be complained of, particularly by the adolescent athlete. The young dancer, for instance, may complain either of clicking due to movement of the iliotibial tract over the greater trochanter, or (more anteriorly) clonking due to snapping of the iliopsoas over the lesser trochanter, the iliopectineal eminence, or the anterior inferior iliac spine (Schaberg 1984). Patients may need to be reassured of the benign nature of these irritating conditions. When a stress injury occurs in the region of the pelvis, much patience is required by the patient (and his physician!), as conditions tend to be refractory to specific therapeutic modalities; spontaneous resolution often occurs over many months.

Applied anatomy and biomechanics

The pelvis is a ring structure, a fact that is just as relevant to a study of overuse injury as it is to the management of pelvic fractures. Stress or weakness at one site in the ring (of which the lumbosacral joint as well as the sacroiliac joints should be considered to be an integral part) will inevitably impart stress to the remaining structures. The hip joints are central to the study of the biomechanics of the pelvis, as an essential function of the pelvis is to provide a mechanism for transmission of forces and mobility from the lower limbs to the trunk.

There are no muscles which are attached to both the sacrum and the ilium. The erector spinae, iliopsoas, and piriformis muscles overlie, and therefore exert an influence on, the sacroiliac joints (SIJs). The SIJs are also influenced indirectly by other powerful muscles (for instance, the glutei and abdominals) acting on the lumbar spine and pelvis to reduce the lumbosacral angle. The sacroiliac joints are synovial joints, well supported by tough ligaments: anterior sacroiliac, posterior sacroiliac, and interosseous (Fig. 6.1). Additional strength is provided by the sacrospinous and sacrotuberous ligaments. The iliolumbar ligament also may be considered to be functionally supportive. The surfaces of the joint are made up of irregular humps and hollows, which contribute to its stability. Joint mobility has been studied extensively: both Weisl (1955), who used cineradiographic studies, and Colachis et al. (1963), who embedded Kirschner wires into the posterior iliac spines, found approximately 5 mm of movement.

Posterior rotation (nutation) of the ilium on the sacrum results in elevation of the anterior superior iliac spine (ASIS) and depression of the posterior superior iliac spine (PSIS) (Grieve 1976). Anterior rotation (contranutation) results in a reversal of these movements. The plane of movement is usually described as posteromedial to anterolateral. Such rotational movement is important in gait when reciprocal rotation in a figure-of-eight pattern occurs with each leg movement. Equal movements of the sacroiliac joints occur in trunk flexion and rotation: in flexion, for instance, there is a relative posterior movement of the ilia on the sacrum.

When there is persistent unilateral posterior rotation, pelvic torsion (or 'distortion') occurs. Lewit (1985) states that, in this (one-sided nutational) situation, rotation of one ilium occurs around a horizontal axis, and rotation of the other ilium occurs around a vertical axis. He considers it to be a common condition. During posterior rotation, the acetabulum rises, and functional leg shortening occurs. This apparent leg-length inequality (as detected by the relative positions of the medial malleoli) is observed in the supine position; leg-lengthening occurs in the sitting position.

The natural history of the mobility of the SI joints is for them to become stiffer, with gradual obliteration of the synovial joint with increasing age. However, *hypermobility* may be a problem in younger athletes. As a result of ligamentous incompetence, increased rotation occurs and may give rise to acute *dysfunction*, in which apparent *hypomobility* may be demonstrated. Dysfunction in which an SIJ is 'stuck', most often in posterior rotation, responds to manipulation, though the basic hypermobility problem remains, with the additional risk of symptoms from chronic ligamentous strain. The innervation of the posterior ligaments is from L5, S1, and S2; thus pain may be referred to the posterior leg as far as the heel. The anterior ligaments have a more extensive innervation, from L3 to S1. Symptoms may then be felt in the groin.

The pubic symphysis is a cartilaginous joint, with the joint surfaces separated by a fibrocartilaginous disc. There are no muscles overlying the symphysis, though several muscles attach

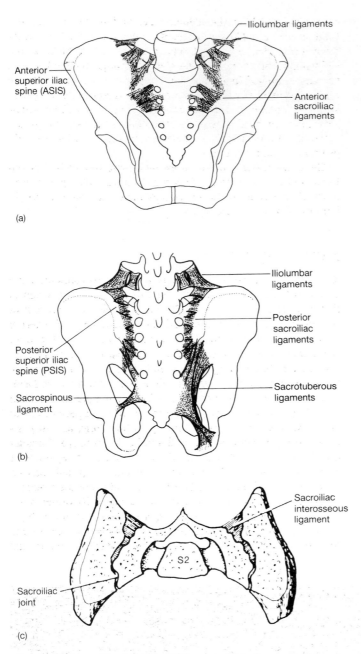

FIG. 6.1 The sacroiliac joints are well supported by ligaments: (a) anterior view; (b) posterior view; (c) transverse section at S2

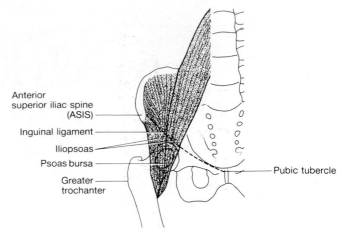

FIG. 6.2 The surface anatomical markings of the hip joint (overlaid by the psoas bursa).

is also found at the midpoint of an imaginary horizontal line from the pubic tubercle to the greater trochanter. An anterior approach to the hip joint for intra-articular injection or aspiration may be made lateral to the femoral neurovascular bundle (see Fig. 12.20, p. 229). Alternatively, a lateral approach immediately above the greater trochanter may be used. The term femoral anteversion refers to the angle made by the femoral neck to the femoral condyles—that is, the degree of forward projection of the neck from the coronal plane (Fig. 6.3). Excessive ('fetal') anteversion in the adult leads to excessive medial femoral rotation and squinting patellae (see Fig. 11.6, p. 198). It is one of a number of aetiological factors involved in overuse injury in the lower limb.

The capsular pattern of the hip, indicating articular pathology, is early restriction of medial rotation, flexion, and abduction. The loss of some degree of medial rotation, in particular, is a sensitive guide to early degenerative disease. The powerful muscles acting upon the hip arise from the pelvis and lumbar spine. Hip flexion is controlled largely by iliopsoas, with additional support from rectus femoris. The iliopsoas tendon is immediately adjacent to the anterior aspect of the hip joint, separated from it by a bursa (Fig. 6.2). The buttock muscles control hip extension (in which they are aided by the hamstrings) and abduction. There is an extensive attachment of gluteus medius to the femur distal to the greater tuberosity. These are strong postural muscles; medius and minimus help to stabilize the hip

to each pubic bone. The triad of joints making up the pelvic ring (that is, SIJ—pubic symphysis—SIJ) have a strong shock-absorbing function. The hip joint, formed from three separate centres of ossification (ilium, ischium, and pubis), is a ball-and-socket joint, allowing movement in all directions. The strengthening of the capsule by ligaments positioned anteriorly (iliofemoral ligament) and medially (pubofemoral ligament) helps restrict overextension and abduction. However, the main stability arises from the depth of the acetabulum and the strength of the muscles acting upon the joint.

Familiarity with the position of the hip joint from surface anatomical markings should be gained (Fig. 6.2). The head of the femur is positioned immediately inferior (and posterior) to the middle one-third of the inguinal ligament. The femoral head

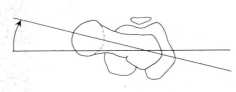

FIG. 6.3 Axial view of right femur. Femoral anteversion refers to the angle made by the femoral neck to the femoral condyles — that is, the degree of forward projection of the neck from the coronal plane.

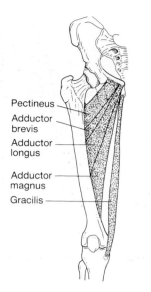

FIG. 6.4 The hip adductors are a powerful group of muscles involved in kicking and running.

Pectineus
Adductor brevis
Adductor longus
Adductor magnus
Gracilis

in running, and maximus is active in the backward thrust of the leg in uphill running. Injuries to the gluteal muscle bellies occur infrequently; insertional tendinitis (particularly of gluteus medius) and bursitis (between the muscle layers) are rather more common. Tensor fascia lata, which inserts into the iliotibial tract, is also an abductor: bursitis, caused by repetitive movement of the tract over the underlying bone at a proximal level (overlying the greater trochanter) or distal level (overlying the lateral femoral condyle), may reflect its tightness.

The adductors are a powerful group of muscles arising from the pubis and puboischial rami; they are inserted into the linea aspera, adductor tubercle of the femur (adductor magnus), and the medial tibial condyle (gracilis) (Fig. 6.4). Adduction of the thigh is one of a sequence of movements that takes place in running and kicking; the adductors flex and internally rotate the thigh as well as adduct, movements which are carried out vigorously in kicking a football. The combination of kicking, the sudden movements which take place in change of direction, and the stress applied in tackling are responsible for the relatively high incidence of chronic adductor strain and anterior pelvic strain in footballers. Internal rotation is produced as an accessory function by the iliopsoas, the adductors, and the glutei; external rotation is produced by the smaller muscles (gemelli, piriformis, and obturators).

There are a few acute injuries giving rise to localized symptoms, and a large variety of overuse injuries which give rise to more diffuse ache in the lower abdomen, anteromedial thigh, buttock, or trochanteric region.

Acute injury

'Groin strain'. In the skeletally mature, the most common acute injury to the soft tissue attachments to the pelvis is a strain of the origin of adductor longus. The patient feels a sudden pain in the groin on stretching the thigh into abduction and external rotation—for example, on turning quickly in soccer (Fig. 6.5). Discomfort is felt on attempted pivoting, sprinting, or kicking. The examination findings are discomfort on passive abduction of the thigh, and pain on resisted adduction. Tenderness is localized to the origin of the cord-like adductor longus tendon from the inferior pubic ramus. The essentials of management are to allow this potentially chronic injury to heal fully, and to postpone resumption of training until a full painless range of abduction is achieved and normal adduction power is regained. A minimum period of three weeks is usually required. Steroid injections should not be used for fear of weakening the tendon.

Rupture of the adductor longus may occur at its origin, midbelly, or insertion on the linea aspera. Weakness and pain, if rupture is incomplete, are elicited on resisted adduction; usually soft tissue swelling and bruising become extensive in the medial

FIG. 6.5 Injuries to the adductors of the thigh are common in soccer players.

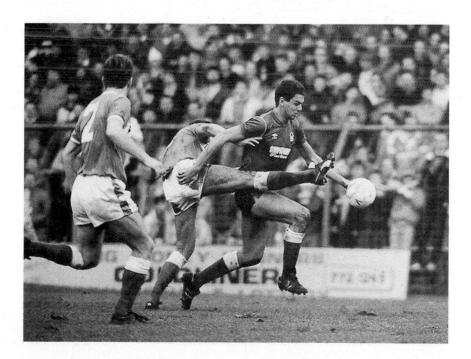

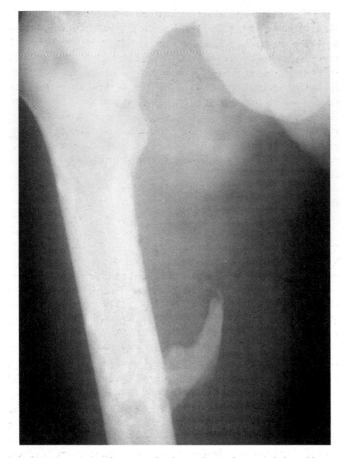

FIG. 6.6 Myositis ossificans in the femoral attachment of the adductor longus

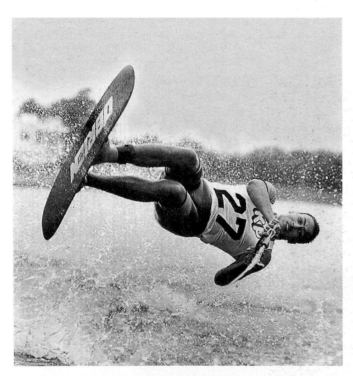

FIG. 6.7 Gluteal muscle tears may result from forced hip flexion in accidents at high speed, such as may occur in water-skiing.

and posterior thigh. Healing without complications may be anticipated unless premature resumption of activity is allowed, in which case myositis ossificans may occur, either proximally or distally (Fig. 6.6). At a later stage, the defect and proximal muscle swellings are palpable, though adductor function is unaffected. Symeonides (1972) advocates a surgical approach for midbelly and distal ruptures. In the author's experience, however, an uneventful recovery may be expected following a conservative approach.

Acute strain of iliopsoas also occurs. The pain is then felt in the groin on hip flexion—for example, during walking or attempted running. Passive hip extension is uncomfortable. The pain is reproduced on resisted flexion and medial rotation of the thigh. Deep tenderness is felt over the musculotendinous junction which is in close proximity to the anterior aspect of the hip joint. For accurate localization, the hip should be supported in slight flexion. Uneventful recovery is to be expected inside two weeks or so.

Muscle tears in the gluteal group are uncommon. They normally result from forced hip flexion in accidents at high speed—for example, while water-skiing (Fig. 6.7). However, the hamstrings are more likely to be injured under these circumstances (see Chapter 9).

Overuse injury

A plethora of conditions exist, for the assessment and management of which a knowledge of aetiological factors is necessary.

Chronic adductor strain. An enthesitis at the origin of the adductor longus may develop from an acute strain that has been managed inappropriately, either by the patient or his physician. Alternatively, a more insidious onset is recorded in the absence of an acute phase. Hockey and soccer players are primarily affected. Pain is felt in the groin and medial thigh on sprinting, turning quickly, or kicking. The signs are similar to an acute sprain: there is no capsular pattern, merely signs of a lesion in a contractile structure. It is tempting to inject steroid around the tendon origin, though, if this is done, it is imperative that adequate stretching and strengthening exercises continue to be undertaken for several weeks thereafter. If an acute-on-chronic strain occurs, the underlying condition may take many months, even a year, to respond. X-ray and bone scan are advisable in the refractory case, to distinguish from stress fracture of the puboischial rami. Adductor tendinitis due to chronic overload may also occur at the origin of gracilis and adductor brevis. In patients who do not respond to a conservative regime, partial tenotomy appears to be a viable alternative management (Martens *et al.* 1987). Ectopic ossification in the adductor longus tendon ('rider's thigh') is a response to overactivity, and is seen particularly in horse-riders.

Osteitis pubis ('pubic symphysitis'). The earlier descriptions of this condition associated it with chronic urinary or prostatic infection, hence the '-itis'. As a sports injury, the condition is manifested by exercise-dependent pain felt in the lower abdomen and medial thighs, gradually increasing in severity and eventually preventing exercise. It is due to excessive stress from those activities which involve running and twisting, and is precipitated particularly by overuse of the abdominal muscles, principally the rectus abdominis. Adams and Chandler (1953) postulate that recurrent microtrauma causes thrombosis and aseptic necrosis of the bone and cartilage. There is evidence that the condition is more likely to arise in the presence of restricted movement and/or reduced resistance to stress in other parts of the pelvis. Muckle (1982) has drawn attention to the association between osteitis pubis and spinal abnormalities. Williams (1978) has noted an association with tilt deformity of the femoral head. The author's experience is of a high correlation between degenerative change in the hip joint and osteitis pubis.

When taking a history, it is necessary to assess the extent of abdominal muscle activity that preceded the onset of symptoms. A typical patient is a sportsman who augments his daily long-distance running by several games of squash and sessions of circuit training each week, with additional daily sit-ups and press-ups performed at home—by no means an unusual situation. Females may substitute aerobics for circuit training, and develop the same overload problem. The examination signs are those of chronic strain at the pubic attachments of both the abdominal and adductor muscles: pain on resisted contraction and discomfort on stretch. Although there is some tenderness at the adductor attachments to the inferior pubic rami, *maximal* tenderness is found on palpating the pubic symphysis. Instability of the symphysis may develop in a severe case owing to shear forces secondary to powerful muscle contraction, particularly of the adductors.

AP X-rays of the pelvis taken while weightbearing, first on one leg and then the other (flamingo views), will reveal any supero-inferior instability. Gross irregularity, moth-eaten erosions, and sclerosis of the margins of the symphysis pubis are stress-related changes; however, they correlate poorly with the presence or severity of symptomatology. Severe changes may be found on routine X-ray—for example, during pre-employment examinations in professional soccer players in the absence of symptoms (Fig. 6.8). In one review, Harris and Murray (1974) found that radiographic changes at the symphysis were present in 76 per cent of professional soccer players on routine X-rays. In a group that included footballers and other athletes, sacroiliac stress changes were also present in 55 per cent. Bone scan is a supplementary test: increased uptake at the symphysis is shown in symptomatic cases.

Management is by stress reduction, which may, in the fully developed syndrome, necessitate complete rest from sport for several months. Localized treatment initially is to little avail, although steroid injections to the superior aspect of the pubic symphysis may be helpful at a later stage. Flexibility exercises, particularly for the hip joints and the muscles acting upon them, are instituted once symptomatic improvement has been gained. Very occasionally, surgical stabilization of the symphysis may be considered if symptoms persist for over six months in the presence of demonstrable instability. More often, even in the presence of instability, symptoms gradually resolve during six to twelve months.

Stress fractures. Stress fractures of the puboischial rami or the femoral neck may present as gradually worsening exercise-dependent pain in the groin. The importance of diagnosis in the case of femoral neck fracture is the possibility of the development of a frank fracture, with its inevitably more serious consequences. There is often no particular pattern of discomfort on hip movement. Localized tenderness may be detected in an anterior pelvic stress fracture. X-rays may not be positive for a couple of months: bone scanning is essential for diagnosis in the early case. Treatment is again by complete rest from exercise for three to six months.

Sacroiliitis. Sacroiliitis may occur as an inflammatory condition—for instance, as a component of one of the spondyloarthritides such as ankylosing spondylitis. It is not a mechanical problem, though it is mentioned here to differentiate it from sacroiliac stress. Although most common in young men, it may also occur in females. The history, of low backache, alternating sciatica, and morning stiffness which are uninfluenced by exercise, should raise suspicions. Sacroiliac stress tests are positive, and the diagnosis confirmed by the typical features on X-ray and a positive HLA B27 antigen test (Fig. 6.9). Referral to a rheumatologist is advised: spinal flexibility exercises are the mainstay of management.

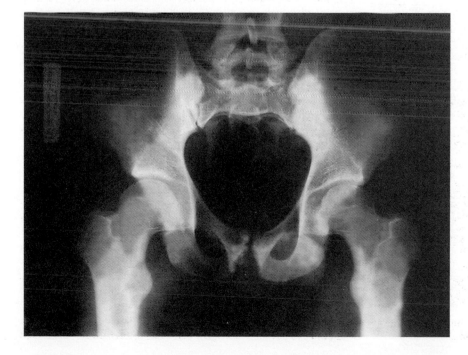

FIG. 6.8 'Osteitis pubis'. These severe erosive changes at the pubic symphysis were found at routine pre-employment screening in a professional soccer player. The player incidentally denied any past history of groin pain, and was asymptomatic at the time of examination.

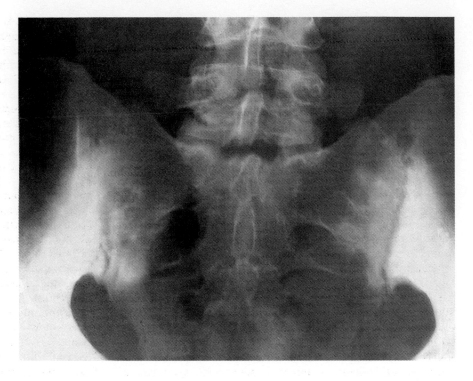

FIG. 6.9 Sacroiliitis: the typical erosive changes associated with sclerosis at the sacroiliac joints.

Sacroiliac stress has a biomechanical aetiology. The shock-absorbing function of the sacroiliac joint may become inadequate as a result of repetitive stress in sports such as the steeplechase in athletics. Although presently there is little supporting evidence, it is possible that muscle imbalance may play a part—for instance, greater strength of the rectus femoris and relative weakness of the gluteals, giving rise to chronic anterior rotational strain. Discomfort is felt typically over the SIJ, radiating through the buttock to the thigh and lower leg, and commonly also to the groin. Unlike the inflammatory condition of sacroiliitis, the symptoms are aggravated by exercise and arise progressively earlier during exercise as the condition worsens. Stress tests are painful, and X-rays reveal increased sclerosis (though no other changes) around the SIJs. Serological testing is negative. Intra-articular steroid injections may be helpful. However, reduced stress is necessary for some months, and muscle imbalance requires correction if present.

Conjoined tendon strain. The conjoined tendon is formed principally from the inferior fibres of the internal oblique and the aponeurosis of the transversalis; it is inserted medially into the pubis, and reinforces the posterior aspect of the superficial inguinal ring. A strain of the medial attachment should be considered with a history of discomfort in the inguinal region, extending to the perineum, felt during and after activity. There are no definite signs on hip movement or resisted muscle contraction. However, there is localized tenderness at the pubic tubercle and in adjacent soft tissues. The integrity of the fibro-muscular components of the walls of the inguinal canal should be assessed specifically; impulse bulge, tenderness, and dilatation of the superficial inguinal ring detected by examination that requires finger invagination of the scrotum indicate the development of Gilmore's groin, in which there is a torn external oblique aponeurosis and a dehiscence between the inguinal ligament and the torn conjoined tendon. X-rays and bone scan are negative. Rest and a steroid injection may help the relatively minor injury, but the more established case requires surgical repair. Occasionally, a frank hernia is detectable by impulse swelling. Inguinal and femoral hernias in athletes should always be referred for surgery, whether symptomatic or otherwise.

Psoas bursitis. This is caused by repetitive hip flexion as in hurdling and in ultramarathon running. Discomfort is localized to the anterior aspect of the groin and thigh and, when severe, may be accompanied by soft tissue swelling. Because of its anatomical proximity to the anterior aspect of the hip, it needs to be differentiated from pathological conditions arising from the hip joint. In psoas bursitis, passive hip flexion is painful because the bursa is squeezed in this position. In addition, other passive movements, such as external rotation, may be uncomfortable, though a non-capsular pattern prevails. Resisted muscle contraction is painless. Tenderness is present over the anterior aspect of the hip. In the less pronounced case, induction of local anaesthesia may be necessary to establish a diagnosis. The addition of steroid is therapeutic: ultrasound also helps.

Hip conditions. 'Sprains' of the hip joint manifesting as synovitis are uncommon, unless accompanied by other pathology—for example, osteoarthritis. When confronted by symptoms and capsular signs suggesting intra-articular pathology, investigation by X-ray and blood tests should be undertaken to exclude conditions which, if unrecognized, are potentially disastrous. Thus Perthes' disease between the ages of five and twelve, slipped femoral epiphysis between twelve and sixteen, and relatively uncommon conditions such as avascular necrosis in the adult should all be considered. Occasionally, inflammatory joint disease, such as that associated with ankylosing spondylitis, is present. In the adult, a 'frozen hip' analogous to 'frozen shoulder' has been described (Chard and Jenner 1988). Nevertheless, synovitis is usually an accompaniment of early degenerative change, and may be caused by excessive exercise.

Hip pain is felt principally in the groin and anterior thigh. Patients commonly fear that discomfort felt over one or both of the greater trochanters ('the hips') indicates hip disease; they need reassurance, should hip pathology be excluded, that this is not the case. The capsular pattern (in which loss of medial rotation is an early feature—see p. 104) is found on examining the passive range of movements in a patient with synovitis of the hip. Resisted muscle contraction is painless. There may be slight tenderness overlying the hip joint. Aspiration for microscopy and culture, erythrocyte sedimentation rate, and white-cell count may be necessary to exclude infection. In the absence of any other significant pathology, an intra-articular steroid injection (on a 'one off' basis) may be useful. Resolution, aided by stress reduction, usually takes place over several months; non-steroidal anti-inflammatory drugs may be tried, though the results are disappointing. Shortwave diathermy may be helpful.

Osteoarthritis (OA) of the hip is a condition that is seen primarily in the over-45s, though it is by no means uncommon in athletic males in their thirties. In the relatively young, this may be due to old Perthes' disease or previous trauma. Although the aetiology is incompletely understood, it is logical to assume that repeated physical stress, probably stemming from childhood, is a major factor. Males who have played team sports such as soccer for many years, particularly at professional level, appear to be at much greater risk than long-distance runners, in whom the increased risk appears minimal. Athletes with symptomatic degenerative disease should be counselled, as the symptoms, and possibly the progression of the condition, may be controlled. However, it is notoriously difficult to prognosticate on either the level of symptomatology or its progression from radiological analysis. Some patients with radiological changes of advanced OA complain of nothing more than a little stiffness; others have pain associated with early degenerative changes only (Fig. 6.10). If there is a history of sharp twinges, a loose body should be considered in the diagnosis.

Established OA increases the likelihood of low back problems. Sports such as squash, which demand repetitive flexion and rotatory movements of the trunk and lower limbs, are particularly demanding on the lumbar spine if hip mobility is reduced. Patients should be encouraged to take up non-weightbearing exercise such as swimming and cycling. In the early case, stretching exercises may be helpful, and a few weeks of treatment by shortwave diathermy may give relief for a longer period of time.

Nerve entrapment: the lateral cutaneous nerve of the thigh. Entrapment may occur at the level at which the nerve passes under the lateral aspect of the inguinal ligament; repetitive pressure or direct trauma is the usual cause in athletes. Paraesthesiae and numbness are felt over the anterolateral aspect of the thigh; this condition is known as *meralgia paraesthetica*. There is no motor involvement, and spontaneous resolution is anticipated.

Gluteal bursitis. Haemorrhagic bursitis has been recorded, possibly secondary to muscle trauma. More commonly, gluteal bursitis is due to overuse, and occurs particularly in long-distance runners. It is more common in the mature athlete. Discomfort is felt in the buttock, with occasional reference to the posterior thigh, and is most troublesome after exercise. Prolonged sitting often is very uncomfortable. Examination reveals what Cyriax has labelled 'the sign of the buttock': pain on both passive hip flexion and on the straight leg raise test (Cyriax 1982). There may be discomfort on performing other passive hip movements, though in no particular pattern. Resisted muscle contraction is usually painless. Deep tenderness is usually present, though it may be difficult to find.

Gluteal bursitis is a difficult condition to treat. Deep frictions, ultrasound, laser therapy, and localized injections may all be tried. Reduction of exercise intensity is required, and a flexibility programme for the hip joint and the hip extensor muscles in particular is instituted.

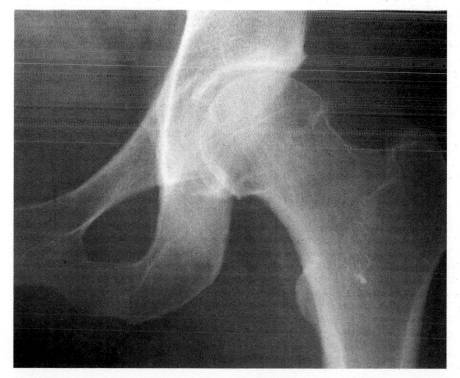

FIG. 6.10 Osteoarthritis of the hip: the typical early features of narrowing of the joint space, subchondral sclerosis, and osteophytes.

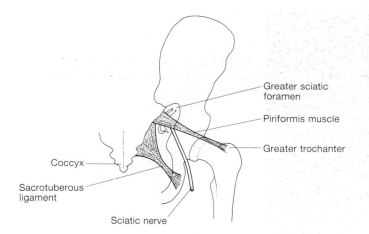

FIG. 6.11 Posterior view of the pelvis: in the piriformis syndrome, tenderness may be detected on palpation of the muscle medial to the greater trochanter.

Piriformis syndrome. This condition is probably due to stretching and tearing of fibres of the piriformis muscle (Kirkaldy-Willis 1983). Pain is felt in the buttock and posterior thigh. On isometric contraction of the external rotators, pain and weakness are found. Tenderness is present on palpation of the muscle medial to the greater trochanter (Fig. 6.11). Marked tenderness of the muscle may also be detected by rectal or vaginal palpation just medial to the ischial spine. Treatment is by localized injection of local anaesthetic and deep transverse friction massage, subsequently progressing to graded stretching exercises. In the past, the author has not recognized the existence of the condition as frequently as it is purported to occur in a number of other texts.

Trochanteric bursitis. This is a common condition, usually an overuse injury, and is found in both young and old. It is prevalent particularly in long-distance runners and in ballet dancers. Discomfort is felt in the lateral buttock and trochanteric region, and is often referred to the posterolateral thigh. Examination

reveals a full painless range of passive movements of the hip except for pain on adduction in flexion. The iliotibial tract may be shown to be taut on Ober's test, in which passive adduction in 0° hip flexion is assessed in the side-lying position (Fig. 6.12). There is no pain on resisted muscle contraction. Tenderness is extremely well localized to the superolateral aspect of the greater tuberosity. Although conventional physiotherapeutic modalities may be employed, there tends to be a better response to localized steroid injections—for example, 10 mg of triamcinolone hexacetonide mixed with 4 ml of 1 per cent lignocaine, combined with regular stretching exercises for the iliotibial tract (see Fig. 11.14, p. 208). The cause of trochanteric bursitis in ballet dancers may be training regimes which favour flexibility in abduction, external rotation, and flexion (Reid *et al.* 1987). A more balanced stretching programme, which includes adduction and medial rotation flexibility exercises, may be necessary.

Gluteal trigger point. Myofascial pain associated with deep tenderness in the buttock (frequently referred to as a TP—trigger point—when the tenderness is exquisite) may be a manifestation of secondary hyperalgesia. The primary site of dysfunction is usually the low lumbar spine, sometimes the sacroiliac joint. Although common enough in the population at large, and certainly not specific to the sporting community, secondary hyperalgesia should always enter the differential diagnosis of buttock pain in the athlete.

The cardinal features are pain on gluteal stretch (combined hip flexion, adduction, and—importantly—external rotation), localized tenderness (sometimes with a 'jump' sign), and palpable muscle hypertonus. The FABER test—in which external rotation is again an important component (see 'examination of the pelvis')—may be painful. The muscle tenderness is often laterally disposed, not uncommonly adjacent to the greater trochanter. Accurate localization, however, will differentiate from trochanteric bursitis. Differentiation from piriformis spasm is made by noting discomfort on stretching the flexed, adducted thigh into external rotation rather than into internal rotation. Trigger point therapy includes deep ('ischaemic') pressure, IMS (intramuscular stimulation with an acupuncture needle), injection of

FIG. 6.12 The position of the examiner and patient on performing Ober's test (assessment of tautness of the iliotibial tract) is demonstrated.

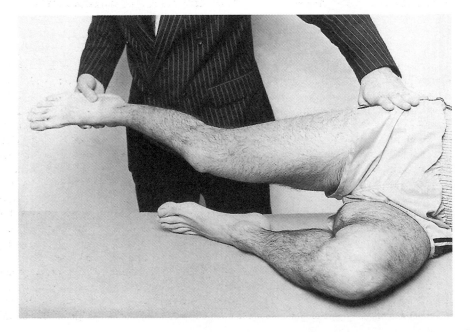

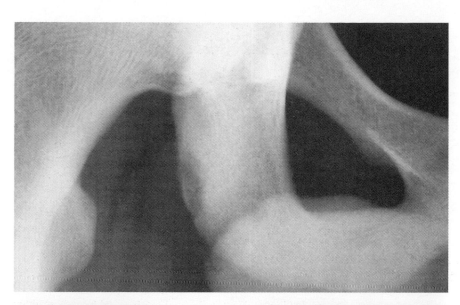

FIG. 6.13 Pelvic X-ray revealing an ischial erosion due to stress at the hamstring origin.

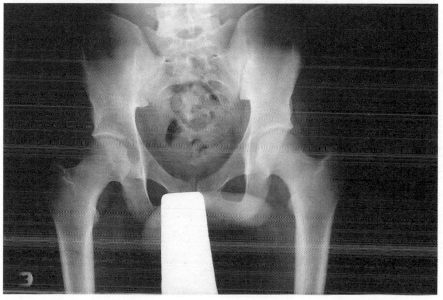

local anaesthetic, and, importantly, stretching exercises. A search for a primary site of dysfunction in the lower back, and its subsequent management, is essential for successful treatment.

Ischial bursitis. This is a friction bursitis, and does not occur too often in athletes. In the same region, a *chronic strain of the origin of the hamstrings* from the ischial tuberosity is more common. In this condition, discomfort is felt in the inferior buttock and posterior thigh, and must be differentiated from sciatic root pain. Both are painful on straight leg raise. In hamstring-origin strain, however, some degree of weakness and discomfort on resisted knee flexion will be found. In addition, localized tenderness is present. Occasionally, an acute tear at the origin fails to settle adequately, and develops into a more chronic injury. Alternatively, overload, and/or excessive stretching of the hamstrings, may give rise to a traction injury. X-rays are usually negative, though they occasionally reveal a localized erosion in the tuberosity (Fig. 6.13). Diagnostic ultrasound and bone scanning may be helpful to differentiate from sciatic root irritation. Surgical excision of granulomatous and fibrotic tissue at the muscle origin may be required to promote healing.

Puranen and Orava (1988) have coined the term 'hamstring syndrome' to describe a condition of persistent pain felt over the inferior buttock and radiating down the back of the thigh, which resulted from tight tendinous structures within the hamstring attachment to the ischial tuberosity. Surgical division of these structures resulted in complete relief in fifty-two out of fifty-nine patients. They suggested that the condition may be secondary to excessive stretching.

The differentiation from sciatic pain is worthy of further comment. Occasionally, a situation arises when an athlete is disabled by exercise-related posterior thigh pain, though examination reveals no definite signs. Diagnostic caudal epidural injections of procaine may be required to assist in the diagnosis. Students of musculoskeletal medicine used to be taught that chronic hamstring pathology does not exist, and that posterior thigh pain should be considered to be sciatica unless proved

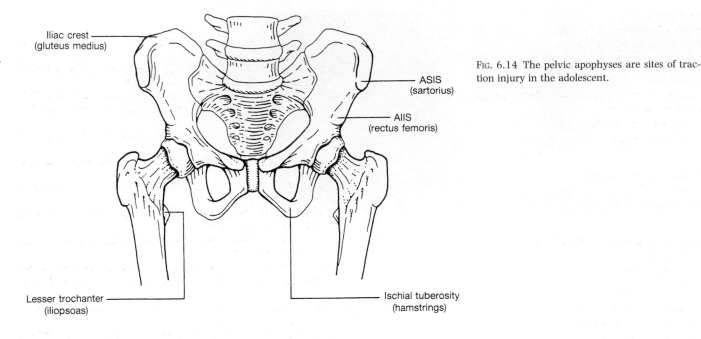

Iliac crest
(gluteus medius)

ASIS
(sartorius)

AIIS
(rectus femoris)

Lesser trochanter
(iliopsoas)

Ischial tuberosity
(hamstrings)

FIG. 6.14 The pelvic apophyses are sites of traction injury in the adolescent.

otherwise. Clearly, in athletic injury, this is not the case. Taking a thorough history is desirable, as an acute incident may be recalled by the athlete when the hamstring is at fault.

Adolescent injuries. The apophyses of the pelvis are sites of traction injury in the adolescent (Fig. 6.14). The patho-anatomical lesion is basically an avulsion fracture (traction separation) of the apophysis (Metzmaker and Pappas 1985). Injuries occur at the following sites:

iliac crest—origin of gluteus medius and oblique abdominal muscles
ASIS—origin of sartorius
AIIS—origin of straight head of rectus femoris
ischial tuberosity—origin of hamstrings (see Fig. 1.13, p. 13)
lesser trochanter—insertion of iliopsoas.

Avulsion results from the same intrinsic stress (vigorous muscle contraction during lengthening) that causes intramuscular injury in the adult. The signs on examination are those of acute injury to a contractile structure: restricted passive stretch, and pain on resisted contraction of the affected muscle. Localized tenderness and firm swelling are found: X-rays confirm. These injuries heal quickly, and almost invariably without complications. The length of time required for healing prior to resumption of early training is approximately four to six weeks.

Summary of examination procedures

Initially a suitable examination of the thoracolumbar junction and lumbar spine should be undertaken to determine any loss of segmental mobility or exacerbation of pain on movement (see Chapter 5).

Examination of the pelvis

Gait
Antalgic
Trendelenburg

Standing
- Observation of the relative heights of ASIS and PSIS
- Sacroiliac mobility (gliding of ilium):
  - loss of ipsilateral downward movement of the PSIS on hip flexion occurs when the SIJ is 'hypomobile' (see Fig. 5.11, p. 96)
  - ipsilateral PSIS is higher on flexion of the trunk when 'hypomobile'
- active weightbearing hip movements
  - squat (hip flexion)
  - groin stretch (abduction)

- cough impulse (inguinal hernia)

Supine
Passive hip movements:
- flexion
- abduction in flexion
- adduction
- medial rotation in 45° flexion
- lateral rotation in 45° flexion
- FABER test—combined flexion, abduction, and external rotation, with the heel resting on the contralateral knee

Sacroiliac stress:
- backward pressure on ASISs
- passive adduction and axial compression of the flexed hip

Sacroiliac mobility (sitting up with legs outstretched and leaning forward). This is also a test for neural tension
- Piedallu sign: PSIS is elevated ipsilaterally on leaning forward when the SIJ is hypomobile (Piedallu 1952)
- apparent leg-length inequality in the supine position, reversed in the sitting position, is noted when the SIJ is hypomobile. Discomfort in the lower back or leg, particularly with superadded neck flexion, indicates neural tension

Resisted muscle contraction (hip):
- flexors
- abductors

- adductors
- medial rotators (in flexion)
- lateral rotators (in flexion)
- abdominals (bilateral SLR/sit up)

Tenderness:
- pubic symphysis/pubic tubercle/conjoined tendon (± defect)
- puboischial rami
- anterior aspect of hip joint
- adductor origin and muscle belly

Prone

Passive hip movements:
- extension
- medial rotation
- lateral rotation

Resisted muscle contraction (hip):
- extensors
- medial rotators
- lateral rotators

Resisted muscle contraction (knee):
- extensors (quadriceps)
- flexors (hamstrings)

Tenderness:
- overlying SIJ
- lateral sacral margin
- gluteal
- ischial tuberosity

Side-lying

- iliotibial tract tautness: the degree of adduction of the hip under gravity (Ober's test)
- tenderness of the tensor fascia lata, trochanteric bursa, and proximal lateral femur (insertion of gluteus medius)

References

Adams, R. J. and Chandler, F. A. (1953). Osteitis pubis of traumatic aetiology. *J. Bone Jt. Surg.*, **35A**, 658.

Chard, M. D. and Jenner, J. R. (1988). The frozen hip: an underdiagnosed condition. *Br. Med. J.*, **297** (6648), 596.

Colachis, S. C., Warden, R. E., Bechtol, C. O., and Strohm, B. R. (1963). Movement of the sacroiliac joint in the adult male. *Arch. Phys. Med. Rehabil.*, **44**, 490.

Cyriax, J. (1982). *Textbook of orthopaedic medicine*, Vol. 1 (8th edn). Baillière Tindall, London.

Grieve, G. P. (1976). The sacroiliac joint. *Physiotherapy*, **62** (12), 384–400.

Harris, N. H. and Murray, R. G. (1974). Lesions of the symphysis in athletes. *Br. Med. J.*, **4**, 211–14.

Kirkaldy-Willis, W. H. (1983). *Managing low back pain*, pp. 96–7. Churchill Livingstone, Edinburgh.

Lewit, K. (1985). *Manipulative therapy in rehabilitation of the motor system*. Butterworth, London.

Martens, M. A., Hansen, L., and Mulier, J. C. (1987). Adductor tendinitis and musculus rectus abdominis tendopathy. *Am. J. Sports Med.*, **15** (4), 353–6.

Metzmaker, J. N. and Pappas, A. M. (1985). Avulsion fractures of the pelvis *Am. J. Sports Med.*, **13**, 349–58.

Muckle, D. S. (1982). Associated factors in recurrent groin and hamstring injuries. *Br. J. Sports Med.*, **16** (1), 37–9.

Piedallu, P. (1952). *Problèmes sacro-iliaques*. Homme Sain, no. 2. Bière Édition, Bordeaux.

Puranen, J. and Orava, S. (1988). The hamstring syndrome. *Am. J. Sports Med.*, **16** (5), 517–21.

Reid, D. C., Burnham, R. S., Saboe, L. A., and Kushner, S. F. (1987). Lower extremity flexibility patterns in classical ballet dancers. *Am. J. Sports Med.*, **15**, 347–52.

Schaberg, J. E., Harper, M. C., and Allen, W. C. (1984). The snapping hip syndrome. *Am. J. Sports Med.*, **12**, 361–5.

Symeonides, P. P. (1972). Isolated traumatic rupture of the adductor longus muscle of the thigh. *Clin. Orthop. Relat. Res.*, **88**, 64–6.

Weisl, H. (1955). The movements of the sacroiliac joint. *Acta Anat.*, **23**, 80–91.

Williams, J. G. P. (1978). Limitation of hip joint movement as a factor in traumatic osteitis pubis. *Br. J. Sports Med.*, **12** (3), 129–33.

7 Injuries to the knee joint

M. A. HUTSON

In this chapter, acute injuries to the knee joint are considered; overuse problems are dealt with in Chapter 9. The majority of acute knee injuries presenting to the sports physician result from a valgus and/or twisting strain. Most commonly they involve the medial joint structures and the anterior cruciate ligament, which has a crucial role in the functional integrity of the tibiofemoral joint. Other types of strain exist, however, so that no ligament is exempt from injury. The menisci and patellofemoral joint mechanism are also frequent sites of injury. The use of the arthroscope for diagnostic and therapeutic purposes has improved knowledge and aided management considerably in acute knee injuries. Magnetic resonance imaging is another useful investigative tool. However, it should not be assumed that all painful knee conditions which give rise to an effusion warrant arthroscopy or expensive imaging. Although recognition of the different types of ligamentous instability demands some experience, it should be within the capabilities of the sports physician to make a provisional diagnosis in the 'acute knee' and to determine when referral to a specialist knee surgeon is necessary. A thorough examination regime should be adopted for all patients, and this is summarized at the end of the chapter.

Applied anatomy and biomechanics

The *tibiofemoral joint* is a modified hinge joint that allows a restricted amount of gliding and rotation in addition to flexion/extension. Lateral rotation of the tibia takes place in the 'screw-home' mechanism at the extreme of extension. The synovium communicates with many of the bursae around the joint, and is so arranged internally that the cruciate ligaments are extrasynovial. Folds of synovium known as 'plicae' are present in most knees, and are classified as suprapatellar, mediopatellar, or infrapatella (Hardaker *et al.* 1980). When traumatized, a plica may become symptomatic and give rise to a condition known as the plica syndrome (see Chapter 9).

The menisci are attached to the tibia, held in place peripherally by the coronary (meniscotibial) ligaments. They act as shock-absorbers, dispersing stress over the articular cartilage, and make the joint surfaces more congruent (Fig. 7.1). Together with the collateral and cruciate ligaments, they play an important part in the provision of stability to the knee: the combination of meniscectomy and anterior cruciate ligament loss is often disastrous with respect to functional instability, and leads to early degenerative change.

The medial (tibial) collateral ligament (MCL) is composed of a superficial layer and a deep layer (the medial capsular ligament) (Fig. 7.2). It is strengthened further by the posterior oblique liga-

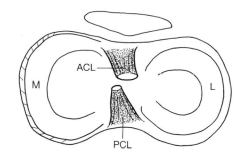

FIG. 7.1 Right tibial plateau from above: the lateral meniscus is circular and is not attached to the capsule, and the medial meniscus is C-shaped and is attached to the capsule and medial ligament: ACL, attachment of anterior cruciate ligament; PCL, attachment of posterior cruciate ligament.

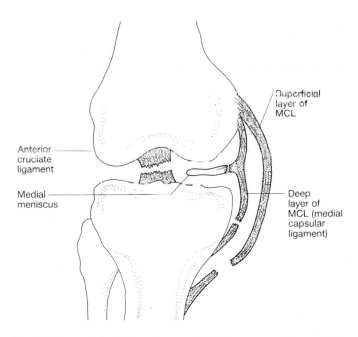

FIG. 7.2 The medial collateral ligament (MCL) is composed of superficial and deep layers. O'Donoghue's triad is shown: rupture of MCL and ACL, and tear of medial meniscus.

ment that merges with the posterior capsule. The superficial layer of the MCL extends from the adductor tubercle of the medial femoral condyle to the tibial metaphysis, approximately 6 cm below the joint line. The deep layer is composed of menis-

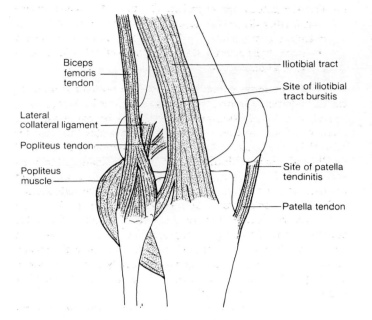

Biceps femoris tendon

Lateral collateral ligament

Popliteus tendon

Popliteus muscle

Iliotibial tract

Site of iliotibial tract bursitis

Site of patella tendinitis

Patella tendon

FIG. 7.3 The lateral ligamentous complex of the knee. The sites of overuse injury also are shown.

cotibial and meniscofemoral elements. The lateral collateral ligament (LCL) is attached superiorly to the lateral femoral epicondyle and inferiorly to the head of the fibula. It is rounded, and may be felt in one's own knee when sitting with the lateral aspect of the ipsilateral ankle resting on the contralateral knee, allowing the thigh to rotate laterally, in which position it is prominent. The lateral ligamentous complex (Fig. 7.3) comprises the LCL reinforced by the iliotibial tract, the biceps femoris tendon, the popliteus tendon, and the arcuate ligament (a thickening of the capsule). The anterior and posterior cruciate ligaments are named by the relationship of their attachments to the tibia (Fig. 7.1). The anterior cruciate ligament (ACL) is composed of an anteromedial and posterolateral bundle positioned in a spiral fashion. The specific functions of the ligaments, as determined by their actions as primary restraints, have been outlined by Marshall and Rubin (1977). A working knowledge helps with interpretation of physical signs, and provides an understanding of the type of instability found upon rupture.

Medial stability is provided initially by the superficial MCL then by the ACL and, in extension, by the posterior capsule. The deep MCL appears to play a minor role.

Lateral stability is provided by the LCL and its associated structures within the lateral ligamentous complex, reinforced by both cruciates.

Anterior stability (that is, restraint against anterior displacement of the tibia on the femur) is provided principally by the ACL.

Posterior stability is provided by the PCL.

Hyperextension stability is provided principally by the ACL, supported by the posterior capsule and PCL.

External rotation stability is provided principally by the superficial MCL and the ACL.

Internal rotation stability is provided by both the ACL and PCL and, to a lesser extent, the lateral supporting structures. In extension, the ACL is the main restraint.

From the foregoing, it can be seen that the anterior cruciate ligament must be taut in most, if not all, positions of the joint. This is explained by the fact that it is a multifascicular structure, with two identifiable portions which are distinguishable both anatomically and functionally. The anteromedial bundle is taut in flexion and is the primary restraint to anterior stress, whereas the posterolateral bundle is taut in extension.

The *patellofemoral joint*. The main biomechanical function of the patella is to increase the effective lever arm of the quadriceps in effecting knee extension, or resisting knee flexion, by distancing the patella tendon from the axis of movement (Hungerford and Barry 1979). It allows the components of the quadriceps muscle to act under as stable a situation as possible in the intercondylar groove of the femur, thereby functioning effectively as a frictionless pulley. The articular cartilage on the back of the patella withstands high compression loads—stresses that tendon is poorly designed to withstand (Ficat and Hungerford 1977). It has been estimated that a pressure of seven times body-weight is exerted upon the patellofemoral joint during a deep knee bend (Cailliet 1983). A similar pressure may be applied on *descending* stairs, compared with a twofold increase on ascending stairs. The patella also protects the anterior aspect of the tibiofemoral joint from direct trauma.

Studies on patellofemoral loading reveal different contact areas on the patella facets in different degrees of flexion (Goodfellow *et al.* 1976; see also Fig. 9.6, p. 155). The overall contact area is increased with greater degrees of flexion. It is of some significance that extension resistance exercises performed in the sitting position (that is, from knee flexion to extension) have been shown to load the articular cartilage in a non-physiological fashion. However, loading in extension—that is, straight leg raising against resistance—creates no patellofemoral compression and provides the basis for strengthening exercises in patellofemoral problems (see Chapter 11, Quadriceps femoris exercises, p. 200).

Stability of the patella is provided by the vastus medialis (or vastus medialis obliquus (VMO)) and the congruency between the lateral patella facet and the articular surface of the lateral femoral condyle (Wiberg 1941). The Q-angle (see Fig. 9.5, p. 155) is the angle between the quadriceps muscle (measured by a line from the anterior superior iliac spine to the midpoint of the patella) and the patella tendon (measured from the midpoint of the patella to the tibial tubercle). The normal range is stated to be 13°–18°. An increase in the Q-angle is often associated with patellofemoral disorders.

Haemarthrosis

It is essential to distinguish clinically between a haemarthrosis and a serous joint effusion. The initial clue lies in the history: swelling that occurs within an hour or two of injury, giving rise to a feeling of joint tightness, is most likely due to bleeding—that is, a haemarthrosis. By contrast, a joint effusion develops overnight, and is noticed by the patient the morning after injury. The size of the joint swelling is another factor—a haemarthrosis is a tense joint containing up to 100 ml of blood. Unless the patient has a chronic or recurring rheumatological problem, a serous effusion associated with osteochondritis dissecans or a torn meniscus for instance is much smaller.

When haemarthrosis of the knee results from acute injury in sport, the likely diagnoses are rupture of the ACL, peripheral meniscus tear, or patella dislocation. Of these the most common is ACL rupture. Noyes *et al.* (1980) found that ACL rupture occurred in 72 per cent of cases of traumatic haemarthrosis without significant collateral ligament injury on clinical examination. Clues to the nature of the intra-articular pathology may be obtained from the history—for example, recognition by the patient of patella dislocation and relocation. A 'pop' from within the joint may be experienced if the ACL tears. Clinical examination is followed by X-rays looking particularly for evidence of osteochondral injury to the patella, when small avulsed fragments may be observed (see Fig. 10.16, p. 187), and for evidence of avulsion fracture of the distal attachment of the ACL to the tibia. Management strategies are dependent upon establishment of the underlying cause of the haemarthrosis. Aspiration may be performed for confirmation of the haemarthrosis and/or for patient comfort. The presence of fat globules within the aspirate indicates an intra-articular fracture.

In the differential diagnosis of a swollen knee due to trauma, the presence of substantial soft tissue swelling may indicate that the joint derangement includes collateral ligament (and therefore capsular) rupture, allowing extravasation of blood into the subcutaneous tissues. ACL rupture remains the most likely diagnosis when the examiner is faced with traumatic haemarthrosis (and therefore with an intact capsule) and negative X-rays.

Patella dislocation

Lateral dislocation of the patella is usually caused by valgus stress to the knee. Although it is often an isolated injury, it may be associated with more extensive derangements of the knee joint such as MCL tear. Normally, patients are taken to the nearest Accident and Emergency department, particularly when relocation has not occurred spontaneously. However, relocation often occurs before medical attention is sought, and the patient presents with a history of valgus or rotational stress, pain over the anterior aspect of the knee, and swelling. The presence of a haemarthrosis is noted, and signs of recent patellofemoral (PF) trauma (due to osteochondral injury) are present.

1. Manipulation of the patella provokes discomfort.
2. There is marked tenderness along the length of the medial retinaculum that has torn during lateral dislocation.
3. Attempts at gentle laterally directed pressure upon the patella evoke discomfort and apprehension.
4. There is tenderness of the medial margin of the medial articular facet of the patella.

If the injury was ignored or unrecognized initially, and the patient presents some weeks or months afterwards, the signs of *patellofemoral dysfunction* may still be present.

(a) Positive patella compression. Manual compression of the patella against the femur is painful.
(b) Tenderness on palpating the margins of the patella facets, particularly the medial facet. This should be differentiated from adjacent tenderness, which is more likely to indicate a painful plica or resolving retinaculitis.
(c) Positive Clarke's sign. Contraction of the quadriceps while the examiner presses the patella into the trochlea causes pain. It is an insensitive test.
(d) Pain on attempting the squat position may be helpful in identifying PF pain when other tests are largely negative. It is unnecessarily painful for confirmation in recent injury or in PF arthritis.

(e) Positive patella apprehension. The patient is apprehensive that further dislocation or subluxation will occur when the examiner exerts a laterally directed force on the patella with the knee slightly flexed. It is pathognomonic of patella instability, or at least recent dislocation.

A thorough examination of the tibiofemoral joint is made to exclude additional injury. Further assessment is by X-rays—AP, lateral, and patella (skyline) views should be requested. The presence of an intra-articular fragment indicates the need for referral for a surgical opinion. The combination of a relocated patella and a haemarthrosis may otherwise be managed by joint aspiration followed by application of a POP cylinder, from groin to ankle, for three weeks, to allow the torn medial retinaculum to heal. For aspiration, a 50 ml syringe and a 20 G 2- inch needle are required. Although there are a number of suitable puncture sites, including the suprapatellar pouch and over the lateral joint line, a recommended and reliable route is the medial approach. The needle is inserted approximately 1 cm posterior to the midpoint of the medial border of the patella and directed laterally (see Fig. 12.21, p. 230).

Physiotherapy is instituted after cast removal. The emphasis initially is on isometric muscle contraction and range of motion exercises. Considerable care is taken not to introduce isotonic exercises too quickly, to reduce the risk of chronic patellofemoral pain.

Tears of quadriceps expansion and patella tendon

Complete loss of extensor function results from a tear of the quadriceps expansion, a complete tear of the patella tendon (syn. quadriceps tendon, infrapatellar tendon, patella ligament), or a transverse fracture of the patella. The mechanism is the same as that causing quadriceps muscle-belly tear: vigorous contraction, usually against resistance, from the flexed position, or on stumbling forwards onto the knee. The supportive function of the quadriceps in the stance phase is lost and the leg collapses. Diagnosis is normally straightforward, as straight leg raise is impossible. Loss of muscle strength is due to intrinsic muscle dysfunction, and not pain inhibition. There may be a palpable gap at the level of the tear or fracture, though surrounding soft tissue swelling may obscure this. When the patella tendon is ruptured, X-rays often reveal a 'high-riding' patella (see Fig. 10.5, p. 181). Surgical referral is indicated.

Medial collateral ligament injury

The commonest injury to the knee is to the MCL, resulting from the combination of valgus and external rotation force. In certain sports such as alpine skiing and rugby football, MCL sprain represents a significant proportion of recorded lower limb injuries. It represents 25 per cent of all recorded alpine ski injuries in some statistical surveys. External rotational forces are magnified by the presence of the attached ski, invoking risk of injury despite improvements in binding-release in recent years (see Fig. 1.7, p. 5). A common cause is 'catching an inside edge'. External rotation is then augmented by reduction in speed and altered direction of the ski, whilst forward body momentum remains unchecked. In rugby football, a blow to the lateral aspect of the knee in a tackle creates a valgus stress to the medial aspect of the joint.

There are three grades of MCL injury.

Grade I: Sprain of the superficial MCL in which there is no demonstrable laxity.

Grade II: Partial tear of the superficial MCL in which laxity may be demonstrated though the deep layer is intact (a firm end-point on valgus stress in 30° flexion).

Grade III: Complete tear of the MCL, involving both superficial and deep layers. A mushy end-point is felt on valgus stress in 30° flexion; frequently over 15° of laxity is present.

The secondary restraints against medial instability—the ACL and the posterior capsule with the knee extended—may also be injured. Therefore, examination of the knee includes relevant tests for the PF joint, the cruciate and collateral ligaments, and both menisci, as indicated in the examination summary at the end of the chapter. The significant findings in MCL injury are described further.

Grade I injury

There is no effusion or it is minimal. A full range of movement is found, with discomfort only at the extreme of flexion. On stressing the MCL in 30° flexion, there is discomfort, though no instability. Tenderness and minimal soft tissue swelling are present at the site of the sprain (usually the femoral attachment). Treatment by anti-inflammatory modalities, maintenance of dynamic stabilization by resisted quadriceps contraction, and early range of motion exercise may be instituted without the need for structural support. Immobilization, for instance in a splint which restricts knee flexion, is contraindicated.

Grade II injury

The signs on examination depend upon the length of time which has elapsed since the injury. The traumatic synovitis causes a small effusion and restriction (to 90°) of passive flexion of the knee, maximal on day 2, resolving over ten days. Extension initially is uncomfortable. The knee is stable to valgus stress in extension. In 30° flexion, there is medial laxity of 10°–15° (increased medial joint opening up to 10 mm) with a firm painful end-point. There is a small swelling, approximately the size of a half walnut, overlying the tear, usually at the femoral attachment. Tenderness is localized to the tear; diffuse tenderness along the whole length of the MCL is more likely to indicate grade III injury. Quadriceps wasting is not as profound as when the knee is locked, though it is sufficient to warrant isometric exercises as soon as passive extension is comfortable. X-ray examination is advisable, and in the child may be combined with stress films to detect epiphyseal injury.

Management principles are common to collateral ligament injuries at both knee and ankle. The combination of functional support for acute ligamentous instability and early mobilization are the cornerstones of therapy. An ambulatory cast-brace may be used: a suitable arrangement is a thigh cast connected through medial and lateral knee hinges to a lower leg cast that in turn is connected to a plastic heel cup (see Fig. 12.1, p. 204). Thereby valgus/varus and rotational movement at the knee are controlled. This should be maintained for three weeks, and then the cast-brace should be removed and the patient referred for flexibility, strengthening, and proprioceptive exercises.

In a less severe grade II injury, crutches may be used for several days, during which time range of motion exercises are instituted and isometric quadriceps contraction commences as soon as possible (within 48 hours). Local therapeutic measures include the use of ice and ultrasound. Normally, isometric contraction against resistance is commenced within a few days. A cycling programme may be started as soon as a full range of motion has been regained (usually inside a week), and isokinetic exercise soon afterwards. A progressive rehabilitation programme is continued until full power and endurance have been regained.

If mobilization following grade II injury is allowed to take place without functional support, there is a risk of the development of ectopic calcification at the site of the injury—namely, the femoral attachment of the MCL (see Fig. 9.10, p. 149). This condition, the Pelligrini–Steida syndrome, is associated with mild laxity of the MCL and may be intermittently painful. However, it usually responds to localized steroid injections. When untreated or unrecognized, the presence of MCL laxity increases the likelihood of further injury, and when combined with ACL rupture it often results in functional instability.

Grade III injury

This may be an isolated injury, although frequently it is associated with medial meniscus tear, ACL tear, or patella dislocation (Fig. 7.2). The patient is aware of significant functional disturbance, and finds that the knee tends to give way unless locked into extension. Diffuse swelling due to bleeding and oedema forms periarticularly. The additional features which suggest a complete tear are an empty feeling—that is, a mushy end-point—on performing the valgus stress test in 30° flexion. However, the knee is stable in full extension, unless the posterior cruciate or posterior capsule has been disrupted. Tenderness is often felt along the entire length of the MCL.

If stress X-rays in valgus are taken, medial laxity is found to be 15° or more. Referral should be made to an orthopaedic surgeon for further management. A surgical approach is usually chosen, although cast immobilization alone for four to six weeks is an alternative management. A peripheral meniscus tear is often associated with complete MCL rupture. Therefore, a minimal therapeutic requirement is a period of immobilization sufficient to allow healing of a secondary structure. Intensive physiotherapy follows (see under ACL tears below).

Anterior cruciate ligament tears

Recognition of the incidence of ACL tears has been facilitated by the widespread use of arthroscopy and/or MRI (see Fig. 10.18(a), p. 178). It is a common injury, though frequently missed by inexperienced clinicians (Noyes *et al.* 1985). Unfortunately, it gives rise to considerable morbidity following initial injury, followed by a significantly increased risk of symptomatic instability and early joint degeneration. A study of the restraining function of the ACL allows an understanding of the biomechanical stresses which are involved in the acute tear. The two commonest situations are first rotational stress applied to the flexed knee, and secondly excessive hyperextension. There are a number of sports in which flexion–rotation stress is common, particularly when the participant descends from a jump and is then jostled, either 'legally' or 'illegally', as, for example, in soccer, rugby, netball, and basketball. ACL tears are also common in skiing. Sometimes a 'popping' sensation is experienced at the moment of injury. Rapid onset of swelling (haemarthrosis) is a further feature.

Assessment of the injury, following the history, is made by a full examination of the knee. Positive physical signs in the acute case are as follows.

1. The presence of a haemarthrosis.

2. The signs of an intense traumatic synovitis: passive flexion restricted to approximately 90° and loss of full extension. This pseudolocking in, for example, 10° of flexion mimics the true locking found in bucket-handle tears of the medial meniscus, and may not be differentiated fully until arthroscopy.

3. Positive Lachman's test. Anterior displacement of the tibia is detected in approximately 10° of flexion (Fig. 7.4). This test relies on the ability of the physician to grasp the patient's thigh above the knee with one hand and the lower leg just below the tibial tuberosity with the other, and thus is not easy for doctors

with small hands or in patients of heavy build. Alternatively, it can be performed with both hands cupping the upper calf and an assistant stabilizing the thigh.

4. Positive pivot shift or jerk test (Hughston *et al.* 1976; Ireland and Trickey 1980). Demonstration of anterolateral instability depends on anterior subluxation of the lateral tibial plateau (Fig. 7.5). This is a rotatory movement. The patient's leg is rotated internally, and a valgus force applied to the knee. Passive flexion and extension are then performed. A positive pivot shift is recorded by a thud when the lateral tibial plateau is relocated when passing from the fully extended position through approximately 20° flexion. A positive jerk test relies on manoeuvring the knee from flexion into extension: at approximately 20°, a jerk is recorded when subluxation and then relocation are felt and observed. The test is facilitated by forward pressure on the fibula head by the examiner's thumb (Fig. 7.6). The critical degree of flexion is the one at which the function of the iliotibial band changes from a restraint to flexion to a restraint to

FIG. 7.4 (a) The positions of the examiner and patient when performing Lachman's test are demonstrated. (b) The position of the examiner's hands is shown.

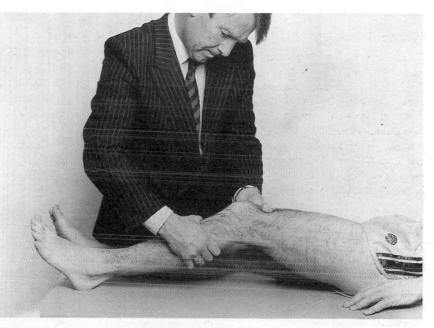

(a)

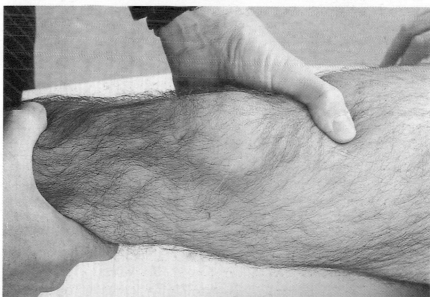

(b)

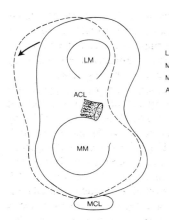

FIG. 7.5 Anterior subluxation of the lateral tibial plateau occurs in anterolateral (rotatory) instability.

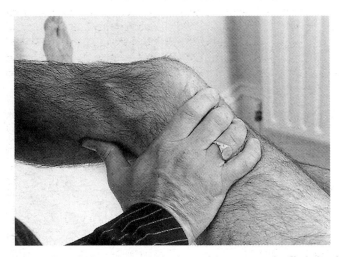

FIG. 7.6 The jerk test is facilitated by forward pressure on the fibula head by the examiner's thumb.

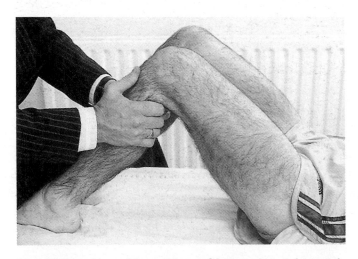

FIG. 7.7 The positions of the examiner and patient when performing the anterior and posterior drawer tests in 90° knee flexion are demonstrated.

extension (or vice versa). Positive Lachman's and jerk tests are usually obtainable in the acute knee with careful handling of the patient. They are pathognomonic of ACL deficiency.

5. Positive anterior drawer sign at 90° flexion (Fig. 7.7). The anterior drawer test, performed with the knee in 90° flexion (maintained by sitting on the patient's feet) and the tibia in neutral rotation, assesses the integrity of the ACL. An abnormal degree of anterior laxity, due to anterior subluxation of the *lateral* tibial plateau, indicates ACL insufficiency. This laxity is also present in external rotation of the tibia, though it is reduced in internal rotation. Interpretation may not always be clear-cut, however. It is sometimes difficult to decide whether anteroposterior instability is due to a positive posterior drawer sign (indicating injury to the posterior cruciate ligament) or to a positive anterior drawer sign. Anterior subluxation of the *medial* tibial plateau with the tibia in neutral (anteromedial instability) indicates MCL injury; this is accentuated when the anterior drawer test is performed with the tibia in external rotation. It is accentuated further by combined ACL and MCL insufficiency.

It should be recognized that an ACL tear is often associated with injury to the menisci or collateral ligaments (Hughston 1983). Therefore, a combination of a grade II or III MCL and an ACL tear is not uncommon. Debate in the past has centred upon whether it is feasible biomechanically for an isolated ACL tear to exist. Although the author believes this to be the case, nevertheless the knee should be examined fully for the existence of other injuries. The coexistence of additional injury increases the likelihood of functional disability at a later stage.

Full assessment necessitates the use of conventional X-rays of the knee prior to consideration of referral for arthroscopy and joint wash-out. X-rays may detect a bony fragment representing avulsion of the distal attachment of the ACL from the tibial intercondylar eminence; a surgical opinion should be sought, as internal fixation is often the treatment of choice. Arthroscopy, if available, is useful to determine the extent of the intra-articular injury: otherwise MRI may be required to confirm the presence of an additional injury such as a meniscus tear. When arthroscopy is used principally for confirmation of diagnosis, it should be borne in mind that preliminary clinical examination may reveal just as much (or more!) information, particularly when the arthroscopist is inexperienced and the cruciate ligaments are poorly visualized.

Management strategy is based on the following facts.

(a) A haemarthrosis requires draining or washing out to facilitate rehabilitation.

(b) Over 50 per cent of patients with ACL deficiency recover sufficiently to participate in sport without surgical intervention (McDaniel and Dameron 1980). However, there is evidence that although the initial functional disability of ACL insufficiency may be minimal, the natural history of the condition is for progressive degenerative change some years later, and for a significantly increased risk of further injury such as meniscus tear (Noyes *et al.* 1983). Thus primary repair has its advocates: however, the consensus of opinion in the UK is to eschew primary repair and to achieve functional stability through intensive rehabilitation.

(c) In recreational athletes, surgical repair or reconstruction should be considered on failure of conservative management after six months—that is, on the presence of the symptoms of functional instability (the knee 'giving away'). In professional sportspeople, the opinion of a knee specialist regarding early surgical management should be sought.

After aspiration, the knee should be given functional support until full extension and adequate quadriceps/hamstring tone have been regained. In this acute phase, there is danger of further damage to the knee. The use of a cast-brace should be considered (Bassett *et al.* 1980); failing this, the use of crutches is advisable for two to three weeks, during which time range of motion and muscle-strengthening exercises are instituted. Initially isometric exercises are emphasized (straight leg raises and sets of static quadriceps contractions). Isotonic exercises for the quadriceps may be started in the seated position when an adequate range of motion has been restored (Fig. 7.8). Repetitions using light weights—for example, 2–5 lbs—are used at the outset; concentric contraction is achieved on slow extension, and eccentric contraction on slow flexion. For rehabilitation of the knee flexors, the patient lies prone or stands, and performs both concentric and eccentric work using a similar range of weights (Fig. 7.9).

The subsequent muscle rehabilitation programme concentrates on the redevelopment in the knee flexors and extensors of strength, power, and endurance. Rapid isotonic repetitions with light weights are necessary to build up power and endurance. Isokinetic exercise may be performed after a few weeks (see Fig. 11.11, p. 203). The capacity of the dynamometer to improve the characteristics of strength (slow speeds—for example, 60° to 90°), power (fast speeds—for example, 240° to 300°), and endurance (repetitions at fast speeds) in both the flexors and extensors makes it a most valuable piece of equipment. In the ACL-deficient knee, it is imperative that the knee flexors (hamstrings) in particular are fully rehabilitated. Inadequate muscle balance in favour of the quadriceps increases the likelihood of functional instability by contributing to anterior subluxation of the tibial plateau.

Subsequently, bicycling, swimming, and then jogging are added to the programme. Care must be taken by the athlete at this stage—around two months after injury—to avoid any cutting movements. Participation in activities including such movements and start–stops should not be allowed until quadriceps and hamstrings are nearly equal in strength to those of the normal limb, and flexion has been restored to full range ± 5°. During rehabilitation, constant evaluation is made, and adaptations to the muscle-strengthening programme are executed if necessary—for example, to accommodate the onset of patello-femoral pain. After sport is resumed, a maintenance programme of exercises should be prescribed to prevent the insidious development of muscle deficit or imbalance. Modification of the intensity of participation in specific types of activity and/or a reduction in competitive standard may be necessary if there are subjective feelings of insecurity or instability.

Established functional instability, manifested by recurrent giving way, pain, and effusion, requires surgical assessment. First, the presence of an associated meniscus tear or mechanical interference by a stump of the ACL should be excluded at arthroscopy. The type of surgical reconstruction for ligamentous

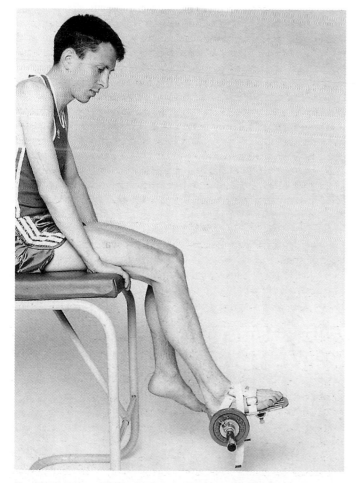
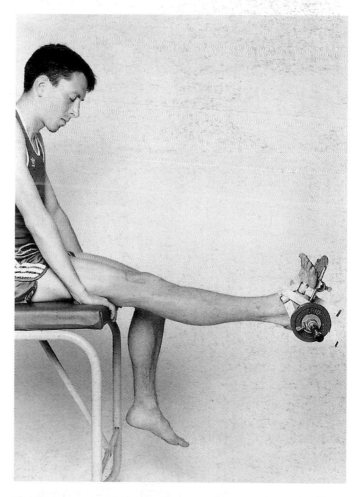

FIG. 7.8 Isotonic exercise for the quadriceps is demonstrated

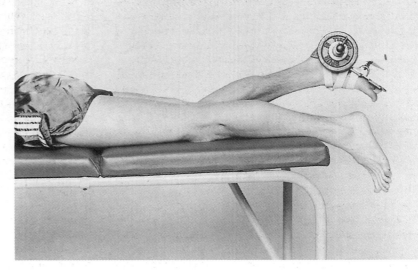

FIG. 7.9 Isotonic exercise for the hamstrings is demonstrated: (right) prone, (below) standing.

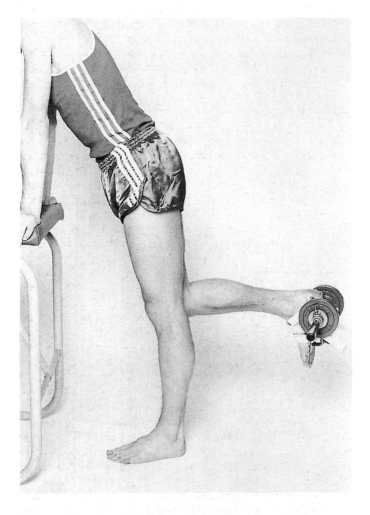

tibial tunnel to the lateral femoral condyle. Paterson and Trickey (1986) have reported good results, and advocate the addition of a MacIntosh extra-articular tenodesis in young sportsmen. An advantage of the use of autografts is the retention of proprioceptive function. A recent vogue is the use of the synthetic material, Gore-tex; an advantage appears to be a reduction of rehabilitation time (although concern is expressed about the presence of intra-articular foreign material). During rehabilitation, the early use of hamstring-strengthening exercises and the cautious use of quadriceps exercises have been advocated by Renstrom *et al.* (1986). The importance of a prolonged well-balanced rehabilitation programme that allows adequate healing and strengthening of the ligament is stressed by Rovere and Adair (1983).

As an alternative to surgery, or in patients who have not benefited from surgery, a knee brace should be considered. Various knee braces are commercially available, including some with derotational constructions such as the Lenox Hill brace (see Fig. 12.2, p. 205). Hunter (1985) states that 'these braces attempt to limit rotation and prevent hyperextension, thereby minimising forward subluxation of the tibia on the femur ... but it is virtually impossible for any brace to mechanically substitute for the function of the cruciate ligaments and prevent excessive rotation of the tibia on the femur ... other braces provide patients with comfort and a feeling of support and serve merely as a reminder to the wearer to exert caution in sport activity.' Normally, surgical reconstruction should be a logical first step in the reversal of functional instability.

Current surgical practice in the management of the torn anterior cruciate ligament—personal view

John Ireland

There has been a considerable increase in the number of operations undertaken in the UK and internationally for knees with a torn or deficient anterior cruciate ligament. However, the management of acute injuries of the ACL, and also of the chronic instability that often follows, remains controversial. The under-

insufficiency depends on the exact nature of the anterior instability. Anterolateral rotatory instability (ALRI) due to isolated ACL rupture, or anteromedial rotatory instability due to a combination of MCL tear and ACL rupture, require different techniques. Autogenous materials such as split grafts from the patella tendon have been used widely for ACL reconstruction; the basic procedure involves passing the graft through a drilled taking of these large numbers of operations by a widening circle of orthopaedic surgeons has, together with a worrying array of new technical possibilities, made the field even more potentially confusing.

Acute ACL rupture is widely recognized as the common cause of knee haemarthrosis resulting from non-contact and contact injury during sporting activities. Even so, the diagnosis is still worryingly elusive in the Accident and Emergency departments of the UK. The diagnosis usually can be made satisfactorily on clinical examination at the time of primary presentation. A positive anterior Lachman sign is the key. Unfortunately this straightforward manoeuvre has not become an established part of the routine clinical examination of injured knees in all circles. If competence in this simple test could be mastered by all front-line physiotherapists, sports injury doctors, and casualty officers, then a far higher proportion of torn anterior cruciate ligaments would be detected at an early stage.

In practice, the popularization of MRI scanning as a means of diagnosis in the injured knee may have had an adverse effect on the refinement of clinical examination skills and acumen. The worrying tendency is the unquestioned acceptance that abnormalities demonstrated by imaging are the cause of the patients' complaints. In order to be of significance, the images must accord with the history and physical signs.

The routine X-ray appearance of the injured knee is usually normal (apart from documentation of the tense haemarthrosis on an under-penetrated lateral view), and the normal appearance may reassure the inexperienced casualty officer, when in fact a caution for the patient, and specialist referral, would be more appropriate.

Aspiration of a knee that is difficult to examine clinically because of tense swelling often facilitates the examination. If haemarthrosis is confirmed in a knee with a normal radiograph, a cruciate ligament injury remains a high probability.

In knees presenting without acute or painful swelling, and which are thus examined more comfortably, the jerk or pivot shift sign must be included. Clinical competence in this test is simple if carried out routinely on large numbers of knees. The test is not difficult to carry out satisfactorily if practised on most knees being examined for any reason.

An informed but conservative approach remains the accepted practice in the UK, when this injury concerns patients whose sporting interests are recreational. Arthroscopy is not generally indicated in the early stages unless there is undue persistence of a block to full extension of the knee or the relatively early development of symptoms which suggest an associated meniscal lesion. Nowadays, it is generally preferred to undertake an MRI scan when meniscal pathology is suspected—it often helps in the planning of a reconstructive procedure, which is being considered. However, if the diagnosis of anterior cruciate injury is clear on clinical grounds, then the MRI scan usually adds little or nothing in the way of useful information concerning the damaged central ligament.

Probably the most important therapeutic event at the outset is the advice for recently injured patients that they should *not* attempt an early return to their sport. This must be delayed until as full a recovery as possible has occurred, and the sporting return should only be made with the approval of an experienced clinician. Premature attempts to return to the football field or tennis court often precipitate early instability when a giving-way episode completes what may have been a partial anterior cruciate rupture or compounds a previously minor meniscal lesion.

When high-class or professional athletes present with an acute anterior cruciate tear, a rather different approach is called for. If their livelihood or lifestyle is threatened by possible instability, early arthroscopy to establish the full diagnosis is advisable. If a worrying degree of instability is confirmed on examination under anaesthesia, primary ligamentous surgery may well have to be considered. Direct repair of a torn anterior cruciate ligament nowadays cannot be supported. Primary reconstructions are usually performed by the same techniques as those used in chronic anterior cruciate instability. Recent technical advances generally have aimed to achieve more secure ligamentous fixation and enabled post-operative immobilization to be largely abandoned, especially in those cases where surgery is undertaken within six weeks of the injury. Even so, problems of so-called arthrofibrosis—an unexpected degree of swelling and stiffness with restricted movement—remain a worry when reconstruction is undertaken during this early phase.

Primary reconstructions may also be indicated where the anterior cruciate ligament is torn in association with a complete rupture of medial structures, in a severe valgus-type injury. In this situation, central reconstruction would be undertaken without surgical repair of the medial ligament, and early mobilization would still be the rule.

In patients presenting with symptoms and signs of chronic knee instability, the high incidence of associated and significant meniscal lesions (75–78 per cent) must be remembered. Some five to ten per cent of these knees will have an asymptomatic posterior peripheral separation of the medial meniscus. These particular meniscal lesions used to be demonstrated clearly by high-quality double-contrast knee arthrograms. Unfortunately, the availability of quality arthrograms is in serious decline, and this particular zone at the meniscal periphery is not well demonstrated by MRI scans which have largely superseded arthrograms. Such meniscal lesions are therefore seen more commonly nowadays arthroscopically, the tip of the telescope being passed through the intercondylar notch to the back of the knee with the view directed medially. These peripheral detachments can usually be repaired by direct open suture through a small posteromedial incision.

There has been a phase of enthusiasm for arthroscopic meniscal suture—nowadays this appears to be in decline in knees with normal ligamentous stability. However, many meniscal lesions are technically repairable by arthroscopic means in knees with anterior cruciate instability, and these meniscal reattachments are generally carried out at the same time as the stabilizing operation. A number of new techniques facilitating the arthroscopic repair have come into practice, but their value in the longer term has yet to be established.

With the widespread improvement of arthroscopic techniques in the knee, open meniscectomy nowadays has no place, especially in the unstable knee. It is not reasonable to remove a torn meniscus by open surgery when there is a considerable chance that it may not relieve the patient's symptoms and may aggravate his instability complaint. Furthermore, a badly sited meniscectomy scar may compromise the surgical exposure for a later stabilizing procedure.

Probably one-third of patients presenting with chronic anterior cruciate instability are likely to require a stabilizing operation. The vast majority of such patients are aged below 40. There has been a tendency to advocate isolated central anterior cruciate ligament reconstruction internationally. Because this type of procedure is associated with lower morbidity than earlier more major operations, there has been a tendency for it to be recommended by relatively junior orthopaedic personnel. The prevalence of MRI scanning, and an associated decline in clinical skills, gives rise to the worry that the operation may be undertaken in inappropriate circumstances. Increasing litigation in this area, arising from complication of inappropriate surgery, is also a cause for concern.

The majority of knees requiring stabilization for severe and chronic anterior cruciate instability will need both central replacement of the deficient ACL and additional reinforcement of the stretched peripheral structures. The ideal choice of material for the central reconstruction remains unresolved. There is no place in a primary stabilizing operation for the use of a purely prosthetic ligament.

The central third of the patellar tendon is the most easily harvested graft option, and offers the convenience of bone blocks at each end for easy, firm fixation using interference screws. Gradual refinement of the instrumentation of these techniques has probably been a factor in the decline of prosthetic ligament usage. However, the relative ease with which patellar tendon type reconstructions can now be undertaken is in itself a worry. Surgeons without sufficient clinical or operative expertise may be tempted to operate on an occasional basis. In my view, this type of surgery should only be carried out by experienced surgeons with a predominant interest in knee surgery.

A less popular recent development is the use of pes anserinus tendons centrally in the joint as an alternative to the patellar tendon. These tendons are more difficult than patellar tendon to harvest satisfactorily in sufficient length. By their nature, tendons cannot be fixed as satisfactorily to bone as patellar tendon with its bone blocks. However, techniques have been developed which are sufficiently secure to allow early mobilization using patellar tendon grafts.

This tendency to immediate post-operative mobilization has, to a large extent, helped to avoid the patellofemoral complications associated with immobilization, and particularly with the former use of patellar tendon grafts. A relatively recent observation following the tendency to early mobilization has been the radiological expansion of the bone tunnels in both hamstring and patellar tendon techniques.

On radiographs taken at six months to a year post-operatively, the tunnel appearances have a trumpet-like shape as they approach the joint. This is assumed to be from movement of the graft within the bone tunnels, hingeing as it were, from its point of attachment—remote from the intra-articular bony surface. This radiological observation has not as yet been associated with clinical failure, but it remains a worry.

In those knees with severe and chronic instability, especially where the jerk or pivot shift sign is gross and sharp, long-lasting and robust stability can only be achieved by the addition of a lateral tenodesis. This serves to obliterate the jerk sign and may possibly protect the central graft in the early stages of healing. This approach is advocated by a minority of UK surgeons, and has largely fallen into disuse in the USA and Europe. It is hard to reconcile the divergence of strongly held opinions on both sides of this argument (Dandy and Hobby 1998).

The author's opinion is that a robust lateral tenodesis carried out in the style of LeMaire (1967), is advisable in selected cases—probably two-thirds of knees undergoing stabilization for severe and chronic instability. The addition of such a tenodesis does not affect the need for post-operative immobilization. This is determined by the security of fixation of the central graft.

In summary, therefore, a cautious and conservative approach is advocated in the management of most acute ACL ruptures. Satisfactory management depends, as ever, on precise anatomical diagnosis. Ignorance of the Lachman and jerk or pivot shift signs remains a diagnostic problem in Accident and Emergency departments and with non-specialized orthopaedic personnel.

The goals of treatment are either:

(i) to advise patients about the hazards of their knee's instability problem, so that avoidable mishaps are prevented; or,

(ii) in those patients who wish to pursue an active sporting lifestyle, satisfactory stability should be achieved by operative means, preferably before meniscal damage occurs. It appears that early stabilization can, in certain circumstances, protect the knee against meniscal damage and the subsequent arthritic consequences.

However, this type of surgery is not without hazard, and requires precision if the patient's expectations are to be met. This type of surgery should be carried out under close scientific scrutiny, and preferably in special centres where the surgeons are concerned predominantly with knee problems of this nature.

Posterior cruciate ligament tears

The PCL has a most important stabilizing function. Unlike the ACL, it is taut principally in the midrange of motion (maximally at 30° flexion). Its primary restraining function is to check posterior displacement of the tibia. When the ligament is ruptured, symptoms are often sufficiently disabling to prevent involvement in body contact sports. Injury is relatively uncommon in sport, however—collision impact to the region of the tibial tuberosity with the knee in flexion is the usual cause. PCL rupture may also be part of a combination injury involving other structures secondary to severe valgus, varus, or rotational stress. The PCL is thus at considerable risk in road traffic accidents (by collision impact against the dashboard) and in those sports in which frontal impact occurs, such as American football.

Immediate pain is felt, and difficulty experienced in weight-bearing. Early swelling is a feature, with the type being dependent upon the extent of the injury. It is not uncommon for concomitant damage to occur to the posterior capsule or collateral ligaments, giving rise to posterolateral or posteromedial instability. The initial findings are extensive periarticular swelling and bruising. In the early stages, there is considerable traumatic synovitis, and corresponding restriction of movements, particularly flexion. The signs that indicate posterior cruciate tear are as follows.

1. Posterior sag sign. With the patient supine, the hip flexed to 45°, and the knee flexed to 90° the tibia drops back on the femur (Fig. 7.10). If both the hip and the knee are flexed to 90° and the heel is supported by the examiner or upon a plinth, the sag may be observed again.

2. Positive posterior drawer test. Posterior laxity is demonstrated when AP stress is applied to the knee maintained in 90° flexion. There is no excessive movement in 0°–10° flexion (negative Lachman's test).

3. Posteromedial or posterolateral instability tests.

   (a) Posterorotatory subluxation of the respective tibial plateaux when posterior stress is applied during rotation with the hip flexed to 45° and the knee flexed to 90°.

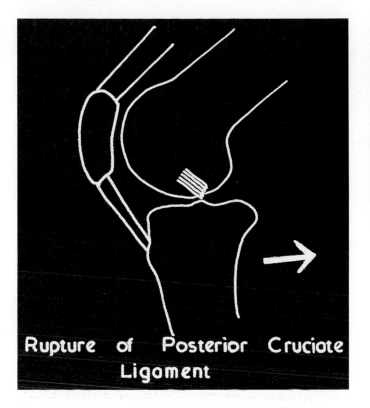

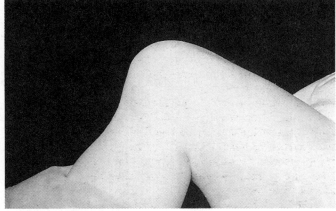

Fig. 7.10 The sag sign is demonstrated in a PCL tear.

(b) External rotation/recurvatum test. When the legs are held by the toes and lifted off the couch, the affected knee slips back into hyperextension and the tibia rotates laterally (giving the appearance of genu varum). A positive test indicates posterolateral instability.

(c) Reverse pivot shift test (for posterolateral instability). The affected limb is held in a similar way to that in which anterolateral instability is demonstrated, though in external rather than internal rotation. The posterior subluxation of the lateral tibial plateau that exists in 90° knee flexion is suddenly reduced as the knee is brought into approximately 30° flexion.

It may not be easy to distinguish clinically between a PCL and ACL tear if the signs of rotatory instability are difficult either to elicit or to interpret. In the presence of abnormal AP laxity at 90° and stability at 10°, one suspects PCL deficiency. X-rays should be taken, as a posterior intercondylar fracture of the tibia may result from PCL avulsion, in which case an urgent surgical opinion should be sought. Management accords to the guidelines for ACL tears. At a later stage, a surgical opinion is required if functional instability develops. It is unusual for the PCL-deficient knee to be compatible with contact sports, particularly those requiring sudden twisting and turning, such as soccer, hockey, rugby football, and American football.

Lateral collateral ligament injury

This injury is also relatively uncommon, as varus stress occurs less frequently than valgus/external rotation stress. The supporting structures to the lateral collateral ligament may also be torn—for example, the biceps femoris tendon and the popliteus tendon. If the injury occurs in extension, the ACL is often torn in addition and demands surgical appraisal.

Varus stress tests are employed in both extension and in 30° flexion (see Fig. 1.11, p. 10). If laxity is found in extension, there is associated cruciate ligament damage. If present at 30° flexion, only the lateral structures are torn. Cast-brace management of lateral tears with intact cruciates may be considered along similar lines to those discussed for MCL tear.

Injury to the superior tibiofibular joint

A fall onto the flexed knee with the leg adducted under the body and the ankle inverted may derange the superior tibiofibular joint. Partial disruption of the proximal tibiofibular ligaments allows anterolateral dislocation of the fibular head to occur. The head of the fibula is found to be excessively prominent and may, in an acute presentation, be relocated by posterior pressure when the knee is flexed. In the subacute case, the patient may accept the presence of minimal symptoms. Turco and Spinella (1985) suggest excision of the fibula head in patients who suffer from recurrent pain from the lax joint. Irritation of the lateral peroneal nerve that winds round the fibula head may be an additional complication.

Meniscus tears

Meniscal tears take many forms, from peripheral tears to midsubstance tears, and from full to split thickness in depth (Fig. 7.11). A vertical tear is common in young athletes; a horizontal tear is more likely with advancing age. Not all tears cause symptoms, particularly in degenerate menisci. The stabilizing function of the menisci has become increasingly recognized, so that if it is possible to leave the damaged meniscus in situ and repair the tear, or at least perform partial arthroscopic meniscectomy rather than total meniscectomy, the likelihood of increasing instability (and of

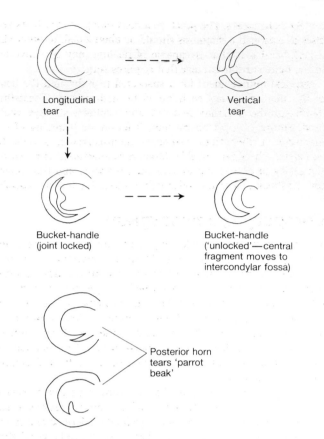

Longitudinal tear

Vertical tear

Bucket-handle (joint locked)

Bucket-handle ('unlocked'—central fragment moves to intercondylar fossa)

Posterior horn tears 'parrot beak'

FIG. 7.11 Different types of meniscus tear may be found.

long-term OA) is reduced. This is particularly important when a meniscus tear arises in the already ACL-deficient knee. The combination of simultaneous ACL rupture and peripheral or posterior horn tear of the medial meniscus is common in an acute injury. The incidence of degenerative change when meniscectomy is performed in an ACL-deficient knee has been referred to already. Jackson (1968) has identified the incidence of degenerative changes twenty years after meniscectomy. In a prospective study, Jørgenson *et al.* (1987) have highlighted the frequency of complaints and incidence of definite OA after meniscectomy for an isolated meniscus injury in an otherwise normal knee.

Injuries to the menisci, of which the medial is considerably more common than the lateral, usually occur when substantial rotational strains are applied to the flexed knee. A common situation is one in which a foot is fixed to turf by a studded boot (in soccer for instance), and thereupon rotational stress is imposed on the leg by the rest of the body. Sudden pain accompanied by a click is felt. A common sequence of events is for there to be initial recovery, followed by further episodes of painful giving way of the joint on twisting. Usually an effusion develops, which gradually resolves but recurs with each acute painful episode. There is often a subjective sensation of inability to extend the knee fully, with a subsequent return of movement on self-manipulation. With a history of this type of instability, the examiner may make a tentative diagnosis of meniscus tear giving rise to bouts of intra-articular derangement.

However, it is necessary to ask for clarification when a patient describes the affected knee as 'giving way' or 'letting him down', as the following circumstances may apply:

(a) meniscus tear (pain on turning);
(b) ACL insufficiency (gives way on turning);
(c) patellofemoral syndrome (anterior pain on weightbearing flexion, such as descending stairs);
(d) loose body (sharp twinges of pain and/or fleeting locking).

As previously recorded, a detached fragment of meniscus may give rise to intra-articular locking and unlocking. In a bucket-handle tear, the joint remains locked—that is, with loss of 5°–10° extension. This situation is not necessarily incompatible with walking or running: regrettably, patients may experience considerable delay before appropriate management is instituted. The diagnosis may have been missed on initial attendance at a busy Accident and Emergency department, and the patient encouraged to exercise; alternatively, the patient may have deferred attendance for advice until some time after the initial incident.

Less dramatic histories may be given by the middle-aged patient who complains principally of recurrent pain; commonly horizontal tears are found. The meniscus rim is then palpable at the joint line, and occasionally is capable of being reduced by digital pressure. Alternatively, a flap is formed that is free to become trapped inside the joint. When this occurs in the lateral meniscus, a type of flap known as a 'parrot beak' may be seen at arthroscopy. Degenerate tears of the menisci, usually the lateral meniscus, may be associated with the formation of a cyst that becomes palpable at the joint line.

Assessment

A history of acute rotational strain and recurrent bouts of pain and swelling is particularly important when a patient has a 'quiescent' knee at the time of examination. When present, the positive signs are due to the mechanical derangement within the knee on meniscus detachment, the associated coronary ligament sprain that inevitably occurs when a meniscus is torn, and the accompanying synovitis. These signs are as follows.

1. A small effusion if injury is recent.
2. A loss of 5°–10° extension with a springy block indicating locking. (Flexion is usually full, though possibly uncomfortable owing to accompanying synovitis.) It may not be possible to differentiate from pseudo-locking in acute ACL tear without arthroscopy.
3. Restricted rotation, particularly external rotation.
4. Localized tenderness and thickening of the coronary ligament on the affected side. (In posterior tears, these localizing signs are less definite.)

Other signs are particularly unreliable: the McMurray test relies on a click or 'clonk' on passive internal and external rotation of the knee in different positions of flexion, and is more likely to be positive with a posterior tear. The Apley test is performed with the patient lying prone and the knee flexed to 90°. The patient's thigh is firmly anchored to the couch by the examiner's knee. Using the patient's foot as a lever, his lower leg is subjected to internal and external rotation, first with distraction and then with compression (Fig. 7.12). Pain during distraction suggests ligamentous injury: pain on compression or 'grinding' suggests meniscus tear. X-rays are advisable to exclude other pathology, such as osteochondral injury. If there is doubt about the diagnosis, particularly in a patient with a quiescent knee and a history of recurrent pain and swelling, an *arthrogram* or

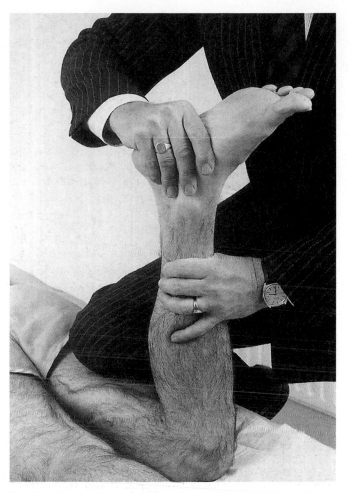

FIG. 7.12 The positions of the examiner and patient when performing Apley's test are demonstrated.

(particularly) an MRI may give positive information (see Fig. 10.19, p. 188). Unfortunately, a negative arthrogram or scan does not definitely exclude meniscus injury, and *arthroscopy* may be required in any event.

Management

In the presence of a locked knee, probably due to a bucket-handle tear, immediate referral to an orthopaedic surgeon is needed. The patient should be supplied with crutches to avoid weightbearing, for comfort, and to reduce further damage prior to surgery. The practice of manipulation, particularly manipulation under anaesthesia, should be eschewed. Even if successful in moving the intra-articular detachment to a position in which extension is freed, the tear is still present and requires excision, not adjustment.

A *peripheral tear* is capable of healing (not so a tear in the avascular body of the meniscus). It is often associated with collateral and ACL tear. When the injury is isolated, there is often a history of a recent twisting strain, and the principal complaint is of pain on certain activities. The signs are a trace or small effusion, localized joint-line tenderness and induration, and discomfort in the last 5° of extension. Nevertheless, extension is of full range. A localized steroid injection to the coronary ligament soon restores painless extension, and quadriceps-strengthening exercises are commenced. Healing may be expected in approxi-

mately eight weeks. The practice of prescribing provocative exercises to establish a diagnosis should be abandoned, or otherwise a peripheral tear that is capable of healing may be converted into a more substantial tear that requires surgery.

Surgical management for a suspected tear through the body of the meniscus may be initiated by arthroscopy. Coexisting damage to the ACL may be noted, and a suitable strategy established. Suture of a peripheral tear, if found, or trimming of the meniscus, rather than extensive meniscectomy, should be employed whenever possible. Modern management is based on the policy of attempting to save the meniscus, and thus maintain its shock-absorbing and stabilizing function if at all possible.

Coronary ligament sprain

The coronary (meniscotibial) ligaments are inevitably sprained during peripheral meniscal tear. However, rotational stress may give rise to coronary ligament sprain without meniscal involvement. Management is as described for peripheral meniscus injury. Coronary ligament sprain, particularly medially, is common in the middle-aged, when there is often no history of acute trauma. Pain is felt during activities requiring frequent knee rotation, such as golf or squash. It is not uncommon for the condition to persist for many months, even if the provocative stress is withdrawn.

On examination, the signs of medial coronary ligament sprain are discomfort on full extension (and sometimes on flexion and external tibial rotation) and very localized tenderness associated with slight thickening along the joint line. There is no effusion (and no history of swelling) and the quadriceps tone is well maintained. Treatment is by localized injection of steroid (for example, 10 mg of triamcinolone hexacetonide (see Fig. 12.22, p. 230)) or by friction massage. If an injection is given, the effect is dramatic: the pain usually disappears entirely within three days. Sport may be resumed within ten days.

Another cause of anteromedial or anterolateral joint line pain is *Hoffa's disease*, in which the alar fat pads adjacent to the patella tendon are traumatized. Tenderness and fullness may be detected on either side of the patella, extending to the anterior joint line, in knee extension. Surgical excision or trimming is required occasionally if symptoms are unremitting.

Osteochondritis dissecans

This condition in juveniles and young adults, in which an area of subchondral bone and overlying articular cartilage becomes non-viable and liable to separation, has been known for centuries. However, the aetiology (and to some degree the management) remains subject to differing views. The consensus of opinion is that the primary fault in osteochondritis dissecans is a fatigue fracture in the subchondral bone. The favoured site in the knee is the lateral surface of the medial femoral condyle, although it may occur elsewhere, including the articular surface of the patella. It affects predominantly the adolescent, whose symptoms are of recurrent swelling owing to effusion, and aching in the knee. A direct relationship to exercise may not be apparent. If separation takes place, with the formation of a loose fragment, symptoms of intra-articular locking may occur. Such a history of locking (owing to a loose body) tends to be different from that caused by a meniscus tear, in that the experience is fleeting, painful, and quickly reversed by a shake of the knee.

Diagnosis relies on an awareness of the possible existence of the condition in an adolescent or young adult with a knee effusion, as localizing signs are absent on examination. Radiological confirmation is necessary to establish the diagnosis (see Fig. 10.17, p. 187), although plain films alone do not reveal the capacity for healing. Scintigraphy (radioisotope scanning) is helpful: the healing potential can be gauged by the level of activity.

Management is by appropriate reduction of stress: weightbearing sports should be excluded. The patient should be monitored by serial X-ray or bone scan over a period of some months. Failure of conservative treatment and/or the establishment of separation are indications for surgery. Revascularization of the fragment by internal fixation is attempted, followed by early joint motion.

Indications for arthroscopy

Arthroscopy may be performed for diagnostic and therapeutic reasons. Referral to an orthopaedic surgeon experienced in the arthroscopic technique may be made for one of the following indications.

Diagnostic

To confirm the presence of a torn meniscus.

To confirm the presence of an ACL tear (partial or complete).

To confirm the extent of an osteochondral lesion.

To confirm the presence of a loose body.

To elucidate the cause of a haemarthrosis.

To elucidate the cause of an unexplained effusion.

To elucidate the cause of unremitting and unexplained knee pain (caused, for example, by a chondral defect).

Therapeutic

To excise or trim a torn meniscus.

To excise a stub of ACL (causing mechanical interference in joint action).

To remove loose bodies or a small osteochondral fragment.

To carry out synovial biopsy (in persistent or unexplained synovitis).

To undertake division or excision of a synovial plica

To repair damage to articular cartilage.

To wash out debris from the joint

Summary of examination procedures for evaluation of acute knee injuries

The following information should be treated as a guide to the procedures to be adopted. As usual, a suitable examination routine should be based on the principles of motion, stress tests, resisted muscle contraction, and then palpation. The division of the knee into tibiofemoral and patellofemoral joints necessitates some overlap during each sequence.

History
Mechanism of injury
Pain location
Locking/unlocking
Giving way
Initial 'pop'
Swelling (immediate/late)

Examination

Standing/walking
Observation
- fixed flexion
- swelling
- limp

Supine
1. Observation
   - fixed flexion
   - swelling? intra-articular or extra-articular
   - bruising
   - femorotibial alignment
   - patellofemoral alignment

2. Assessment of effusion
   - nil (0), trace (1), small (2), moderate (3), tense (4)

3. Range of motion
   - flexion, extension, and hyperextension
   - nature of 'end-feel'

4. Extensor mechanism
   - palpable gap (patella; tendon)
   - manipulation of patella
   - tenderness of patella articular surfaces
   - tenderness of medial retinaculum
   - compression test
   - Clarke's sign
   - apprehension test
   - isometric quads: VMO tone
   - straight leg raise

5. Ligament stress tests
   - valgus/varus at 0°
   - valgus/varus at 30° flexion
   - Lachman's test
   - anteroposterior stress at 90° flexion in neutral, external rotation, and internal rotation
   - pivot shift/jerk test
   - posterior sag sign
   - reverse pivot shift
   - external rotation/recurvatum test

6. Meniscal stress tests
   - McMurray's test
   - limitation of/pain on rotations

7. Palpation
   a) tenderness
   - joint line
   - collateral ligament
   - elsewhere

b) extra-articular swelling
- joint line or collateral ligament
- periarticular haematoma
- swelling elsewhere, e.g. Baker's cyst
- periosteal swelling

8. Mobility assessment of superior tibiofibular joint

Prone

1. Meniscus stress test
   - Apley's test
2. Muscle function (isometric contraction)
   - resisted knee extension (quads)
   - resisted knee flexion (hams)
3. Range of motion
   - confirmation of range of passive flexion

Radiology

AP, lateral, and patella films are requested (augmented if indicated by tunnel views), with particular reference to the following:

- intercondylar area of tibia (avulsion fracture at cruciate attachment)
- tibial plateaux (compression fracture)
- osseous fragments (osteochondral fracture of the patella or osteochondritis dissecans)
- femoral condyles (fracture sprain of MCL or osteochondritis dissecans)

Aspiration

(of haemarthrosis)
- observe blood/fat globules

Arthroscopy

if necessary (referral to orthopaedic surgeon)
- wash out joint
- diagnostic
- arthroscopic surgery

References

Bassett, F. H., Beck, J. L., and Weiker, G. (1980). A modified cast brace: its use in nonoperative and postoperative management of serious knee ligament injuries. *Am J. Sports Med.*, **8** (2), 63–7.

Cailliet, R. (1983). *Knee pain and disability* (2nd edn). F. A. Davis, Philadelphia, PA.

Dandy, D. J. and Hobby, J. L. (1998). Anterior cruciate ligament reconstruction—editorial. *J. Bone Jt. Surg.*, **80B** (2) 189–190.

Ficat, R. P. and Hungerford, D. S. (1977). *Disorders of the patello-femoral joint*. Williams and Wilkins, Baltimore, MD.

Goodfellow, J. W., Hungerford, D. S., and Zindel, M. (1976). Patellofemoral mechanics and pathology. *J. Bone Jt. Surg.*, **58B**, 287–91.

Hardaker, W. T., Whipple, T. L., and Bassett, F. H. (1980). Diagnosis and treatment of the plica syndrome of the knee. *J. Bone Jt. Surg.*, **62A**, 221–5.

Hughston, J. C. (1983). Editorial: anterior cruciate deficient knee. *Am. J. Sports Med.*, **11** (1), 1–2.

Hughston, J. C., Andrews, J. R., Cross, M. J., and Moschi, A. (1976). Classification of knee ligament instabilities. *J. Bone Jt. Surg.*, **58A**, 159–79.

Hungerford, D. S. and Barry, M. (1979). Biomechanics of the patellofemoral joint. *Clin. Orthop. Relat. Res.*, **144**, 9–15.

Hunter, L. Y. (1985). Braces and taping. *Clin. Sports Med.*, **4** (3), 439–54.

Ireland, J. and Trickey, E. L. (1980). MacIntosh tenodesis for anterolateral instability of the knee. *J. Bone Jt. Surg.*, **62B**, 340–5.

Jackson, J. P. (1968). Degenerative changes in the knee after meniscectomy. *Br. Med J.*, **5604** (2), 525–7.

Jørgensen, U., Sonne-Holm, S., Lauridsen, F., and Rosenklint, A. (1987). Long-term follow-up of meniscectomy in athletes. *J. Bone Jt. Surg.*, **69B**, 80–83.

Lemaire, M. (1997). Ruptures anciennes du ligament croise anterieur du genou. *J. Chir.*, **93**; 311–20.

McDaniel, W. J. and Dameron, T. B. (1980). Untreated ruptures of the anterior cruciate ligament. *J. Bone Jt. Surg.*, **62A**, 696–705.

Marshall, J. L. and Rubin, R. M. (1977). Knee ligament injuries—a diagnostic and therapeutic approach. *Orthop. Clin. North Am.*, **8** (3) 641–68.

Noyes, F. R., Matthews, D. S., Mooar, P. A., *et al.* (1983). The symptomatic anterior cruciate deficient knee. Part I: the long-term functional disability in athletically active individuals. *J. Bone Jt. Surg.*, **65A**, 154–62.

Noyes, F. R., Bassett, R. W., Grood, E. S., and Butler, D. L. (1980). Arthroscopy in acute traumatic haemarthrosis of the knee. *J. Bone Jt. Surg.*, **62A**, 687–95.

Noyes, F. R. *et al.* (1985). The anterior cruciate deficient knee. *Orthop. Clin. North Am.*, **16** (1), 47–67.

Paterson, F. W. N. and Trickey, E. L. (1986). Anterior cruciate ligament reconstruction using part of the patellar tendon as a free graft. *J. Bone Jt. Surg.*, **68B**, 453–7.

Renstrom, P., Arms, S. W., Stanwyck, T. S., Johnson, R. J., and Pope, M.H. (1986). Strain within the anterior cruciate ligament during hamstring and quadriceps activity. *Am. J. Sports Med.*, **14** (1), 83–7.

Rovere, G. D. and Adair, D. M. (1983). Anterior cruciate-deficient knees: a review of the literature. *Am. J. Sports Med.*, **11** (6), 412–19.

Turco, V. J. and Spinella, A. J. (1985). Anterolateral dislocation of the head of the fibula in sports. *Am. J. Sports Med.*, **13** (4), 209–15.

Wiberg, G. (1941). Roentgenographic and anatomic studies of the patellofemoral joint. *Acta Orthop. Scand.*, **12**, 319–410.

8 Injuries to the ankle and foot

M. A. HUTSON

The common acute soft tissue injuries to the ankle and foot are described here. Overuse injury is described in Chapter 9. Ligamentous injuries are particularly common; it has been estimated that over five thousand inversion injuries of the ankle are seen each year in the Accident and Emergency department at the University Hospital, Nottingham, alone (Muwanga *et al.* 1986). Although the majority are capable of healing naturally and uneventfully, it is often (incorrectly) assumed that the 'sprained ankle' may be safely managed by strapping or Tubigrip support. The frequency of injury is such that complications contribute significantly to the work-load of the sports physician. The 'weak ankle syndrome' is common. This, and other conditions which result in a prolonged period of rehabilitation, are potentially avoidable, however.

Applied anatomy and biomechanics

The foot and ankle combine flexibility with stability, thus providing two main functions—propulsion and support. The propulsion that is required in walking, running, and jumping takes place in the various joints of the foot as a result of a complicated series of movements involving rotation and gliding. Stability is offered by the ankle and the foot in its pronated position. The *inferior tibiofibular* joint is a fibrous joint supported by the anterior tibiofibular, posterior tibiofibular, inferior transverse, and interosseous ligaments. Although the movements are minimal, there is a little expansion when the ankle joint is fully dorsiflexed.

The ankle (talocrural) joint is a hinge synovial joint, consisting of the articular surfaces of the medial malleolus, distal tibia and lateral malleolus of the fibula (forming a mortise), and the articular surface of the talus. The talus is wedge-shaped, being approximately 2.4 mm wider anteriorly than posteriorly, thus allowing little or no inversion or eversion at the ankle joint in dorsiflexion. The lateral malleolus is situated posterior to the medial malleolus, thus creating an axis of rotation that is approximately 18° to the coronal plane. A greater range of dorsiflexion than plantarflexion is found. The capsular pattern of the ankle joint is limitation more of plantarflexion than dorsiflexion. Medially, the joint is supported by the deltoid (medial collateral) ligament, and laterally by the three components of the lateral ligament.

The *subtalar (talocalcanean) joint* is a synovial joint, allowing movements around an average axis of motion that is 42° to the transverse plane and 16° to the sagittal plane (Fig. 8.1). It is supported by medial and lateral ligaments, in addition to the interosseous talocalcanean ligaments. Inferior to the medial malleolus may be palpated the sustentaculum tali (a projection of the os calcis), immediately above which is the medial opening of the sinus tarsi; this canal divides the joint into anterior and posterior parts. The lateral opening is found below the lateral

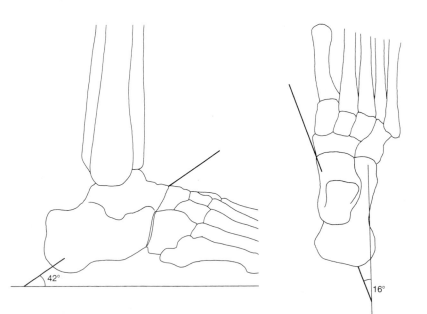

FIG. 8.1 The subtalar joint: axes of motion are 42° to the transverse plane and 16° to the sagittal plane.

malleolus. The triplanar movements that take place are as follows:

(i) inversion/eversion in the coronal plane;
(ii) abduction/adduction in the transverse plane;
(iii) dorsiflexion/plantarflexion in the sagittal plane.

Pronation of the foot is a combination of eversion, abduction, and dorsiflexion. Supination is a combination of inversion, adduction, and plantarflexion. Clinically the degree of eversion/inversion at the subtalar joint may be gauged by moving the calcaneum when the ankle joint has been locked into dorsiflexion.

The *midtarsal joint* consists of the talonavicular joint medially and the calcaneocuboid joint laterally. The two axes (longitudinal and oblique) allow pronation and supination of the forefoot on the rearfoot to take place (Fig. 8.2). The oblique axis makes an angle of 52° from the transverse plane, and 57° from the sagittal plane. The longitudinal axis angulates 15° from the transverse and 9° from the sagittal planes. The midtarsal joint is functionally 'unlocked'—that is, a greater range of movement is allowed, thereby enabling the forefoot to accommodate to uneven surfaces, when the subtalar joint is pronated. At the interconnecting joints with the cuneiform bones, further gliding and rotational movements occur. In the forefoot are the tarsometatarsal joints, at which gliding occurs, the intermetatarsal joints (gliding only), the metatarsophalangeal joints, which allow flexion, extension, abduction, and adduction, and the interphalangeal joints, at which flexion and extension take place.

Inversion injury

The causative stress is usually a combination of plantarflexion and inversion, although true adduction stress occasionally may occur. The primary restraints at the ankle are the ligaments of the lateral ligament complex (Fig. 8.3): the anterior talofibular ligament, the calcaneofibular ligament (intimately bound to the peroneal tendon sheath), and the posterior talofibular ligament. The stability given by these ligaments is under threat in plantarflexion, when the relatively narrow posterior part of the dome of the talus becomes positioned in the ankle mortise. Up to 10° of talar tilt into inversion may be seen in the plantarflexed position in the normal ankle—thus it is important when considering abnormality to compare with the contralateral normal side.

The initial injury at the ankle as a result of inversion is a sprain of the anterior talofibular ligament; with increasing stress, rupture occurs, followed by rupture of the calcaneofibular ligament (Fig. 8.4). Further rupture of the posterior talofibular ligament results in dislocation. The importance of the establishment of an accurate diagnosis lies in the fact that untreated or mistreated ligament rupture may give rise to mechanical instability, proprioceptive insufficiency, or persistent capsulitis. Prolonged rehabilitation and/or the weak ankle syndrome are the consequences.

Assessment

A patient with a moderately severe ankle sprain may hobble or be carried into the consulting room on a stretcher. The stoic may attend with a flat-footed limp. However, a patient who retains a heel–toe gait has not sustained a recently ruptured ankle ligament. A history of the ankle 'going over' into inversion is usually obtained, although the ankle that is injured in an 'over the ball' tackle on the soccer field may suffer from direct trauma from an opponent's boot as well as indirect strain, and the history may be somewhat inexact. Early swelling and bruising, difficulty in weightbearing, and pain felt throughout the ankle region, though tending to be maximal laterally, are features.

Observation of the ankle and foot when the patient is comfortable in the supine position reveals swelling over the lateral aspect of the ankle extending into the forefoot, and bruising in the same region often extending to the toes. Soft tissue swelling may be seen circumferentially around the ankle due to infiltration of oedema. The active ankle movements are uncomfortable and limited in range. Examination of the passive movements of the ankle in the sagittal plane reveals restriction of both dorsiflexion and plantarflexion, particularly the latter, due to traumatic synovitis. All findings are compared with the noninjured side, which should be examined first.

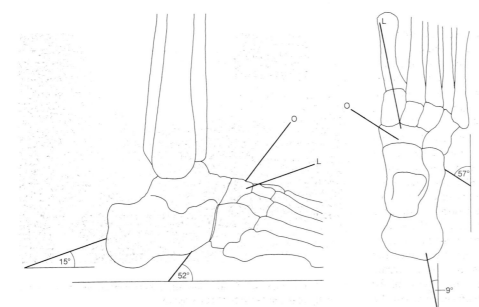

FIG. 8.2 The midtarsal joint. There are two axes of motion, oblique (O) and longitudinal (L).

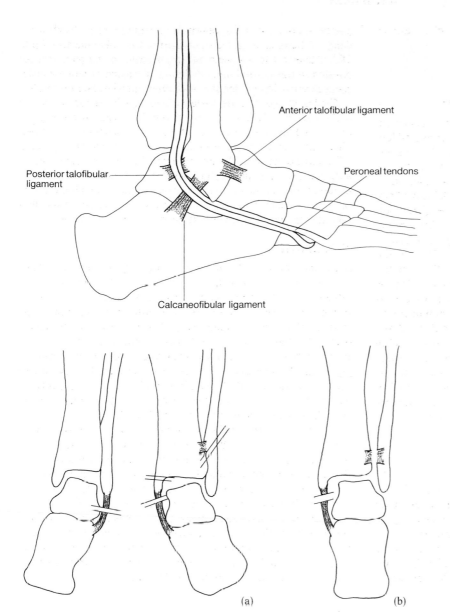

FIG. 8.3 The lateral ligamentous complex of the ankle joint. The peronei are superficial yet intimately bound to the calcaneofibular ligament.

Anterior talofibular ligament

Posterior talofibular ligament

Peroneal tendons

Calcaneofibular ligament

FIG. 8.4 Diagrammatic representation of inversion and eversion injuries at the ankle. (a) Inversion injury: rupture of calcaneofibular ligament. (b) Eversion injury: the possibilities are

- rupture of deltoid ligament
- rupture of tibiofibular ligament
- oblique fracture of fibula
- fracture of medial malleolus
- wide joint space on X-ray.

(a)   (b)

The *anterior stress test* is then employed to assess the integrity of the anterior talofibular ligament. One of the examiner's hands firmly grasps the leg above the ankle whilst the other grips the heel, so that with the foot in the neutral position force is applied to draw the heel (and therefore the talus and the rest of the foot) anteriorly (Fig. 8.5). If the anterior talofibular ligament has been sprained, the anterior stress test provokes discomfort, though it does not reveal excessive laxity. If the ligament has been ruptured, however, the *anterior drawer sign*, in which anterior displacement of the talus in the ankle mortise leads to laxity which is both seen and felt, is positive. In common with the findings on clinical stress tests of complete ligament tears in other joints, there is often minimal discomfort on stress-testing a ruptured anterior talofibular ligament; on careful examination, the experienced examiner is often confident in his judgement in the non-anaesthetized patient. The *inversion stress test* determines the integrity of the calcaneofibular ligament (Fig. 8.6). In moderate plantarflexion, the foot is passively inverted. This is painful for the patient with a sprain, and is often uncomfortable when the ligament is ruptured, possibly as a result of further traction on

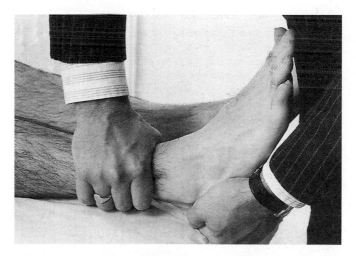

FIG. 8.5 Examination of the ankle: the anterior stress test assesses the integrity of the anterior talofibular ligament.

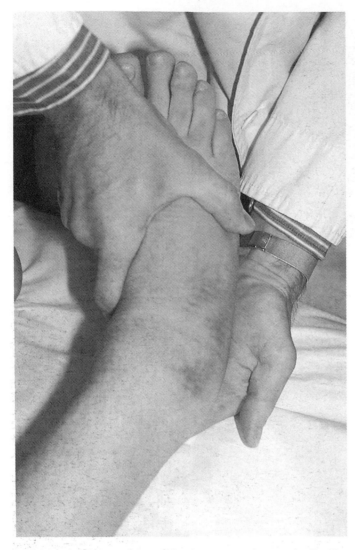

FIG. 8.6 Examination of the ankle: the inversion stress test (for the integrity of the calcaneofibular ligament) may require a peroneal nerve block or local anaesthesia.

adjacent structures. Nevertheless, with experience, laxity may be detected by the examiner. Alternatively, anaesthesia (for example, peroneal nerve block or extensive local anaesthesia) may be necessary: should this prove to be the case, it should be combined with stress radiography.

Resisted muscle contraction is used to detect abnormality of the peroneal tendons. Even if the peroneal tendon sheath is ruptured, as happens in association with rupture of the calcaneofibular ligament, there should be full painless muscle power (resisted eversion of the foot). However, when examining a patient with a 'subacute ankle', that is, one recovering from previous injury, it may be found that the evertors are weak. One of the differential diagnoses in the recurrently painful ankle is subluxation of the peroneal tendons anteriorly over the lateral malleolus, owing to rupture of the restraining retinaculi, and this should be excluded.

Palpation reveals maximal tenderness over the lateral ligamentous complex, although the associated capsulitis often results in additional tenderness felt medially. Tenderness in the surrounding tissues—for example, those overlying the distal fibula—is usually due to extravasation of blood and oedema, though at least AP and lateral X-rays may be required to exclude a fracture.

Since there is capsular rupture in severe ligamentous injury and much soft tissue swelling in any event, a haemarthrosis does not occur and intra-articular aspiration is pointless. However, if there is little soft tissue swelling or bruising in the presence of diffuse bulging over the posterior aspect of the joint on either side of the Achilles tendon, indicating a joint effusion, this is a different situation, which is described on p. 146. (Haemarthrosis associated with osteochondral injury to the talus).

Further investigations. If the patient walks into the surgery and there is minimal or very localized swelling over the lateral ligaments of the ankle, associated with no laxity on stress tests, a sprain may be confidently diagnosed and X-rays are not indicated. However, a suspicion of ligament rupture, and therefore instability, may arise from the following:

inability to bear weight;
inability to walk with a heel–toe gait;
substantial soft tissue swelling and tenderness;
laxity on ligament stress tests.

Under these circumstances, AP and lateral X-rays are compulsory. Stress X-rays should be undertaken under local anaesthesia (at least for the inversion stress test) when the extent of the injury is uncertain following clinical examination. If facilities are not available the above suspicions indicate probable ligament rupture, and the patient is treated accordingly (Jackson and Hutson 1986). To avoid undue exposure to the clinician, the radiological anterior stress test may be performed with the patient comfortable in the supine position, the heel resting on a small plinth, and a sandbag of weight approximately 4.5 kg applied to the anterior distal tibia; this creates a posterior distracting force to the tibia at the ankle, and thus an anterior distracting force to the talus (Fig. 8.7). Two minutes are allowed for the patient to relax his leg, after which a lateral X-ray is taken and compared with the non-injured side. A positive *anterior drawer* sign (Fig. 8.8) is one in which the measured distance between the posterior articular surface of the tibia and the most adjacent articular surface of the talus is 6 mm or more (Lindstrand and Mortensson 1977). Local anaesthesia or peroneal nerve block with 0.25 per cent bupivacaine or 1 per cent lignocaine may be required for the inversion stress test, in which the clinician passively inverts the foot; if local anaesthesia alone is used, this remains an uncomfortable procedure, and care is required. AP X-rays are taken, and once more comparison is made with the non-injured side. Talar tilt, when present, is usually quite obvious, being at least 10° greater than on the other side (Fig. 8.9), and indicates a positive inversion stress test.

One of four situations may be found and the following conclusions drawn:

(i) no instability = a sprain only;
(ii) positive anterior drawer sign + normal inversion stress test = rupture of the talofibular ligament;
(iii) positive anterior drawer sign + positive inversion stress test = biligamentous rupture—that is, of the anterior talofibular and calcaneofibular ligaments;
(iv) normal anterior drawer sign + positive inversion stress test = isolated rupture of the calcaneofibular ligament (rare).

Confirmatory investigations historically have included ankle arthrography or peroneal tenography. The basis of either investigation is that a tear of the calcaneofibular ligament inevitably tears the capsule and adjacent peroneal tendon sheath. Dye

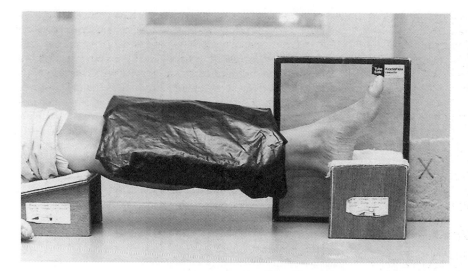

FIG. 8.7 The technique used for the radiological anterior stress test is demonstrated.

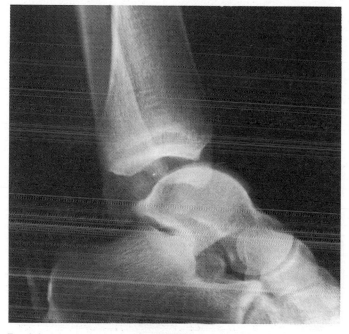

FIG. 8.8 A positive anterior drawer sign is present: the distance between the posterior articular surface of the tibia and the most adjacent articular surface of the talus is over 6 mm.

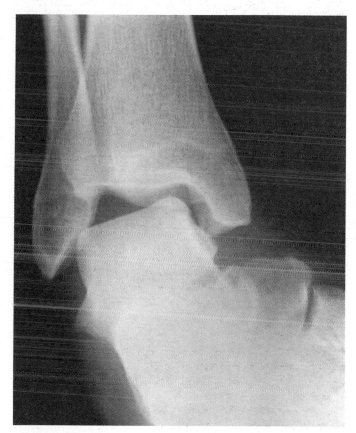

FIG. 8.9 A talar tilt of 20° is present.

introduced intra-articularly or into the sheath thus extravasates into the other compartment and may be detected when the extent of the injury is uncertain following clinical examination. If facilities are not available, radiologically. The author's experience is that the peroneal tenogram does indeed confirm biligamentous tear, though the need for this definitive confirmation in the presence of firm suspicions and stress radiological evidence should be critically questioned. To reduce the incidence of false negatives on stress radiology, it is highly recommended that maximal patient relaxation is obtained in the manner described. It will be recognized that at the turn of the millenium, the use of invasive investigative techniques such as the peroneal tenogram or ankle arthrogram has been superseded by MRI scanning, when available. However, even in relatively advanced state-funded Health Services, the priority accorded to such ubiquitious injuries as the sprained ankle is low, and is likely to remain so. Accordingly, the use of relatively invasive techniques should remain a valid option for some time yet in many countries.

Management

Sprain. Mobilization techniques are imperative to attain the goal of an early return of normal function. The resumption of heel–toe gait, if this has been temporarily lost, and reduction of oedema are encouraged by the therapist. Otherwise the adverse effects of periarticular swelling and immobilization are particularly disadvantageous in soft tissue injuries around the ankle. The application of ice, ultrasound, and effleurage are usually employed. Friction massage is useful after three or four days. Strapping, for example double Tubigrip, frequently is applied to help reduce oedema and temporarily improve proprioceptive deficit. The efficacy of its mechanical supportive role is questionable, and the current literature does not support its widespread use (Wilson and Cooke 1998).

Acute ligamentous instability. Although biligamentous rupture is more likely to give rise to the weak ankle syndrome, comprising recurrent episodes of giving way, pain, and swelling, uniligamentous rupture alone may have the same effect. Therefore, it is imperative for functional support to be supplied. Historically, orthopaedic surgeons have favoured surgical repair followed by plaster of Paris immobilization in the young athletic patient in whom there is definite evidence of recent tear (Freeman 1965; Brostrom 1966; Staples 1975). However, virtually all observers admit that the prolonged rehabilitation time is a major disadvantage. Ruth (1961) reviewed the results of surgical repair and found a high percentage of patients with residual symptoms. Early mobilization and strapping, on the other hand, run the risk of recurrent symptoms from ligamentous insufficiency. Brostrom (1966) found that 25 per cent of patients with primary tears treated conservatively complained of subsequent instability. If used, eversion strapping should be reapplied daily to accommodate the gradually decreasing ankle girth resulting from reduction of oedema.

Experience with a cast-brace for ankle ligament tears at the Sports Injury Clinic, General Hospital, Nottingham over several years (Jackson and Hutson 1986) has suggested a number of advantages of this form of treatment. A well-fitting Scotchcast cast is applied from below the knee to the ankle. This is followed by the application of a plastic heel cup attached to medial and lateral plastic hinges (Fig. 8.10) and held by a Velcro strap. This arrangement allows a limited amount of plantarflexion, though no eversion/inversion. It is applied for three weeks; removal is followed by proprioceptive rehabilitation. The most gratifying initial effect is that patients are immediately very comfortable and resume a normal gait spontaneously. Other than comfort, the following advantages embrace the very essence of early mobilization with functional support.

1. Muscle tone is maintained, thus avoiding the muscle wasting seen after immobilization.
2. Articular cartilage nutrition is maintained, thus preventing degeneration (Salter and McNeil 1965).
3. Sound ligament healing is encouraged, thus reducing the likelihood of reduction of strength (Noyes *et al.* 1974). With the advent of MRI, studies have confirmed that the most severe lateral ligament tears heal with early mobilization (Renstrom and Konradsen 1997).
4. Skin hygiene is improved if the brace is constructed in such a way that the hinges can be removed from the cast, thus allowing washing.
5. Early return to work is possible, as the patient is able to walk with comfort. Safe and comfortable car driving may also be possible (not so in a POP splint).
6. Early rehabilitation follows, thus allowing the earliest possible safe return to specific sports training.

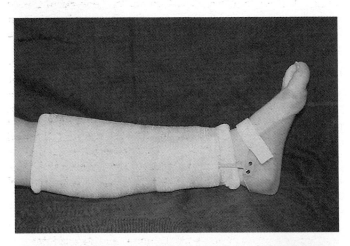

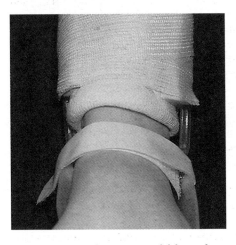

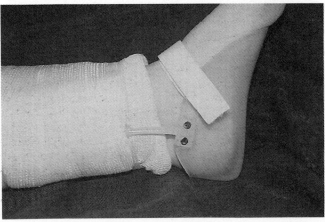

FIG. 8.10 A cast-brace is a useful form of treatment for lateral ligament tears of the ankle. Views from the medial and anterior aspects are shown.

The Nottingham trial suggested that the results are no worse, and may be better, than with surgery and/or immobilization. Forty-one out of forty-two patients with radiological instability returned to sport, including a number of international athletes and soccer players. One patient failed to resume sport because of pain (though her ankle became 'radiologically normal'). Nineteen per cent commented on occasional giving way, though this was not disabling, and 29 per cent complained only of occasional twinges of pain. Of significance was that no athlete required further attention as a result of the 'weak ankle syndrome'.

An Aircast inflatable stirrup brace is a commonly used alternative to a cast-brace, and avoids the need for a plaster-room setting.

Proprioceptive, strengthening, and flexibility exercises are commenced after removal of a cast or cast-brace. They should also be undertaken as soon as possible after a sprain, and when an athlete presents with the weak ankle syndrome. Manual resistive (isometric) exercises are performed in all planes of movement, with particular emphasis on maintenance of the strength of the ankle dorsiflexors and evertors. Subsequently, isokinetic exercises are employed; when testing reveals a return to at least 75 per cent of normal muscle strength, jogging may be allowed.

Limitation in joint-capsule mobility is detected by manual testing, and corrected by active and passive exercises. Active range of motion exercises are started immediately. The use of passive exercises and mobilization techniques for the ankle and foot joints are particularly important after immobilization; they will be required to a much lesser degree otherwise. Anterior and posterior gliding movements at the ankle joint are particularly useful, and are performed during traction of the talus from the tibia.

Deep friction massage mobilizes the affected ligament as soon as reduction of oedema allows. Proprioceptive exercises have a crucial role. They include the use of the wobble board (an invaluable piece of rehabilitative equipment) and frequent tip-toeing exercises (Fig. 8.11). Taping is thought to help prevent re-injury in the early stages of rehabilitation, probably as much for its proprioceptive as for its mechanical effect. Finally, weight-bearing stretching exercises, particularly for the calf muscles, are demonstrated to the patient.

Complications of inversion injury. Patients who suffer from recurrent giving way, pain, and swelling (the *weak ankle syndrome*) following injury should be examined carefully for evidence of mechanical instability. Absence of ligament laxity indicates the need for proprioceptive rehabilitation; a short course of treatment may improve function dramatically. A significant degree of laxity, particularly inversion laxity, should be managed initially by exercises, and eversion strapping should be applied during sport. It is likely that, under such a regime, sufficient function will be restored to allow further participation in sport; functional stability is present, despite demonstrable (clinical) instability. If rehabilitation does not control the symptoms adequately—that is, if functional instability persists—referral to an orthopaedic surgeon should be considered for surgical reconstruction. The results of extra-articular carbon fibre, for instance, have been encouraging. The more traditional method of functional reconstruction, using the peronei, continues to be applied successfully.

Occasionally, the signs of persistent *capsulitis* are apparent. Slight restriction of passive dorsi- and plantarflexion of the ankle, often associated with synovial tenderness or thickening, are found. An intra-articular injection of steroid—for example,

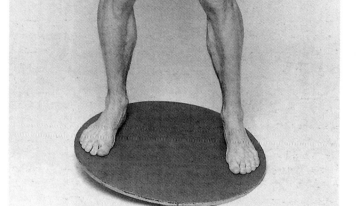

FIG. 8.11 The wobble board is an invaluable piece of equipment for use during rehabilitation of ankle injuries.

20 mg of triamcinolone hexacetonide—is a worthwhile technique. A suitable approach is between the tendons of tibialis anterior and extensor hallucis longus (see Fig. 12.23, p. 230). A 21 gauge needle is introduced in a slightly cephalic direction to accommodate the dome of the talus.

Occasionally a traumatic *capsulitis of the subtalar joint* complicates an ankle injury. This is not surprising, perhaps, when it is appreciated that a considerable percentage of patients with positive tenograms are found to have contrast medium in the subtalar joint (Blanchard *et al.* 1986). Furthermore, instability of the subtalar joint as a result of inversion injury has been described (Brantigan *et al.* 1977). Detection of subtalar joint capsulitis is made with the ankle in the plantigrade position; inversion/eversion movements at the subtalar joint are assessed using the heel for leverage, and found to be restricted (comparison is made with the normal side). Injection of steroid is usually helpful; a 23 gauge needle is introduced in a slightly cephalic direction from the superior aspect of the sustentaculum tali into the joint (see Fig. 12.25, p. 231).

Other inversion injuries. Straight X-rays may reveal an avulsion fracture of the tip of the lateral malleolus. This should be managed as a ligament tear. A common injury is a sprain of the *calcaneocuboid ligament* in which localized swelling and tenderness, and pain on passive inversion and plantarflexion of the tarsus, are found. Occasionally it is associated with a flake fracture. It usually responds well, over two or three weeks, to local anti-inflammatory measures and instep support. *Avulsion fracture* of the *base of the fifth metatarsal* gives rise to localized pain, swelling, tenderness, and pain on passive inversion. X-rays confirm its presence (see Fig. 10.7, p. 182). A lightweight below-knee walking cast for between two and four weeks is advisable for pain control, though some athletes may be sufficiently comfortable in Elastoplast strapping alone. *Subluxation* of the peroneal

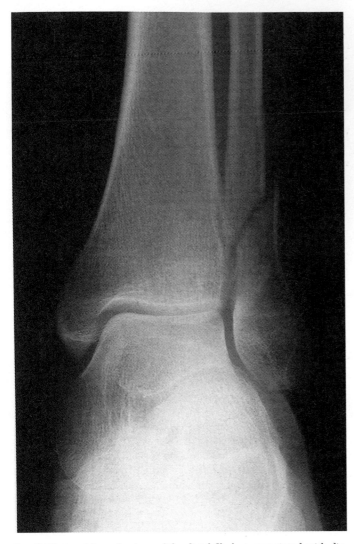

FIG. 8.12 An oblique fracture of the distal fibula is associated with disruption of the distal tibiofibular ligament.

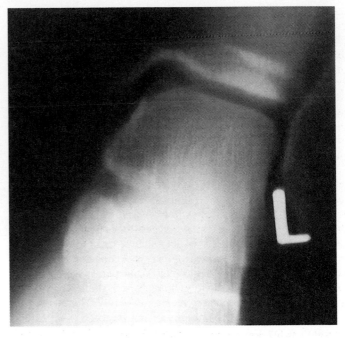

FIG. 8.13 Tomogram revealing an osteochondral injury to the anteromedial aspect of the dome of the talus (resulting from ankle inversion)

tendons may cause temporary localized pain; it is not always recognized as such by the patient, and therefore must be looked for specifically if there is no evidence of ligament injury. Surgical relocation is indicated if recurrently troublesome. Compression injury to the talus may be a further complication of inversion stress (see 'Osteochondral injury to the talus').

Eversion injury

The tough deltoid ligament supports the medial aspect of the ankle. It is stressed by a combination of eversion and dorsiflexion. There is a range of relatively serious injuries of the fracture-dislocation type involving the malleoli and/or metaphysis of the tibia which are associated with deltoid ligament rupture or fracture of the medial malleolus (Fig. 8.4). They require the attention of the orthopaedic surgeon, otherwise the inadequately treated diastasis causes substantive morbidity. An 'isolated' oblique fracture of the distal fibula (Fig. 8.12) is associated with some degree of disrup-

tion of the distal tibiofibular (syndesmotic) interosseous ligament. If there is no involvement of the medial ankle structures, however, it usually heals well in a B/K walking plaster applied for four to six weeks. Straight X-rays are necessary to exclude a medial malleolus fracture. In the presence of NBI (no bony injury), localized soft tissue swelling and tenderness should not automatically be dismissed, as they may indicate deltoid ligament tear, that is an unstable ankle. Orthopaedic surgical referral is then indicated. A partial tear of the deltoid ligament is recognized by a mild degree of lateral talar tilt on stress films and, when unaccompanied by a fracture, may be managed by a cast-brace in a similar way to lateral ligament tear. A sprain should be mobilized without a brace, though an instep support to prevent heel eversion may be useful.

Occasionally an isolated syndesmotic sprain (involving the distal tibiofibular ligaments) is encountered, and is identified by reproduction of pain on the combination of passive dorsiflexion and eversion at the ankle. In the absence of any other structural injury, it settles quickly. In collision injuries, for instance in block tackles on the soccer field, a syndesmotic sprain is often associated with a partial tear of the deltoid ligament, and with a compression injury to the articular surfaces of the ankle joint. In this situation, resolution occurs much more slowly, often over several months. Subsequently, heterotopic calcification of the interosseous membrane may be visible on X-ray.

Osteochondral injury to the talus

A jarring injury to the ankle, such as is sustained by landing heavily on the foot, may result in chondral or osteochondral injury to the dome of the talus (Fig. 8.13). Inversion of the ankle is a common cause of fracture of the posteromedial aspect of the dome (Mukherjee and Young 1973). There may be periarticular swelling, though haemarthrosis within the ankle joint is more likely to have been sustained; it is recognized by observing the diffuse bulging in the para-Achilles depressions. Passive ankle movements are restricted in the capsular pattern, though there are no signs of instability and no pain on resisted muscle contraction. Tenderness is localized to the injury site, usually the medial or lateral margins of the articular surface of the dome of the talus; on careful palpation, it is differentiated from tenderness related to the ankle collateral ligaments. In the subacute stage, discomfort is usually felt upon the extreme of passive dorsiflexion. Initially X-rays may not reveal a fracture, and the patient may not seek attention until a later date, complaining then of recurrent pain on attempted running or jumping. AP X-rays should be taken with the foot plantarflexed as well as in the neutral position, when the typical lesion on the dome may be seen (Thompson and Loomer 1984). Further investigations by tomogram, CT scan, or arthrography may be necessary. Haemarthrosis has also been reported after stumbling with no evidence of chondral injury, presumably due to rupture of a small synovial vessel.

In the absence of major fracture, the haemarthrosis should be aspirated using the technique described on p. 147 for intra-articular injection; immediate improvement in symptoms is to be expected. Subsequent management depends on the severity of the injury . Healing may occur over some months, though radiological evidence of separation and history of repeated impingement may indicate the need for surgical intervention.

Rupture of the Achilles tendon

Achilles tendon rupture has been well documented, though cases are regularly missed, particularly in the middle-aged and elderly. The sudden onset, with no history of extrinsic trauma (though the patient often suspects that he has been struck in the back of the ankle), should make one suspicious. It should be recalled that the action of the other plantarflexors of the ankle and foot, for instance tibialis posterior, may allow the patient to maintain the upright walking posture (after a fashion). Standing or walking on tiptoe is impossible; there is often excessive dorsiflexion of the ankle, and Simmond's (otherwise known as Thompson's) squeeze test (loss of plantarflexion at the ankle on squeezing the calf) is positive. Careful palpation will reveal the defect, usually felt some few centimetres above the insertion into the os calcis. If necessary, MRI confirms (see Fig. 10.20(b), p. 188).

Debate continues on the relative merits of conservative and surgical management (Gillies and Chalmers 1970; Lea and Smith 1972; Nistor 1981). If the non-operative approach is used, a prolonged period of plantarflexion of the ankle by POP immobilization is necessary. The value of surgery lies not so much in the tendon suturing as in the removal of haemorrhagic material to allow closer approximation of the frayed ends of the tendon. Subsequent cast revisions to allow graded repositioning of the ankle into the plantigrade position are necessary, followed in due course by physiotherapy. Referral for orthopaedic surgical opinion is thus indicated. Patients should be advised that full recovery will take six months at the very least.

If the initial diagnosis has been missed, *partial* recovery of function is to be expected. However, the extensive fibrous union often results in permanent weakness of the calf that is noticed by the patient when attempting vigorous weightbearing exercise.

Summary of examination procedures

Standing/walking

1. *Observation*
   - limp
2. *Weightbearing ankle dorsiflexion* (squat)
   - except in 'acute' ankle injury

Supine

1. *Observation*
   - swelling? localized
     - ? diffuse
     - ? effusion within ankle joint
   - bruising
2. *Active movements*
   - dorsiflexion of the ankle
   - plantarflexion of the ankle
3. *Passive movements*

ankle
   - dorsiflexion
   - plantarflexion

subtalar
   - inversion
   - eversion

midtarsal
   - dorsiflexion
   - plantarflexion
   - inversion
   - eversion
   - abduction
   - adduction

4. *Stress tests*

ankle
   - anterior stress test (anterior talofibular ligament)
   - inversion stress test (calcaneofibular ligament)
   - eversion stress test (deltoid ligament)
   - peroneal subluxation
5. *Resisted muscle contraction*
   - ankle dorsiflexion
   - ankle plantarflexion
   - inversion
   - eversion
6. *Palpation*
   - localized tenderness

Prone

1. *Observation*
   - ankle effusion
   - Achilles swelling
2. *Palpation*
   - Simmond's (Thompson's) squeeze test
   - Achilles defect

References

Blanshard, K. S., Finlay, D. B. L., Scott, D. J. A., Ley, C. C., et al. (1986). A radiological analysis of lateral ligament injuries of the ankle. *Clin. Radiol.*, **37**, 247–51.

Brantigan, J. W., Pedegana, L. R., and Lippert, F. G. (1977). Instability of the subtalar joint. *J. Bone Jt. Surg.*, **59A**, 321–4.

Brostrom, L. (I966). Sprained ankles; treatment and prognosis in recent ligament rupture. *Acta Chir. Scand.*, **132**, 537–50.

Freeman, M. A. R. (I965). Treatment of ruptures of the lateral ligament of the ankle. *J. Bone Jt. Surg.*, **47B**, 661–8.

Gillies, H. and Chalmers, J. (1970). The management of fresh ruptures of the tendoachillies. *J. Bone Jt. Surg.*, **52A**, 337–43.

Jackson, P. J. and Hutson, M. A. (I986). Cast brace treatment of ankle sprains. *Injury*, **17**, 251–5.

Lea, R. B. and Smith, L. (1972). Non-surgical treatment of tendoachilles rupture. *J. Bone Jt. Surg.*, **54A**, 1398–1407.

Lindstrand, A. and Mortensson, W. (1977). Anterior instability in the ankle joint following acute lateral sprain. *Acta Radiol. Diagn.*, **18**, 529–39.

Mukherjee, S. K. and Young, A. B. (1973). Dome fractures of the talus *J Bone Jt. Surg.*, **55B**, 319–26.

Muwanga, C. L., Quinton, D. N., Sloan, J. P., Gillies, P., et al. (1986). A new treatment of stable lateral ligament injuries of the ankle joint. *Injury*, **17**, 380–2.

Nistor, L. (1981). Surgical and non-surgical treatment of Achilles tendon rupture. *J. Bone Jt. Surg.*, **63A**, 394–9.

Noyes, F. R., Torvik, P. T., Hyde, W. B., et al. (1974). Biomechanics of ligament failure. *J. Bone Jt. Surg.*, **56A**, 1406–18.

Renstrom, P. A. F. H. and Konradsen, L. (1997). Ankle ligament injuries. *Br. J. Sports Med.*, **31**, 11–20.

Ruth, C. H. J. (1961). The surgical treatment of injuries of the fibular collateral ligament of the ankle. *J. Bone Jt. Surg*, **43A**, 229–39.

Salter, R. B. and McNeill, R. (I965). Pathological changes in articular cartilage secondary to persistent joint deformity. *J. Bone Jt. Surg.*, **47B**, 185–6.

Staples, O. S. (1975). Ruptures of the fibular collateral ligament of the ankle. *J. Bone Jt. Surg.*, **57A**, 101–7.

Thompson, J. P. and Loomer, R. L. (1984). Osteochondral lesions of the talus in a sports medicine clinic. *Am. J. Sports Med.*, **12**, 460–3.

Wilson, S. and Cooke, M. (1998). Double bandaging of sprained ankles. *Br. Med. J.*, **317**, 1722–3.

9 Lower limb muscle and overuse injuries

M. A. HUTSON AND M. J. ALLEN

Muscle injury

M. A. HUTSON

Introduction

Since skeletal muscle contributes approximately 45 per cent of an average individual's body-weight, it is not surprising that, statistically, muscle injury is particularly common in sport. Fibre-type composition in different muscles has some relevance to patterns of injury, injury prevention, and rehabilitation (see Chapter 1).

Research has shown that athletes of national and international standard have fibre-type compositions that would seem to be advantageous for their particular sport. Sprinters have a high percentage of fast-twitch (FT) fibres, and endurance athletes a high percentage of slow-twitch (ST) fibres. Muscles such as the hamstrings, rectus femoris, and gastrocnemius, which require fast propulsive activity, span two joints, and are the most frequently injured by intrinsic trauma.

Quadriceps injury

Injury to the quadriceps femoris may be either extrinsic or intrinsic in origin. Extrinsic injury is common: the frequency of direct contusion is related to the relatively exposed nature of the anterior aspect of the thigh. Intrinsic injury is also common, as overload is frequently applied in sports involving kicking: the kicker is usually injured when unexpected resistance is met—for example, in kicking a heavy ball, the ground, or an opponent. Jumping is another activity in which excessive stresses are applied to the quadriceps.

The site of injury is usually the rectus femoris, which is the only component of the quadriceps that spans both the hip and the knee joints. A complete tear of the rectus femoris is not unusual, though subsequent loss of function is often only slight. The defect in the muscle may not be palpable initially, as swelling soon occurs. It becomes obvious after some weeks, when the swelling of the muscle belly (on contraction) adjacent to the scar may be confused by the unwary with a myosarcoma (see Fig. 1.5, p. 4).

Little difficulty is experienced normally in the diagnosis of muscle tears. Pain is localized to the anterior thigh, and dysfunction is immediate. Pain is felt and weakness is demonstrated on resisted contraction of the knee extensors; passive stretching is painfully restricted (Fig. 9.1). The basic principles of RICE (rest, ice, compression, and elevation) apply to early management. Of special importance during rehabilitation is the establishment of normal elasticity prior to resumption of training. Therapists and trainers should not allow their players to proceed to unsupervised training, particularly if joining other squad members in team sports, until the two 'Ss'—stretch and strength—have been restored.

The 'charley horse' injury is caused by direct contusion to the anterior aspect of the thigh. In its mild form, it is well known to many sportsmen as a 'dead leg', which happily usually recovers inside five to seven days. In its more severe form, however, there is much swelling of the anterior thigh, and often a sympathetic effusion of the knee joint. Flexion of the knee with the hip extended is less than 90°—often 30°–45° only on day 2. Dysfunction is obvious, and the risk of myositis ossificans is very high. Subsequently, if myositis is suspected, X-rays are taken at least two weeks after injury. Acute quadriceps contusion is one of the few musculotendinous injuries which justify immobilization in a cast: a long leg cast for two weeks to rest the quadriceps appears to be effective in prophylaxis. A severely contused quadriceps may require up to six to eight weeks to settle and for restoration of the physiological parameters necessary for commencement of training. Surgical drainage is rarely indicated in the acute stage; subsequently, if an encysted intramuscular haematoma develops, a surgical approach may be necessary.

If myositis ossificans develops, immobilization is pointless and the time for resolution extends to three to six months. Although serial X-rays which reveal increasing bone maturity and contraction may be used to monitor progress, clinical appraisal is preferable. Occasionally an area of ectopic ossification may require excision if residual symptoms are still present after six months.

In the growing child, the anterior inferior iliac spine (AIIS), the apophysis to which rectus femoris is attached, may sustain

FIG. 9.1 The positions of the examiner and patient when assessing both contraction and stretch of the quadriceps femoris, and performing the femoral stretch test, are demonstrated.

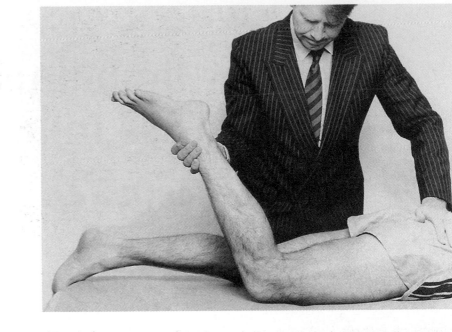

FIG. 9.2 Avulsion of the anterior inferior iliac spine is demonstrated in a child.

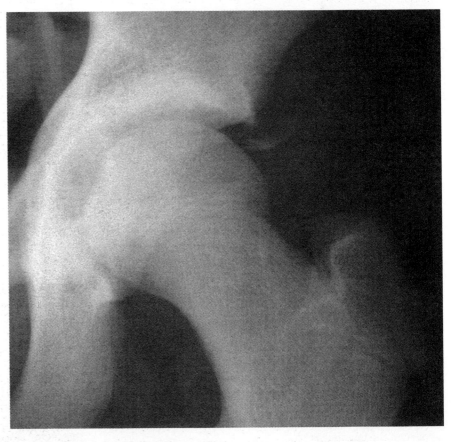

avulsion fracture (Fig. 9.2). Therapy other than rest is to little avail in the first few weeks; thereafter healing occurs rapidly, and should be augmented by stretching exercises.

Tears of the quadriceps tendon and patella tendon are discussed in Chapter 7.

Hamstring injury

Injury is almost entirely by overload when the hip is flexed and the knee extended, as in hurdling and sprinting. The degree of injury varies from a strain which prevents full stretch of the muscle to a more severe tear that may cause pain on walking. The site of the injury is usually mid-belly, sometimes more proximally close to the origin from the ischial tuberosity. Pain on resisted contraction (Fig. 9.3) and restricted painful stretch are features of acute injury;

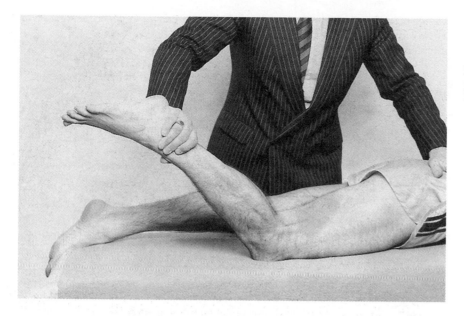

FIG. 9.3 The position of the examiner and patient when assessing contraction of the hamstrings is demonstrated.

prognosis is improved by the appearance of early bruising. The poor reputation that muscle injuries have for recurrence is epitomized by the hamstring tear. The usual cause is inadequate rehabilitation. On the question of predisposition, it is unfortunately only too common to find that either hamstring stretch or strength is poor on routine 'screening' examination of the asymptomatic athlete. As indicated previously (Chapter 1), those muscles which have explosive capacities require preloading by stretching for maximal performance and for protection from injury. Any biomechanical deficiency, such as hamstring–quadriceps imbalance, will lead to a tendency to recurrent breakdown.

Some patients complain of recurrent 'niggles' in their hamstrings, though overall function is adequate. This may be due to an increasing percentage of scar tissue resulting from previous tears; irritable foci may be treated satisfactorily by transverse friction massage.

Avulsion fracture of the ischial apophysis may occur in the child (see Fig. 1.13, p. 13): rapid healing over six weeks is to be expected. At the same site in the adult, chronic traction injury, sometimes associated with an osseous erosion, may be caused by inadequate resolution of an acute tear in the muscle adjacent to the hamstring origin (see Fig. 6.13, p. 121).

Both sprinting efficiency and incidence of injury may be improved by eccentric conditioning of the hamstring muscle group. The knee flexors undergo eccentric contraction in the late recovery phase of sprinting (before foot-strike); the biceps femoris undergoes maximal stretch. The elitist sprinter generates propulsive forces earlier during the support phase, suggesting that the critical phases are late recovery and early support (when the foot descends rapidly and then moves back rapidly) (Wood 1987). Appropriate hamstring training is thus essential for sprint running.

Distally, the biceps femoris tendon may be avulsed as a component of an injury that causes rupture of the posterolateral structures of the knee (see Chapter 7).

Adductor injury

This is principally an injury of the adductor longus. Rupture (partial or complete) may occur mid-belly, at the origin from the

pubic ramus, or at the insertion on the linea aspera. Extensive bruising distal to the site of the lesion may be observed. Initially, a boggy swelling is usually palpable when a significant tear has

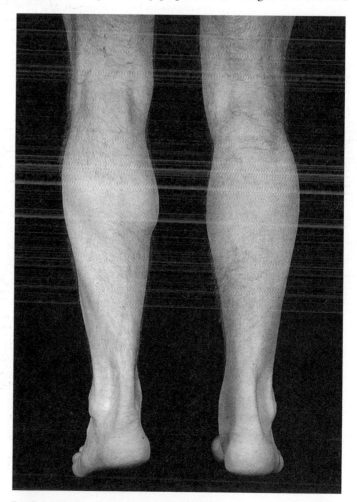

FIG. 9.4 Wasting of the medial belly of the right gastrocnemius within a week of rupture is demonstrated in this patient who is attempting to rise onto tiptoe.

occurred. Passive abduction of the thigh is restricted, and resisted adduction is virtually impossible. Although surgical management has been propounded by some authorities for distal avulsions, uneventful resolution may normally be expected following a conservative regime. Referral to an experienced therapist is advisable, as overenthusiastic mobilization may give rise to ectopic ossification (see Fig. 6.6, p. 106).

Calf muscle injury

The triceps surae comprises the gastrocnemius and soleus muscles which unite through the Achilles tendon. The medial and lateral heads of the gastrocnemius arise from the posterior aspect of the femoral condyles; the origin of the soleus is the posterior aspect of the tibia and fibula. Whereas the soleus is a postural muscle containing a high proportion of type I (ST) muscle fibres, the gastrocnemius component of the triceps surae contains a high percentage of FT fibres and spans three joints (knee, ankle, and the subtalar joint). Injury usually occurs when a sudden explosive contraction is undertaken: the patient feels a sudden 'rifle shot' in the calf. Initially the only method of ambulation is on tiptoe. The medial belly of the gastrocnemius is nearly always affected, the usual site being a few centimetres proximal to the musculotendinous junction. Dysfunction is immediate, though maximal discomfort is not usually felt until the second day. Active heel raise on standing (and therefore normal ambulation) is usually impossible for ten days. Bruising and oedema tracking to the ankle are observed within a few days of injury. Wasting of the medial belly becomes obvious within a week or so (Fig. 9.4).

Initially, a heel raise is required for ambulation. Various proprietary materials or pads are available. After ten days, this may be dispensed with, and graded stretching exercises instituted. Unlike other muscles, non-weightbearing strengthening exercises are virtually useless. The function of the gastrocnemius is propulsion during weightbearing, and recovery takes place as ambulation gradually becomes more comfortable. It takes a month or more for the endurance capacity of the muscle to have recovered sufficiently for jogging to be resumed. At this stage, weightbearing strengthening may be accomplished by overload—for example, by repeated jumps whilst holding dumbells.

A tear of the medial belly of the gastrocnemius used to be known as 'tennis leg' and was thought to be due to rupture of the plantaris muscle—this is not the case. Less severe strains also occur at the proximal attachment of gastrocnemius, masquerading as (and therefore requiring differentiation from) posterior knee or hamstring insertional strain. The diagnosis should be made by the establishment of pain on stretching the calf, either in the standing position (leaning forward) or when supine (the foot is passively dorsiflexed), with the knee extended.

At the musculotendinous junction, injuries tend to take longer to resolve. (It should be recalled that the Achilles tendon is much longer than might be supposed from its colloquial appellation of 'heel cord'.) At this site, just inferior to the muscle bellies, injury may be best treated by a course of friction massage and graded stretching.

Overuse injuries of the knee

M. A. HUTSON

Introduction

A wide variety of conditions resulting from overuse are responsible for those leg and foot pains which frequently occur in many athletic activities. Some are sufficiently common to have received colloquial names such as 'runner's knee', 'jumper's knee', and 'shin splints'. The signs on examination are often subtle. All require pathoanatomical identification and an understanding of the aetiological factors involved in their pathogenesis. Of these exercise risk factors, biomechanical considerations, particularly involving the patellofemoral and subtalar joints, are of prime importance. Risk factors are identified and summarized at the end of the chapter.

Patellofemoral function and dysfunction

The classification and aetiology of anterior knee pain have for long been confused, though they are gradually becoming clearer with a greater understanding of patellofemoral biomechanics. One reason for the confusion is to be found in the origins of the term 'chondromalacia patellae'. In the past, 'chondromalacia patellae' ('CP' or 'CMP') has been used as an all-embracing term to describe those clinical conditions giving rise to anterior knee pain which are categorized by the presence of the classical patellofemoral examination findings of compression pain, facet tenderness, etc. Since it is established that patellofemoral pain often exists in the absence of arthroscopically detectable chondromalacia, it is accepted that 'chondromalacia patellae' should be reserved for the histopathological condition that includes such features as softening and fissuring of the articular cartilage of the patella. Patellar and peripatellar pain are associated more frequently with a number of detectable abnormalities of patellofemoral function, which may be more fully understood by reference to the biomechanical function of the patella.

In extension, the patella lies proximal to the trochlea. As the knee flexes, the patella enters the trochlear groove from the lateral side, owing to the Q-angle that has been established by

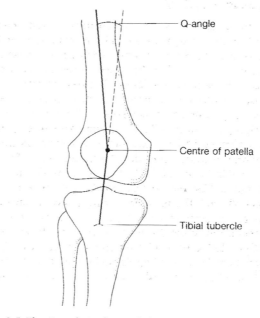

FIG. 9.5 The Q-angle is the angle between the line of the femur and the line of the patella tendon.

the screw-home mechanism of terminal extension (Fig. 9.5). During flexion, the patella is maintained within the trochlear groove by the combination of the relatively increased height of the lateral femoral condyle, the contraction of the oblique fibres of the vastus medialis (VMO), and the ligamentous support of the patella retinaculi. The contact areas on the articular patella facets vary as flexion proceeds to 90° (Fig. 9.6). Medial and lateral contact is equal at 90°. Thereafter, as flexion increases further, the patella describes a somewhat lateral course again—the medial facet enters the intercondylar notch and the 'odd' facet contacts the lateral margin of the medial femoral condyle (Goodfellow et al. 1976).

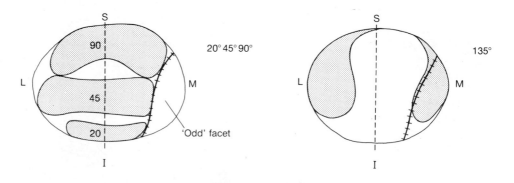

FIG. 9.6 Contact areas of the patella during flexion (after Goodfellow et al. 1976).

During extension, the lateral shift of the patella in the later stages of the movement is accentuated by the abnormal Q-angle that is associated with external tibial torsion (see Patellofemoral stress syndrome). Alternatively, excessive lateral pressure upon the patella may be associated with abnormalities of the patellofemoral articulation, such as hypoplasia of the lateral femoral condyle, hypoplasia of the patella (Wiberg–Baumgartl classification III, IV, and V; see also Wiberg (1941) and Baumgartl (1964)), patella alta, and abnormalities of the supporting structures such as tightness of the lateral retinaculum, laxity of the medial retinaculum (for example, owing to previous dislocation/subluxation), and weakness/atrophy of vastus medialis. Such functional lateralization of the patella has been termed *excessive lateral pressure syndrome* (ELPS) by Ficat and Hungerford (1977).

The presence of wasting of the VMO is often secondary to prolonged patellofemoral pain. However, it may be a primary aetiological factor, and thereby may play a significant role in the development of this condition in a percentage of patients, particularly adolescent girls. The specific functions of the different muscle groups within the quadiceps femoris complex are highlighted in long-distance cyclists, in whom patellofemoral pain may be exacerbated (or caused) by the fact that full knee extension rarely occurs, with the resultant relatively poor development of VMO, despite hypertrophy of vastus intermedius, vastus lateralis, and rectus femoris.

The pathological condition of *chondromalacia patellae* is characterized by the progressive features of softening, fissuring, fasciculation, and subsequently erosion to subchondral bone. It is often an incidental finding in conditions of the knee; when associated with malalignment syndromes, the articular cartilage is not responsible for the symptoms of pain, which probably originate either in the sensory nerve-endings of the peripatellar soft tissues or in the subchondral bone. It has been considered by some authorities that chondromalacia is found more commonly on the medial patella facet, which is not the facet that is the usual site of osteoarthritis (OA). Therefore, it is doubtful whether the one condition leads to the other: in the younger patient, it is relatively unusual for chondromalacia to develop into OA.

However, *recurrent subluxation or dislocation* of the patella is very likely to give rise to patellofemoral OA. Such patellar instability may progress to a state of permanent subluxation or dislocation, in which case OA is inevitable.

Stress fractures of the patella are occasionally found. They may take the form of a transverse fracture across the patella, or occur in a vertical direction. If vertical separation occurs, the condition may need to be differentiated from a painful bipartite patella, in which recurrent stress changes are found at the fibrous union (Fig. 9.7).

In summary, the known *structural abnormalities* which are associated with the development of anterior knee pain are as follows:

(i)   patella instability;
(ii)   stress fracture patella/bipartite patella;
(iii) congenital hypoplasia of patella or trochlea;
(iv)   patella alta;
(v)   VMO atrophy;
(vi)   lateral retinacular tightness;
(vii) OA patellofemoral joint;
(viii) chondromalacia patellae.

Patellofemoral stress syndrome

Notwithstanding the possibility of structural pathology, the majority of patients who complain of exercise-related anterior knee pain do *not* have any obvious patellofemoral abnormality, and may be considered to be suffering from the patellofemoral stress syndrome. In the absence of patellofemoral pathology, the most likely aetiological factors in those sports which involve running are *training errors*. James *et al.* (1978) consider that 60 per cent of all injuries to (long-distance) runners are due to training errors. When considering the possibility of inappropriate training schedules, it should be borne in mind that the serious athlete, particularly the long-distance runner, may not utilize the degree of common sense that is commensurate with either his running experience or his intelligence. The inexperienced runner may have received little or no advice. In any event, the motivation to continue to maintain accustomed training schedules despite warning symptoms may be formidable. The 'high' that is associated with good physical conditioning in endurance sports does not always promote a healthy detached attitude when decision-making is required in response to the needs of competition, injury, climatic conditions, illness, and a whole host of other situations. During history-taking, it is often

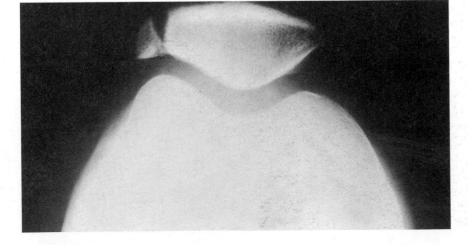

Fig. 9.7 A stress fracture of the patella which may need to be differentiated from a bipartite patella.

necessary to take considerable time over analysis of the training schedule for the purpose of identification of the adverse or potentially destabilizing aspects of training.

In a minority of cases, there is evidence of *malalignment* that is associated with an excessive Q-angle. Genu valgus is one condition in which Q-angle is increased: 'thus runner's knee' is considered to be more common in women. The condition known colloquially as the 'miserable malalignment syndrome' is due essentially to increased femoral anteversion that effectively results in medial femoral torsion, 'squinting' patellae, compensatory external tibial torsion (otherwise 'pigeon toes' would result), and functional equinus and foot pronation (see Fig. 11.6, p. 198). When the syndrome is bilateral, spurious genu varum is observed.

The cause of patellofemoral pain in cyclists may be a *technical* fault in the bicycle. Functional malalignment may result from a worn (or poorly adjusted) bottom bracket axle, excessive play on the pedal spindle bearings (or a bent spindle), or a loose connection between the crank and the bottom bracket.

Assessment

History. Irrespective of its cause, *pain* is usually located at the patella or the posterior surface of the patella. Other symptoms commonly complained of are 'clicking' or 'creaking' related to the patellofemoral joint. Although, when marked, this is a feature of patellofemoral arthritis, it is often present to a greater or lesser extent in the normal knee. Sharp twinges from the patellofemoral joint on weightbearing flexion—for example, on ascending or descending stairs—may give rise to a sensation of 'the knee giving way'. This should be differentiated from temporary locking, either due to a loose body or from ligamentous instability. Typically, prolonged sitting is accompanied by increasing patellofemoral discomfort.

Examination of the patient with chronic anterior knee pain should commence with the lumbar spine and pelvis. Hip disease and L4 root pressure both give rise to anterior thigh pain radiating to the knee. Knee pain only may be complained of. Examination of the patellofemoral joint often reveals varying degrees of tenderness along the medial margin of the patella and pain on posterior patella compression in anterior knee pain from whatever cause. A sideways 'hitch' of the patella may be observed on either active or passive flexion of the knee in the supine position, indicative of maltracking. Increased lateral mobility of the patella suggests the possibility of recurrent subluxation. Patella alta may be suspected clinically and confirmed radiologically. The Q-angle may be measured using a marker pen and goniometer. Wasting of the vastus medialis becomes obvious to the naked eye and is confirmed by palpation of the muscle undergoing isometric contraction. Further investigations include the use of radiographic techniques and occasional use of scintigraphy. The patella is viewed by AP, lateral, and skyline projections. The benefit of the skyline (tangential) views in different degrees of knee flexion—for example, 30°, 60°, and 90°—is contentious: however, it is clear that in certain patients with ELPS, maltracking of the patella, as well as subluxation, may be detected by this means (Fig. 9.8). Increased patellar uptake on technetium scan is seen in a stress fracture. Arthroscopy is usually required when an effusion accompanies patellofemoral dysfunction—otherwise its usefulness is limited.

Management

The management of patellar instability should be dictated by the specialist knee surgeon. A variety of procedures are available once patellar instability has been established (Kettelkamp 1981). Medial plication and lateral release are acclaimed for their simplicity, though unfortunately they may not control the situation. The disadvantage of further procedures that adjust patellofemoral biomechanics—for example, the Elmslie–Trillat medial transfer of the tibial tubercle—is that they too may be unsuccessful, resulting in an increasingly disenchanted patient. It may be kinder in the long

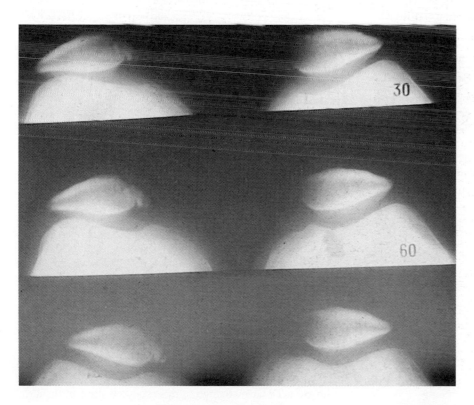

FIG. 9.8 Skyline views of the patella in different degrees of knee flexion may reveal lateral subluxation.

run to advise the patient who is disadvantaged by inadequate patellar biomechanics to resist the desire to pursue exercise that loads the patellofemoral joint excessively.

For a patient with patellofemoral pain (from whatever cause) that is not incapacitating, simple advice to avoid exercises which involve weightbearing flexion of the knee may be helpful. Thus hill running (or cycling) should be avoided, and exercises involving the squat position should be banned from training programmes. Reduction of stress by analysis and subsequent adjustment of the other aetiological factors—outlined later—is often profitable. The mainstay of any management schedule is to *redevelop the VMO*. Whether primary or secondary to the pathological process, wasting of the VMO requires reversal. A suitable isometric strengthening regime must be instituted and maintained for some time (Hungerford and Barry 1979). Abolition of symptoms in the mild case and amelioration in the more entrenched is to be expected. An understanding must be gained by the patient of the difference between isometric contraction (with the knee extended) and isotonic contraction (involving knee flexion, and thereby loading the patellofemoral joint).

The use of patella straps to elevate the patella, and patella supports or taping to control lateral deviation, occasionally may be helpful. However, this should not be a substitute for adequate muscle control. Excessive rotation of the tibia associated with abnormal biomechanics of running may be prevented by the use of orthotics in the running or training shoe. Biomechanical readjustments in cyclists include alteration of the alignment of the cleat on the sole of the shoe, thereby affecting lower limb rotation.

Peripatellar problems

Superior to the patella

Stress fracture of the femur. Gradually disabling and poorly localized pain felt deep in the thigh and related to exercise should raise the possibility of stress fracture of the femoral shaft. Since the femur is well hidden by supporting musculature, there are

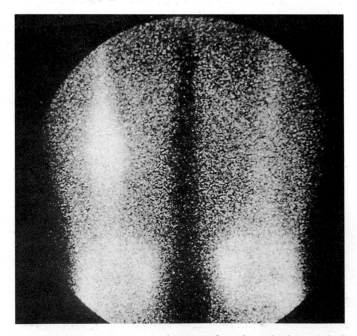

FIG. 9.9 A technetium scan reveals increased uptake in the femoral shaft due to a stress fracture.

no abnormal signs on clinical examination. X-ray is mandatory, though it may not be positive for one to two months. Therefore, a technetium scan must be employed, and this will identify a stress fracture by localized increased uptake (Fig. 9.9). In common with other lower-limb stress fractures, any form of running exercise should be discontinued, though non-weightbearing exercise, such as swimming or cycling, may be substituted as soon as the initial discomfort has settled. It is usually safe to resume running after three months provided that there is no discomfort on walking or jumping.

Quadriceps tendinitis. Discomfort is felt in the suprapatellar region, and may be reproduced on examination by stretching the quadriceps and upon resisted contraction. Crepitus may be present. Localized tenderness confirms the diagnosis, and guides the physiotherapist in the application of anti-inflammatory modalities. Ice, ultrasound, and transverse friction are complemented by quadriceps-stretching exercises.

Medial to the patella

Synovial plica syndrome (syn. synovial shelf or medial shelf syndrome). In the majority of the general population, a synovial plica is palpable, running vertically alongside the medial border of the patella. It may become symptomatic, and give rise to anteromedial knee pain, when hypertrophied, as a result of either trauma or overuse. It is not uncommon in the trailing leg of hurdlers as a result of repeated trauma. Clicking may be complained of, and may need to be differentiated from retropatellar crepitus. Careful palpation reveals marked tenderness of the plica (as opposed to the medial border of the patella). Occasionally, a small effusion may be present. Management by localized steroid injections may be attempted. In the refractory case, arthroscopy confirms the diagnosis, and excision of the plica ('plicectomy') may be curative.

Medial retinaculitis. It is postulated that the retinaculi may be the source of pain in a considerable percentage of patients with patellofemoral pain. The medial retinaculum is torn in acute lateral dislocation of the patella, and is tender for a while afterwards. As an overuse injury, careful palpation may reveal tenderness that is felt in the soft tissues rather than the patella.

Medial coronary ligament sprain. This is a common lesion found in the middle-aged athlete engaged in sports that necessitate frequent knee rotation, such as squash or golf. It is also frequently a source of pain in the osteoarthritic knee. Alternatively, it may be secondary to a torn or degenerate medial meniscus. Pain is usually present after exercise, and may subsequently prevent exercise. When unaccompanied by intra-articular pathology, there is no effusion; discomfort is elicited at the extreme of flexion, and on passive external rotation of the tibia. Slight thickening and tenderness, well localized to the joint line, are found. The condition responds dramatically to one steroid injection—for example, triamcinolone hexacetonide 10 mg—followed by two weeks' rest from exercise (see Fig. 12.22, p. 230). The presence of an effusion increases the likelihood of an underlying degenerate meniscus or OA. Even in the presence of established OA, a low-dose steroid injection may give considerable relief. An alternative remedy is transverse friction massage; however, this takes significantly longer to be effective.

Chronic medial ligament sprain. Although this condition undoubtedly occurs, it is often a mistaken diagnosis for coronary ligament sprain. It occurs in those sports, for instance breaststroke swimming, that involve repeated valgus/external rotation strain to the knee. In the child, this is said to be the cause of 'breast-stroker's knee', though in this condition stress at the distal

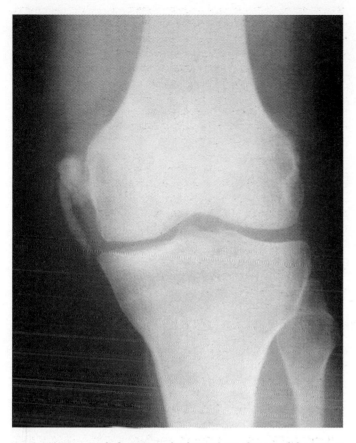

FIG. 9.10 Ectopic calcification in the femoral attachment of the MCL in the Pelligrini–Steida syndrome.

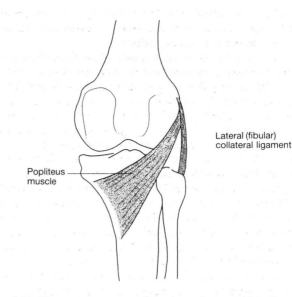

FIG. 9.11 The posterior aspect of the knee demonstrating the attachments of the popliteus.

femoral epiphysis may be an additional factor. An inflammatory reaction at the proximal attachment of the medial collateral ligament (MCL) may be secondary to ectopic calcification (Pelligrini–Stelda syndrome) (Fig. 9.10). A localized steroid injection is usually helpful. Orthotics for the training shoe and temporary avoidance of provocative stress may be required for the chronic MCL sprain that is secondary to excessive tibial rotation.

Anserine bursitis. A bursa usually exists deep to the pes anserinus (combined tendons of sartorius, gracilis, and semitendinosus). A bursitis secondary to overuse causes a nagging medial knee ache. Soft tissue swelling and tenderness are found several centimetres distal to the joint line, and therefore should not be confused with joint line lesions. Movements of the knee and resisted muscle-contraction tests are usually normal. Localized anti-inflammatory measures are required.

Stress fracture of the tibia. This may arise in the proximal metaphysis, particularly in the young adult, and give rise to tenderness of the tibia with overlying oedema (see Fig. 10.11, p. 184). It is said to be more common in patients with genu varum.

Tendinitis of the medial hamstrings. Both hamstring stretch and resisted contraction (knee flexion and medial rotation) may be uncomfortable, though not markedly so. Tenderness is localized to the affected tendon, and is difficult to manage other than by relative rest. If weakness of the hamstrings is found, appropriate strengthening exercises are prescribed.

Lateral to the patella

There are a number of conditions which arise in close proximity to each other (see Fig. 7.3, p. 126).

Iliotibial tract (syn. band) syndrome. This common condition, usually found in long-distance runners, is an inflammatory reaction caused by friction between the iliotibial tract and the underlying lateral femoral condyle. It is more common when the iliotibial tract is tight, and is thus found in patients with genu varum or hyperpronation of the foot, and in runners who persistently run on heavily cambered roads or on banked bends (which causes varus stress on the lower leg) during the indoor sprinting season. When acute, it is accompanied by palpable crepitus. When less severe, tenderness is well localized to the proximal margin of the lateral condyle adjacent to the tract. It usually takes several weeks to resolve, and may be helped initally by anti-inflammatory measures, including steroid injection, and subsequently by stretching the iliotibial tract (see Fig. 11.14, p. 208). Orthotics occasionally are required.

Popliteal tendinitis (tendinitis of the tendon of the popliteus). The tendon of the popliteus is attached proximally to the lateral aspect of the lateral femoral condyle, having an intimate relationship with the lateral meniscus (and its associated popliteal bursa), and for some of its course blending with the capsule of the knee joint and lined by synovium. Its distal muscle attachment is to the posteromedial aspect of the tibia (Fig. 9.11). It medially rotates the tibia, being involved in the early phase of knee flexion from the extended position. It also assists the posterior cruciate ligament in restraining anterior displacement of the femur on the tibia, for instance in downhill running. In this situation, additional stress is imposed on the posterolateral aspect of the knee owing to hyperpronation of the foot. Therefore, overuse injury is often secondary to excessive hill running (Andrews 1983). In common with the medial hamstrings, pain may be reproduced on resisted medial tibial rotation. Tenderness is localized to the tendon attachment, posterior and distal to the source of iliotibial tract pain, and anterior to the biceps femoris tendon. Reduction of abnormal biomechanical stress and localized steroid injections are the mainstays of treatment.

Cyst of the lateral meniscus. Although a lateral coronary ligament sprain, comparable with medial coronary ligament sprain, is relatively rare, a cyst of the lateral meniscus is more common. It is often associated with an abnormal (discoid) meniscus and may require excision. Movements of the knee may be uncomfortable at the extremes of range, though they are largely unrestricted. A palpable cyst is often approximately 1 cm in diameter, though its size varies in different positions of the joint. An inflammatory reaction appears to be involved in the causation of symptoms, as a steroid injection is often helpful and may abolish the need for surgery.

Biceps femoris tendinitis. This apparently affects certain groups of sportsmen, for instance, cyclists, though it does not appear to be very common. Diagnosis and management are similar to that for medial hamstring tendon strain. Cyclists are usually accustomed to adjusting the distance between their seat and the pedals in an attempt to resolve such problems.

Inferior to the patella

Patella tendinitis (jumper's knee). In one form or another, this is an extremely common complaint. In high jumping, excessive knee extensor activity is required to translate the horizontal approach into vertical lift. In volleyball, basketball, and netball, jumping is a repetitive activity. In weight-training and weight-lifting regimes, additional loading is applied to the patella tendon by various forms of hand-held weights. In its mild form, it may be considered to be an enthesitis of the superior attachment of the patella tendon to the inferior pole of the patella (when it is sometimes referred to as 'patella apicitis'). Discomfort is well localized by the patient to the pathological site and, in common with patellofemoral disorders, is felt principally under conditions of weight-bearing flexion. Histologically it affects the calcification front (the so-called 'blue line' transition of fibres) between bone and mature tendon. Discretely localized tenderness and thickening of the proximal tendon are often the only positive signs on examination, though the squat position may become uncomfortable. In common with Achilles tendinitis, a spectrum of pathology is possible, so that in its more severe form partial rupture of the patella tendon may be found. Swelling is then more substantial and dysfunction more profound. Occasionally complete rupture occurs.

A self-perpetuating inflammatory response occurs, so that spontaneous resolution may be extremely slow. Physiotherapeutic modalities are often ineffective. Although intratendinous steroid injections are eschewed, localized injections around the medial or lateral aspect of the lesion are often helpful, and may need to be repeated. However, reduction of stress is necessary. Bodybuilders and weight-lifters who depend on quadriceps loading in knee flexion for good muscle definition and strength find this particularly frustrating, as they need to rely for some time on isometric contraction only. Athletes involved in jumping and racket sports must restrict their levels of activity or consider exercising on a different more resilient surface if appropriate. In common with other enthesopathies, surgical debridement occasionally is required. Cystic lesions within the patella tendon distal to the lower pole of the patella have been described by King *et al.* (1990). CT scanning, MRI, and ultrasound reveal the lesion, which may be treated effectively by excision and paratenon strip. Partial rupture usually responds to conservative measures, though complete rupture requires surgery.

Soft tissue lateral X-rays reveal thickening of the patella tendon in the more severe cases (Fig. 9.12). In the presence of infrapatellar swelling, this may assist in the differential diagnosis between 'jumper's knee' and infrapatellar bursitis. Both infrapatellar and prepatellar bursitis are the result of repeated friction ('housemaid's' or 'beat' knee), and require local anti-inflammatory measures to aid resolution.

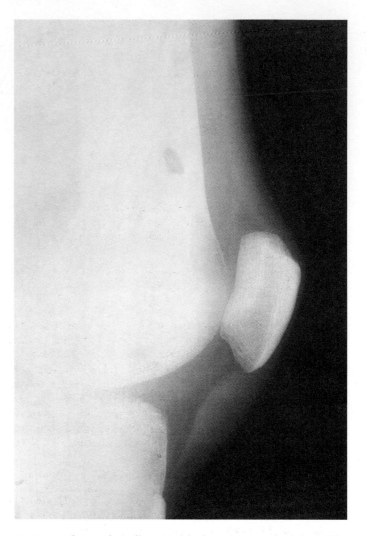

FIG. 9.12 Soft tissue lateral X-rays of the knee may reveal swelling of the patella tendon in partial rupture.

Sinding–Larsen–Johannson syndrome is the juvenile form of jumper's knee. Small fragments of bone from the inferior pole of the patella, representing a chronic traction osteochondrosis, may be seen on X-ray. Reduction (or temporary restriction) of exercise for some months is necessary.

Osgood–Schlatter's disease. This is so common that many parents of affected children have heard of the condition. It occurs mainly in active boys aged 12 to 14, and is a similar traction osteochondrosis to Sinding–Larsen–Johannson syndrome, though occurring at the distal end of the patella tendon, causing fragmented avulsion of the tibial apophysis. Commonly, a talented junior athlete increases his time spent on sport by becoming involved in representative fixtures at the weekends as well as his involvement in the school sports curriculum. Eventually, increasing discomfort prevents his effective contribution.

The diagnosis is usually straightforward. Localized swelling and tenderness are the principal features. X-ray is often not required; if requested, the lateral film reveals fragmentation and separation of the apophysis. Rest or reduction of activity is required for periods lasting a couple of months to a year. Very occasionally, with a failed conservative approach, surgical excision of bony fragments is necessary. Immobilization is rarely required, though it is occasionally used for short periods if this is considered to be the only effective way to reduce involvement in sport.

Shin pain

M. J. ALLEN

Introduction

The name 'shin splints' is most often used by doctors, athletes, and trainers alike as an umbrella term to describe lower-limb pain during exercise. It includes such distinct conditions as:

(1) stress fracture;
(2) chronic compartment syndrome;
(3) medial tibial syndrome (periostitis);
(4) muscle hernia.

These conditions commonly occur in young fit sportsmen and sportswomen, although symptoms may appear in patients of all ages and fitness levels. During the fitness boom of the last two decades, in which more and more people took up running, often unsupervised and without proper training schedules, it became increasingly common. In addition to walkers, casual joggers, and competitive runners, it also occurs in such sports as soccer, rugby, cricket, tennis, and aerobics. It results from the running involved in each particular sport. These conditions are never seen in cyclists or swimmers.

The condition most frequently encountered is chronic compartment syndrome, particularly involving the anterior compartment, which accounts for approximately 75 per cent of all patients suffering from exercise-related pain in the lower leg. Approximately 25 per cent of patients with shin splints have a medial tibial syndrome; approximately half of these syndromes are found in conjunction with a compartment syndrome, when they are an additional irritation rather than the major problem. Both compartment syndromes and medial tibial syndromes are bilateral in 50 per cent of patients. Stress fractures account for less than 5 per cent of problems, and are usually limited to the serious runner or 'pavement pounder' (for example, postmen), often being related to repetitive exercise and hard surfaces. Muscle hernias are extremely rare, accounting for less than 1 per cent of patients.

It should be stressed that none of these conditions is mutually exclusive; any combination of two or three, or even all four together are possible. Sometimes, the patient may progress through each one in turn. This is not entirely surprising, as all can be regarded as 'overuse injuries' due to repetitive loading, sharing the same underlying causes.

Pathophysiology

A stress fracture, as the name implies, is a partial fracture affection only one cortex of the bone which is caused by repeated exercise, often on hard surfaces. This condition is usually self-limiting, because of the acute pain, though if the patient does not rest, it is possible, although extremely rare, for the fracture line to spread across the bone, resulting in a conventional fracture.

A chronic compartment syndrome results from an elevation of pressure in the affected compartment(s). There are four major compartments in the calf (Fig. 9.13), each of which is a separate anatomical entity containing specific muscles, nerves, and blood vessels, and bounded by an osseofascial envelope. The normal compartment pressures in athletes both at rest and during exercise are between 10 and 15 mmHg. In those patients with a chronic compartment syndrome, the pressures during exercise will rise to exceed 50 mmHg. On exercise, the increase in blood flow and retention of fluid by muscle causes swelling which, combined with the relative inelasticity of the fascia, results in an increase in pressure. As the pressure rises, the blood supply to the muscles is compromised, causing ischaemic pain. When exercise stops, the pressure drops, the blood supply returns to normal, and the pain ceases. All this usually takes place within a few minutes.

The pathophysiology of medial tibial syndrome remains unclear. Some authors (for instance, Mubarak 1982) suggest that it may be due to inflammation of the periosteum caused by abnormal or excessive pull of the muscles. However, this has not been borne out by the author's experience, when tissue removed from the periosteum has been examined both histologically and under the electron microscope, and has always been of normal appearance.

A muscle hernia is a defect in which nerves or vessels pass through the fascia. On exercise, the muscle mass protrudes through the defect, and on reaching a certain size becomes strangulated, causing pain.

The reason why some athletes are affected by these conditions and others are not is unknown, though in certain cases it is related to biomechanical factors—for example, overpronation resulting in muscle hypertrophy.

Clinical presentation

Stress fracture. Patients complain of an acute or subacute onset of lower-limb pain of a crescendo type that is well localized, normally to the lower third of the tibia or fibula. There is very well localized bony tenderness. Tapping the affected bone reveals a specific fingertip area of tenderness. Hopping is painful. Palpable callus may be present.

Chronic compartment syndrome. A gradual onset of cramp-like pain is experienced. This may increase over a period of time to such an intensity as to make running impossible. On ceasing exercise, the pain usually subsides over a short period of time (usually minutes or a few hours). Occasionally it may take longer, perhaps even as long as a day. The pain may be localized to the lateral side of the calf (anterior compartment) or to the inner aspect of the calf (posterior compartment) (Fig. 9.13). This occurs in approximately 50 per cent of cases, and in the other half the pain is poorly localized and felt throughout the whole of the calf. It is extremely rare to have a chronic compartment syndrome of the lateral or superficial compartments. Occasionally pain may be accompanied by distal neurological symptoms, such as tingling in the foot during exercise.

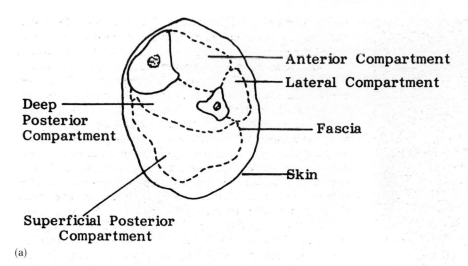

(a)

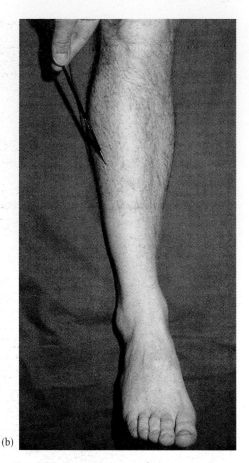

(b)

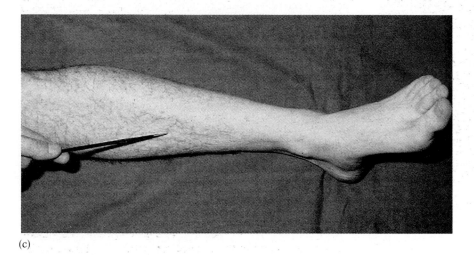

(c)

FIG. 9.13 Compartment syndromes:
(a) anatomy of the calf compartments;
(b) site of localization of pain to the anterior
compartment; (c) site of localization of pain to
the deep posterior compartment

Examination invariably is normal, other than the possibility of some slight lower tibial border tenderness in those with deep posterior compartment involvement.

Medial tibial syndromes. The pain is described as either cramp-like or aching in character, and can occur either during or after exercise. When compared with compartment pain, it usually takes much longer to disappear—periods of days, or even constant pain, are not unusual. It can vary from an irritable niggle to being totally incapacitating. The pain is always felt in the inner aspect of the leg over the inner tibial border, usually the lower third. On examination, there is always an acutely tender area to palpation in the lower third of the inner aspect of the tibia.

Muscle hernia. This produces a localized intense pain around the fascial defect which is directly proportional to the amount of exercise. On ceasing exercise, the pain rapidly disappears. Fascial defects may be papable. They are usually fairly small, about the size of a fingertip, and usually involve the anterior compartment fascia. On stressing the affected muscle (tibialis anterior) against resistance, a noticeable lump is apparent.

Investigations

Plain radiographs are important to exclude other conditions such as bone tumour. A stress fracture will not appear on a plain X-ray until several weeks after the onset of symptoms, when either a transverse fracture line or callus formation may be seen. Hence they are only of use for confirmation of the diagnosis. In all other conditions, the radiograph is normal. Tibial cortical hypertrophy may be present, though this is not a pathological entity, and is seen equally in normal athletes and those complaining of shin splints.

Bone scans are generally unhelpful in the early stages as increased diffuse uptake is relatively non-specific. A stress fracture will show up, earlier than on a plain radiograph, as a 'hot spot.' Often a patchy uptake is seen, which is equally prevalent in normal individuals and those suffering from medial tibial or chronic compartment syndromes (see Fig. 1.3, p. 3). Magnetic resonance imaging has been demonstrated to provide similar sensitivity and specificity to triple phase bone scanning (Batt, 1995).

The increased intramuscular pressure in chronic compartment syndrome may be measured by a variety of techniques (Styf, 1989). Intracompartmental pressure monitoring (ICPM) should be carried out during exercise. This is best achieved by placing a slit catheter into the anterior and deep posterior compartments of both legs and measuring the pressures as the patient runs. Figure 9.14 shows the technique involved. The heparinized-saline-filled catheters are connected to pressure transducers which convert the hydrostatic pressure in the compartment into an elec-

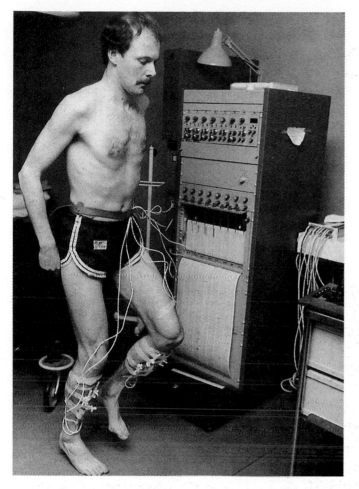

FIG. 9.14 Intracompartmental pressure monitoring during exercise.

trical signal which can then be amplified and displayed on a chart recorder. Figure 9.15 shows a typical recording obtained from a patient with bilateral anterior compartment syndrome.

Management

A stress fracture requires rest from running. Often abstinence from sport is sufficient, though occasionally the patient requires protective weightbearing in the form of crutches or a cast. Training on soft grounds can be resumed after about ten to twelve weeks for tibial fractures and a little sooner for fibular fractures, depending on symptoms and radiological appearance.

Rest should also be prescribed for the compartment syndrome, as undoubtedly some individuals respond to a period of two to three months' rest followed by gradual resumption of activities, which should begin on a soft surface. This is especially true for the so-called 'fresher's leg'—that is, those young students leaving school and going on to higher education who suddenly and dramatically increase their level of sporting activities. Hence all patients with a suspected compartment syndrome of short duration are advised to rest for a few months before any further treatment is undertaken. Physiotherapy appears to be of little help in treating this condition. Surgery, when indicated, takes the form of a subcutaneous fasciotomy of the affected compartment(s). Post-operatively, the patient should be encouraged to commence light activities as soon as possible, to prevent the fascia from closing over and the condition recurring. Athletes should be back to full performance in six to eight weeks after surgery to the anterior compartment, and after a little longer if the deep posterior compartment is involved.

Treatment of the medial tibial syndrome is difficult. If the symptoms are not incapacitating, the athlete should continue activities. Rest is generally unhelpful. Physiotherapy in the form of ice or ultrasound is also unhelpful, and occasionally the ultrasound may aggravate the condition. Steroid injections may be tried, though they tend to be of temporary benefit only. Surgery takes the form of a fasciotomy of the deep posterior compartment, followed by stripping the periosteum off the inner tibial border and drilling three holes in the tibia. The patient should not undertake any strenuous exercise for twelve weeks following surgery. It usually takes approximately six months before the athlete is back to full activities, although results are by no means guaranteed.

Symptomatic hernias should be treated surgically by a subcutaneous fasciotomy of the affected compartment. Closure of the defect should never be undertaken, as it usually gives a poor result and can lead to an acute compartment syndrome.

Differential diagnosis

There are many and varied conditions that may mimic any one of the causes of shin splints.

Sciatica resulting from a prolapsed intervertebral disc or spinal stenosis due to narrowing of the spinal canal may give rise to lower-leg pain. In the spinal stenotic condition, neurological features may present in the lower limbs upon exercise. Such condi-

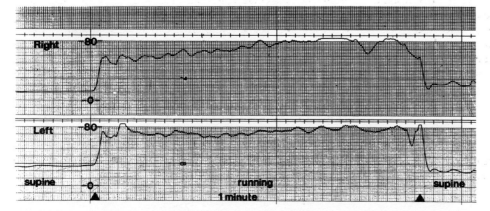

FIG. 9.15 Pressure recording of a bilateral anterior compartment syndrome (values in mmHg).

tions are excluded by careful examination, followed by plain radiographs and computerized tomography or MRI if indicated.

Popliteal entrapment syndrome occasionally occurs, though it is very rare. Owing to the abnormal anatomy of the popliteal artery in the popliteal fossa, temporary occlusion may occur when exercising, giving rise to pain in the lower limbs. This condition is diagnosed by palpating the dorsalis pedis pulse with the knee flexed. If it disappears, it is suggestive of the entrapment syndrome. Confirmation is made by arteriography. When dealing with a population of young patients, it is rare to find intermittent claudication, though this must be excluded by palpation of the distal pulses.

Very occasionally a bone tumour, either benign or malignant, may mimic shin splints. It should be excluded by plain radiographs of the leg.

Occasionally chronic muscle injury or tenosynovitis may be mistaken for shin splints.

Superficial peroneal nerve entrapment may mimic anterior compartment pain. This occurs when the superficial peroneal nerve becomes trapped at the level of its exit through the fascia, giving rise to symptoms in the leg. Diagnosis is often difficult, and EMGs are often not conclusive. Clinically, patients will have a positive Tinel's test. A trial injection of local anaesthetic at the site where the nerve passes through the fascia alleviates symptoms. Once a positive diagnosis has been confirmed, the condition can be relieved by surgery.

Compression of the deep peroneal nerve (in the anterior compartment) may occur with an acute compartment syndrome. This is occasionally seen when a very intensive burst of activity is taken by a normally sedentary person. Alternatively, it follows direct soft tissue trauma (contusion of the muscles in the anterior compartment) or a fracture, or it may occur as a complication of surgery on the tibia. The symptoms are throbbing and paraesthesia, followed by anaesthesia, in the web between the first and second toes. Icing and elevation are required. If there is doubt about the viability of the compartment tissues, particularly if motor weakness develops, referral for decompression should be undertaken.

Overuse injuries of the ankle and foot

M. A. HUTSON

Anterior to the ankle

Anterior impingement syndrome. Pain may result from repeated impingement *in ankle dorsiflexion* of the adjacent articular margins of the tibia and talus (Hontas *et al.* 1986). As the syndrome evolves, osteophytic projections from the adjacent bony margins may develop. Compression of previously avulsed bony fragments from the anterior joint margins may occur, giving rise to a localized capsulitis and periostitis. Alternatively, repetitive stress to the anterior aspect of the ankle in *plantarflexion*—for example, when kicking a 'dead ball' in soccer or rugby

football—may be the initial cause of the osteophytic projections (McMurray 1950). The term 'footballer's ankle' is coined to reflect the presence of such avulsed fragments and osteophytes, which are typically seen in professional soccer players. Anterior impingement may also be seen in dancers, particularly in classical ballet, as a result of the repeated ankle dorsiflexion required by the demi-plie position. Examination findings are reproduction of pain on passive ankle dorsiflexion and localized anterior joint line tenderness. The range of dorsiflexion may become limited owing to intervening fragments. X-ray usually confirms the bony abnormalities (Fig. 9.16). However, the joint space is well

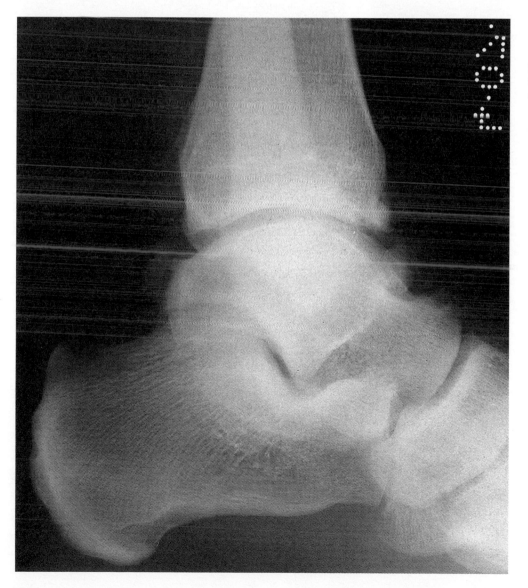

FIG. 9.16 Typical 'footballer's ankle': anterior (and posterior) osteophytes and avulsion fragments.

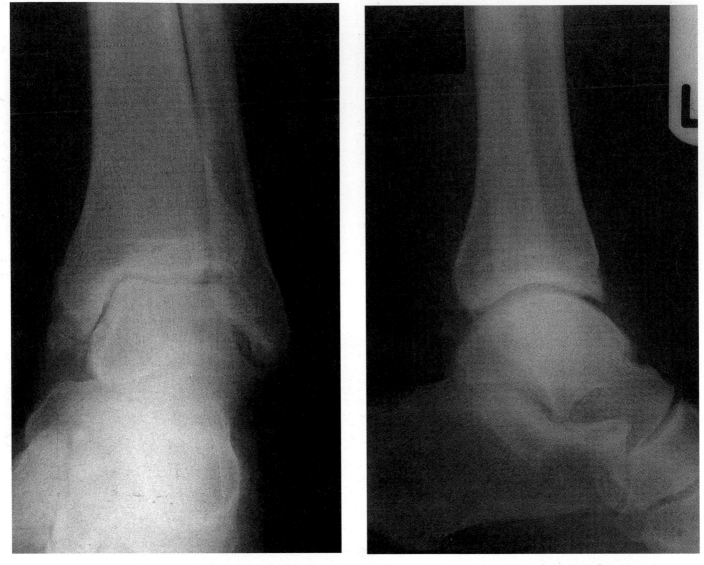

FIG. 9.17 Osteoarthritis of the ankle in an ex-professional soccer player: in comparison with Fig 9.16, there is additional subchondral sclerosis and joint-space narrowing.

maintained. Elastoplast adhesive strapping may control the extent of ankle dorsiflexion in footballers prior to the introduction of a suitable rest period. Occasionally, surgical excision is required.

Care should be taken to differentiate the marginal osteophytosis present in 'footballer's ankle' from osteoarthritis, in which loss of joint space and subchondral sclerosis occur (Fig. 9.17). The prognosis is different, and the former condition does *not* inevitably lead to the latter.

Extensor tenosynovitis. This either results from unaccustomed intensive running—for example, in ultramarathoners—or is secondary to overtight lacing of running shoes. Localized swelling of the extensor tendons may be seen. Passive plantarflexion and resisted dorsiflexion of the foot and/or toes are painful. Local anti-inflammatory measures and reduction of stress are indicated. Surgical release is necessary occasionally in the chronic case.

Posterior to the ankle

Achilles tendon pathology and bursitis

All grades of injury to the Achilles tendon (syn. tendo-Achilles (TA)) are seen and are a common source of pain in sports that require bursts of propulsive activity such as badminton and also in runners. The most common type is *Achilles tendinitis* that is due to repeated microtrauma. Typically, at an early stage, discomfort is felt after running and morning stiffness is a feature. Subsequently, discomfort is experienced at the beginning of a run, though it improves later. However, it soon becomes increasingly difficult to 'run off' the symptoms, at which stage advice is usually sought. Aetiological factors are poor equipment and training errors of all kinds: inadequate footwear, the presence of a whiplash effect on the Achilles tendon due to overpronation of the foot, pressure from a shoe-heel tab, and inadequate elasticity of the musculotendinous unit. Pain is elicited on active contraction (rising on to tiptoe) and, unless the condition is mild, on stretch, either weightbearing or supine. Localized tenderness is found, commonly 4–6 cm from the TA insertion into the os calcis. In more severe cases, thickening of the affected area is noted. The presence of a fusiform swelling may indicate a central (core) degenerative process.

Since the Achilles tendon is surrounded by a paratenon rather than a tendon sheath, an inflammatory reaction in this tissue is described as a *paratendinitis*. It may be secondary to underlying tendinitis, in which case a more diffuse swelling than that found in a tendinitis is observed. It may also develop as a primary response to repeated friction from a shoe or walking boot. Crepitating paratendinitis may be felt: this responds quickly to a steroid injection into the paratenon.

Partial rupture presents as a more acute injury. Pain then prevents active heel raise. A more substantial degree of swelling and tenderness are observed: however, the tendon is intact, as determined by a negative Simmond's (Thompson's) squeeze test. With the patient lying prone, the calf is squeezed—a resulting plantarflexion of the foot takes place in the presence of an intact tendon (a negative test). A positive test indicates complete rupture (see Chapter 8).

Examination of the foot, with particular reference to the biomechanics of subtalar function, is essential. The running or training shoes are examined. An assessment is made of the degree of stretch of the TA by reference to the normal side. Soft tissue lateral X-rays may reveal haziness of the anterior margin of the TA (Kager 1939) or the presence of tendon swelling (Fig. 9.18). Management strategies are based on the following guidelines.

1. A heel lift in the early stages. Shock-absorbing materials such as PPT are useful, both in early management and during later rehabilitation.
2. Ultrasound, ice applications/massage, and deep friction massage.
3. Subsequently, graded stretching.

4. Podiatric assessment and provision of antipronational orthoses, if appropriate.
5. Advice on footwear, with particular reference to a supportive heel counter, an effective shock-absorbing midsole, and a non-irritating (or excised) heel tab.
6. Advice on graded rehabilitation including eccentric loading.

Steroid injections have been implicated in tendon rupture (Mahler and Fritschy 1992). However, the evidence with respect to TA rupture is conflicting. Whilst adhering to the general view that intra-tendinous injections should never be given, the author believes that steroid injections are useful in paratendinitis (see Fig. 12.24, p. 231). In refractory cases of tendinitis, an injection to the paratenon may be considered. In the chronic or relapsing case, an adhesive paratendinitis often complicates tendon pathology; MRI is helpful, and subsequent referral to a specialist surgeon. A variety of measures, which usually include stripping of the paratenon, are often successful.

Sever's apophysitis. In juveniles, repeated stress more commonly manifests itself as a traction osteochondrosis of the

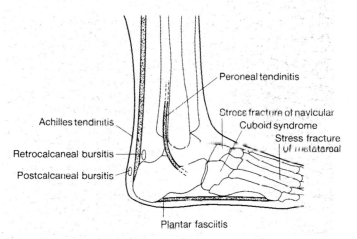

FIG. 9.19 Sites of overuse injury in the ankle and foot.

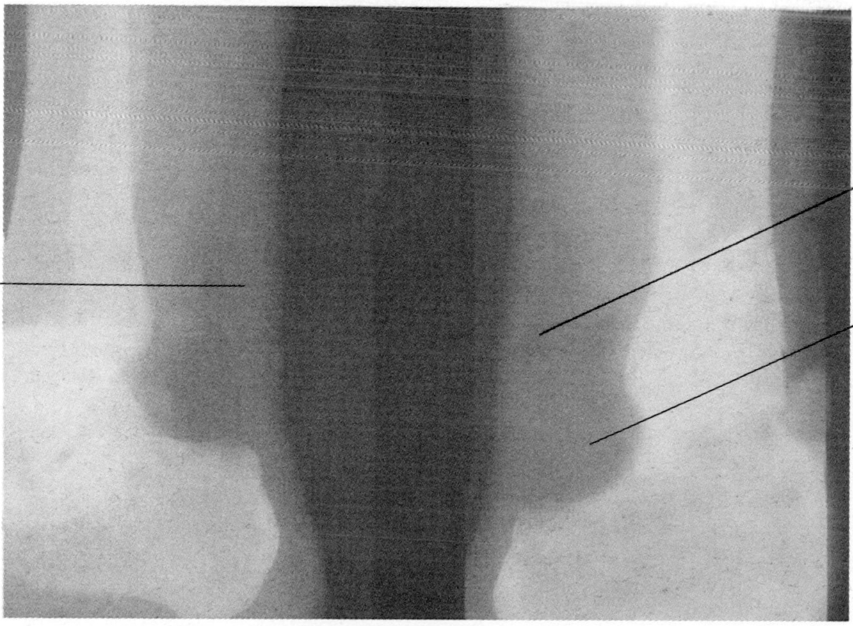

Normal Achilles soft-tissue shadow

Abnormal enlargement of Achilles soft-tissue shadow

Contraction of Kager's triangle

FIG. 9.18 'Soft tissue' lateral X-rays of the ankle may reveal swelling of the Achilles tendon in the presence of Achilles tendinitis or partial rupture.

posterior calcaneal apophysis into which the TA is attached. Localized tenderness is felt over the posterior aspect of the os calcis: the tendon itself is apparently normal. Although X-rays frequently are taken, the normal apophysis often has a fragmented appearance and interpretation may be difficult. Therefore, a clinical diagnosis should be made. Localized physiotherapeutic measures are unhelpful. Reduction of stress is required, with assistance from a shock-absorbing heel cushion.

Retrocalcaneal (pre-Achilles) bursitis. Pain and swelling arise from the bursa that is situated between the Achilles tendon and the superoposterior angle of the os calcis (Fig. 9.19). Although the symptomatology is similar to that caused by tendon pathology, bursitis is characterized by a tender swelling that may be palpated both medial and lateral to the distal TA. In common with plantar fasciitis, retrocalcaneal bursitis may be a manifestation of a rheumatological condition—for instance, one of the spondyloarthritides, especially Reiter's syndrome. Bursitis is very responsive to steroid injections or non-steroidal anti-inflammatory drugs. However, blood tests should be undertaken to exclude an underlying rheumatological condition.

Postcalcaneal (tendo-Achilles) bursitis. A bursa exists between the TA and the skin, and may become inflamed as a result of friction from a running shoe or boot. It is also common in the non-athletic population, particularly in women who wear shoes with close-fitting heel counters. Tenderness and thickening overlying the insertion of the TA is often accompanied by bossing of the os calcis, giving rise to the common 'pump bump'. Haglund described a syndrome (Torg *et al.* 1987) characterized by the combined presence of bursitis, insertional tendinitis, and bossing (Haglund deformity). Shoes should be examined, as simple measures to smooth over any roughened internal surface of the heel counter may be effective. The heel may also be protected by suitable padding around the tender area. Postcalcaneal bursitis is less responsive than retrocalcaneal bursitis to steroid injections.

Insertional tendinitis of the TA. Occasionally an isolated tendinitis is found at the insertion of the TA, where it should be differentiated from bursitis (both pre- and postcalcaneal) and stress fracture. It is an enthesitis, akin to patella tendinitis. Its management follows the guidelines already outlined for Achilles tendinitis.

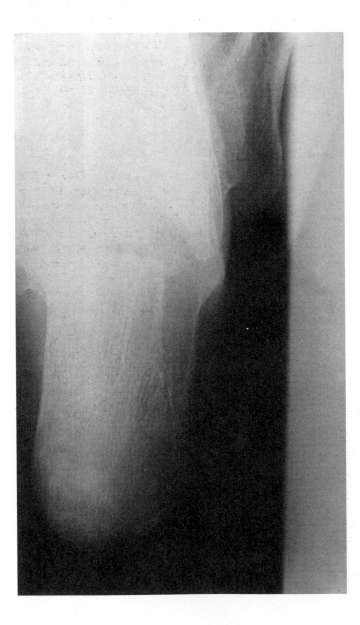

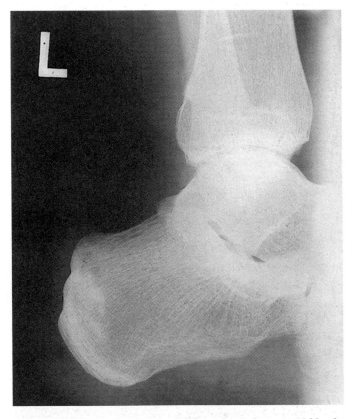

FIG. 9.20 A typical stress fracture of the os calcis is demonstrated by the sclerotic line parallel to the posterior margin of the os calcis on the lateral X-ray, and oblique to the inferior border of the os calcis on the AP.

Non-Achilles pathology

Stress fracture of the os calcis. Although one of the least common stress fractures associated with running, stress fracture of the os calcis does enter into the differential diagnosis of heel pain. A typical crescendo pattern of pain is usually found, so that by the time the athlete is forced to stop running he has discomfort on walking, and particularly on stamping the heel on the ground. In contrast to the other conditions in the heel region, the tenderness is found on compressing the os calcis between thumb and forefinger from the medial and lateral aspects. X-ray is positive after a few weeks, when a sclerotic line may be seen running parallel to the posterior margin of the os calcis (Fig. 9.20). In the meantime, a technetium scan reveals increased uptake. Up to three months' abstinence from all sport involving running is required; other activities such as swimming and cycling are permissible (and encouraged for maintenance of overall fitness).

Tibialis posterior tendinitis. Tendinitis of tibialis posterior and flexor hallucis longus may give rise to posteromedial heel pain, often radiating to the instep. They are more common in pronated feet. Tendinitis of tibialis posterior is characterized by discomfort felt on passive eversion and resisted supination of the foot.

Precipitating situations are those demanding prolonged and repeated inversion, as in speedskating. The condition is also seen in sprinters and long-jumpers if loss of ankle dorsiflexion—for example, owing to tightness of the Achilles tendon—is compensated by eversion of the foot. If a lesion of the flexor hallucis longus exists, discomfort is felt on passive dorsiflexion and resisted plantarflexion of the big toe. It is common in ballet dancers. Tenderness may be felt behind the medial malleolus or more distally—for example, at the insertion of the tibialis posterior into the navicular bone or, in the case of flexor hallucis longus, along the instep. Anti-inflammatory therapy may need to be combined with reduction of pronation by the use of orthotics, or with stretching exercises for ankle equinus.

If tibialis posterior tendinopathy becomes chronic and the tendon attenuated or ruptured, weakness is profound. The power of supination of the foot and maintenance of the medial longitudinal arch are lost; acquired flat-foot is inevitable. Calcaneo-valgus and medial prominence ('bulging') of the ankle are apparent. Forefoot abduction is manifest on the 'too many toes' sign when viewed from the rear. The most useful functional test at this advanced stage of dysfunction is the inability to heel-raise when single limb weightbearing.

Posterior (ankle) impingement syndrome (syn. talar compression syndrome). Repeated impingement of the posterior bony margins resulting from plantarflexion of the ankle may give rise to localized pain (Brodsky and Khalil 1986). It is usually due to impingement of the posterior process of the talus against the posterior lip of the tibia. It is more likely in the presence of an os trigonum (an accessory ossicle behind the talus) which is then caught, much as a nut in a nutcracker, between the tibia and os calcis when the ankle is plantarflexed. Occasionally, either the posterior process of the talus or the os trigonum is fractured.

The condition is common in ballet dancers, as a result of time spent *en pointe*. It is observed in footballers, when it is due to kicking, particularly when kicks are blocked. Javelin throwers and other field athletes are a further 'at risk' group. Passive plantarflexion of the ankle reproduces the pain. Resisted muscle contraction is painless, thus differentiating the condition from tendinitis of tibialis posterior, flexor hallucis longus, the peronei, and the Achilles tendon. Tenderness is localized to the posterior joint margin, detected by palpating from either side of the Achilles tendon. Lateral X-rays may reveal a talar posterior process or os trigonum (Fig. 9.21). Bone scan is positive if a fracture has occurred, though if negative it does not preclude the diagnosis of impingement. Conservative management is instituted initially; a steroid injection may be followed by POP immobilization for a few weeks. Surgical excision of the os trigonum may be necessary in refractory cases, and is usually successful.

Lateral to the ankle

Peroneal tendinitis. This results from overactivity of the peronei, which evert the foot. Frequent running across slopes or in the gutter of a cambered road may be responsible. Pain is felt over the peroneal tendons, and may be accompanied by swelling or crepitus. Passive inversion of the foot is uncomfortable, and pain is reproduced on resisting peronei contraction. Localized anti-inflammatory measures are useful, and recognition of training errors important. A stronger heel counter, if appropriate, may help. Occasionally tendinitis is secondary to an inversion sprain. Lateral ankle soreness is also associated with lateral instability

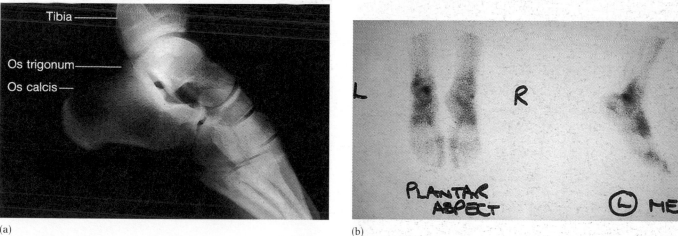

(a) (b)

FIG. 9.21 (a) An os trigonum is demonstrated in a patient suffering from posterior (ankle) impingement: when the ankle is plantarflexed, a 'nutcracker' effect occurs between the tibia and the os calcis. (b) A positive bone scan confirms the diagnosis.

due to previous lateral ankle ligament rupture: proprioceptive exercises are then required (see Chapter 8).

Inferior to the heel

Plantar fasciitis. This common condition arises at the proximal attachment of the plantar fascia to the medial calcaneal tubercle. It is often ascribed mistakenly to the presence of a calcaneal spur (should one exist), though it occurs irrespective of any bony irregularity. It is often associated with a heavily pronated foot when the plantar fascia is overstretched. It may also occur in the rigid cavoid foot (Doxey 1987). The history is of gradually increasing discomfort felt under the heel during running. Examination reveals tenderness that is localized to the medial calcaneal tubercle, just to the medial side of the midline. Occasionally discomfort is reproduced by stretching the plantar fascia (passively dorsiflexing the big toe with the foot also dorsiflexed). The presence of more substantial pain on this manoeuvre, particularly when accompanied by a pronounced limp, indicates the likelihood of a partial tear of the fascia in the instep (Leach *et al.* 1978). Muscle contraction

tests are normal. The differential diagnosis includes stress fracture of the os calcis and nerve entrapment (usually involving the medial plantar nerve deep to the abductor hallucis muscle, when the tenderness is along the medial border of the heel).

Management is by the combination of anti-inflammatory measures and protection of the foot by appropriate antipronational devices. Thus a localized steroid injection at the point of tenderness in fasciitis is very helpful (see Fig. 12.26, p. 231), though it may fail to prevent recurrence unless the heel is protected by a shock-absorbing pad and the fascia is supported by a medial arch support. A suitable appliance is a Rose insole with the addition of a PPT heel. Stretching exercises for the calf muscles, for instance using an adjustable inclined ramp, may be helpful. A 90° polypropylene night splint is a further useful measure for recalcitrant heel pain (Kilmartin, 1999).

Contusion of the heel pad. The heel pad has a shock-absorbing function, and is composed of fatty and fibroelastic tissue divided by septa into compartments. Repeated contusion may give rise to localized pain on heel-strike. Protection is required by additional shock-absorbing heel inserts in the athletic shoe.

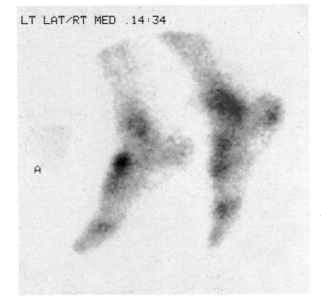

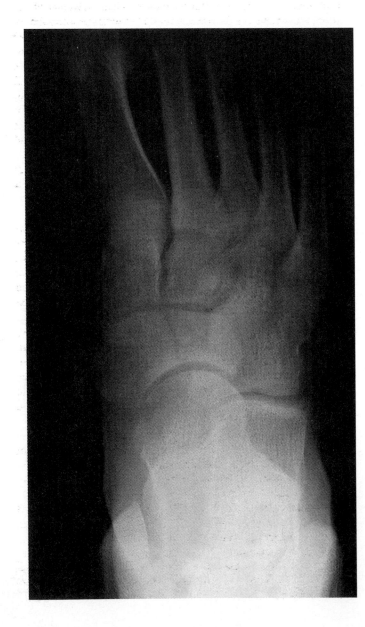

FIG. 9.22 (left) The typical X-ray appearance of a stress fracture of the navicular confirmed by a technetium scan (above).

Injuries to the tarsus

Stress fracture of the navicular (Fig. 9.22). This is uncommon, though it should be suspected when an athlete, often involved in a discipline in which jumping or hurdling are essential elements, complains of instep pain. The pain is worse on weightbearing on the affected foot. Localized tenderness and surrounding oedema are the only abnormal clinical signs. X-rays are often negative in the early stages, so that a technetium scan should be performed for confirmation of the diagnosis. Localized increased uptake is then clearly seen. Management is by rest from weightbearing sport for a disappointingly long period of time. It is not unusual for several months, or even a year or more, of rest to be necessary. If discomfort is felt during everyday activities, a period of non-weightbearing immobilization in a POP cast should be utilized for confirmation of the diagnosis. Further assessment and timing of the reintroduction of training should be predicated on the comfort experienced on everyday activities and loss of tenderness, rather than on a change in the bone scan or X-ray.

An accessory ossicle, the os naviculare, may cause pain at its fibrous union with the navicular bone. If localized anti-inflammatory measures are ineffective, excision may be necessary.

Nerve entrapment. Pain felt along the instep, particularly in association with radiation to the medial aspect of the heel, may be secondary to nerve compression. The tarsal tunnel syndrome, in which the posterior tibial nerve or one of its branches is compressed just posterior to the medial malleolus, is well recognized. Medial collapse of the hindfoot is a common cause. Pain is usually sharp or electric in nature, and is often associated with paraesthesiae and/or numbness felt in the sole. There may be an associated os trigonum. Diagnostic signs are localized tenderness over the groove behind the medial malleolus and a positive Tinel sign. Nerve conduction studies may be performed for confirmation.

Other nerve entrapments occur: compression of the medial calcaneal nerve should be considered in the differential diagnosis of plantar fasciitis, as pain is commonly felt in the medio-inferior aspect of the heel. Instep pain may be due to compression of the nerve to the abductor digiti minimi that courses deep to the abductor hallucis muscle (Murphy and Baxter 1985). Entrapment of the medial plantar nerve close to the calcaneonavicular ligament has also been described. Localized steroid injections may be helpful; otherwise, surgical release is indicated in refractory cases.

Cuboid syndrome. This relatively rare condition behaves as a stress injury to the cuboid, though without the progress to stress fracture that is seen with the navicular. Localized discomfort, tenderness, and soft tissue swelling resolve over a period of a few weeks' rest. The condition does not appear to be related to overactivity of the peronei.

Arch strain. This may be secondary to muscle weakness or fatigue, ligamentous inadequacy, or overstrain of the plantar fascia (when it is felt particularly on toe-off). Inadequate support of the instep from the running shoe is often observed. The pronated foot is at most risk. Although there is minimal muscle activity in the standing position, when aching may predominantly be felt, both extrinsic and intrinsic muscle-strengthening exercises are prescribed to correct any imbalance during running or walking.

Degenerative changes in the tarsus. This may be secondary to previous injury, and gives rise to a loss of mobility of the tarsus. Painful passive rotation and localized dorsal tenderness are the salient clinical features. Superior osteophytic projections may cause localized discomfort in a shoe that is too tightly laced or inadequate in size. Generalized discomfort is felt during or after exercise, and should be controlled by an adequate instep support.

Metatarsalgia and forefoot pain

Stress fracture (see Fig. 10.10, p. 184). One of the most common stress fractures in the lower limb is the metatarsal (MT) stress fracture, usually occurring at the distal metaphysis of MT2 or MT3, although fracture at the base of MT5 is also recorded. Usually it results from increased walking or running activities in the relatively untrained—for instance, in military recruits or inexperienced joggers. Localized tenderness and swelling are found over the distal shaft of the relevant MT. Diagnosis is made on clinical grounds: X-rays may not become positive for two or three weeks. A suitable metatarsal pad (on elastic or on insole) is effective for comfort when combined with four weeks' reduction in activity.

Inadequacy of the transverse arch. This is usually found in the more mature runner, and may be combined with other structural abnormalities, for instance, hallux valgus. Reversal of the superior convexity of the arch is associated with the formation of callosities under the second and third metatarsophalangeal (MTP) joints. In its more severe form it is commonly found in rheumatoid arthritis, when dorsal subluxation of the proximal digits occurs. (It may also be the presenting feature of rheumatoid arthritis.) Localized tenderness under the MTP joints is found. Although the introduction of intrinsic muscle exercises does not influence the structural configuration found on examination, it may help dynamically. An appropriately positioned metatarsal pad—that is, one proximal to the MTP joints—is usually helpful.

Freiberg's disease is an osteochondritis affecting the head of MT2 or MT3 in the skeletally immature. Discomfort may be felt at this time; metatarsalgia is a secondary manifestation in adulthood. A metatarsal pad is required.

Hallux rigidus. Degenerative changes in the first MTP joint give rise to restriction of mobility of the joint—hallux limitus or rigidus. This common condition may be secondary to a previous osteochondritis; at least, there is often a history of synovitis that subsequently settles, only to lead to a more chronic condition in which repeated stress results in pain and increasing restriction of mobility. Pain is felt when the joint is dorsiflexed forcibly—for example, in toe-off on running and in gymnastics or ballet. Examination confirms restricted dorsiflexion and plantarflexion. Osteophytes may be palpated around the joint. Tenderness is felt over the dorsal joint margin. It is a problem which may be difficult to overcome, though the use of a metatarsal 'rocker' in the running shoe may help. In a ballet dancer, it may herald a premature end to a career.

Trauma, as in stubbing the toe, may cause a haemarthrosis of the first MTP joint. Aspiration allows earlier resolution than would otherwise be the case, and thus an earlier return to activity. If an assistant delivers an axial distracting force to the joint, dorsal needle entry is facilitated.

Sesamoiditis. Stress may give rise to pain from the sesamoid bones that are associated with the insertion of flexor hallucis brevis along the plantar aspect of the first MTP joint. This is particularly common in ballet dancers. An inflammatory reaction, chondromalacia, or a stress fracture may develop (see Fig. 10.15, p. 186), occasionally necessitating excision of the affected sesamoid.

Bunions. Bunions (adventitious bursae) may be troublesome over the first and fifth MTP joints. The former often is associated with *hallux valgus*, caused by tight-fitting shoes. There may be a primary metatarsus primus varus and subsequent development of hammer and overriding toes. The choice of adequate shoe-width is essential. Advice from a podiatrist or chiropodist may be required.

Morton's interdigital neuroma. Pain that radiates between the second and third, or third and fourth, toes may be due to a neuroma of a plantar digital nerve. There are accompanying paraesthesiae, and numbness radiating along the adjacent toes. Tenderness may be elicited on pressure applied to the web at the point of division of the nerve to the adjacent digits. A painful click is often demonstrated when the adjacent metatarsal heads are manipulated (upwards and downwards) against each other. Injections of the associated intermetatarsal bursa, accompanied by restriction of activities, may help, though excision is usually required.

Aetiological factors

Identification of the aetiological factors involved in the development of overuse injury in the lower limb is of paramount importance. Following the establishment of the patho-anatomical nature of the injury and recovery therefrom, relapse may be expected unless predisposing factors are corrected. These factors may be considered by reference to the following groups:

   training errors;

   terrain characteristics;

   inadequate flexibility and muscle imbalance;

   pathology elsewhere;

   biomechanical abnormalities;

   inadequate footwear;

   growth characteristics.

Although reference is made particularly to running injuries, the same principles may be applied to all sports that involve weight-bearing activity.

Training errors. Training errors probably account for the majority of running injuries. Although it is understandable that the inexperienced jogger/runner may indulge in an inappropriate training programme, often with too rapid an increase in mileage, the experienced or elitist athlete is by no means exempt. On the one hand, risk may be taken with new or innovative programmes; on the other a lack of common sense may prevail. The body's adaptive process may be compromised by excessive mileage, excessively frequent (for instance, daily with no rest-day) or infrequent activity, addition of extra loading (for example, frequent hill work or fartleking), and excessive incremental increases in training distances. Although it may be a question of being wise after the event in individual cases, the most extraordinary circumstances are reported. The author has interviewed one runner with multiple stress fractures who increased his mileage from 0 to 110 miles per week in three weeks!

Information on suitable schedules for beginners is readily available in other texts, and particularly in the various running magazines. Having overcome the initial phase of muscle soreness, further progression should be at a comfortable pace. Adaptive responses are compromised by the inappropriate targeting of a future race meeting that allows an inadequate amount of training time, thereby imposing excessive musculoskeletal strain.

Terrain. It is clear that the transmission of shock on foot-strike is affected by the nature of the running surface. Exaggeration of shock waves is found on concrete; a marginal improvement may be expected on asphalt. Although it is usually stated that running on grass is desirable, particularly when recovering from injury, there are obvious drawbacks. Wet grass may be too slippery, and dry grass may cover a bumpy surface; in any event, apart from well-prepared recreational surfaces, potholes may be a problem. The best surfaces are perhaps a level dirt track or a prepared bark surface, though in Britain these are rarely available. Sand should normally be avoided, as it imposes a considerable strain on the Achilles tendons. Banked surfaces, such as heavily cambered roads, impose an excessive pronational strain on the higher foot and a varus strain on the lower knee. Competitive athletes often experience problems in the spring and autumn—that is, between running seasons—when adjustments are required from road or cross-country running to running on tartan tracks, and vice versa. Tartan surfaces vary in their shock-absorbing quality, depending to some degree on their thickness. Transitional programmes should be as graded as possible.

Flexibility/muscle balance. Sprinters, who often have the benefit of advice on training programmes from qualified coaches at club level, are usually diligent in performing stretching exercises. However, both their longer-distance club colleagues and 'fun-runners' have in the past been notoriously negligent in this respect. Yet loss of musculotendinous flexibility contributes to the development of many injuries, such as Achilles tendinitis and iliotibial tract bursitis. Elsewhere in the text, it has been suggested that restricted flexibility around the hip joint, often due to tight soft tissues, contributes to chronic pelvic and back strains.

Not enough data are available on muscle imbalance to be certain how significant this is in the development of injury. It appears to be a logical concept, however, so that clinical appraisal should always be made of the strength of the major muscle groups in the legs.

Pathology elsewhere. The presence of (a) ligamentous instability, for example at the ankle, (b) structural deformity, for example after previous tibial fracture, and (c) joint stiffness, for example as a result of degenerative change, increases the stress applied to the leg during running. This increased loading may cause stress symptoms some distance away from the affected site. Examination of the lumbar spine, pelvis, hips, and knees, as well as the lower legs, should be carried out routinely.

Biomechanical abnormalities. Traditionally, convention has dictated that foot shape be described by reference to the longitudinal arch on standing. Thus the 'flat foot' or pes planus is easily recognizable, as is the rigid cavoid (supinated) foot. Of these, the most common abnormality is the pronated *pes planus*, which may be either a congenital variant or developmentally acquired. Usually, however, such a foot will be capable of revealing a substantial longitudinal arch when standing on tiptoe.

Dynamic biomechanical studies have demonstrated that during the foot contact (stance) phase of running, the foot has the ability to change from a rigid lever in the supinated state to a mobile adaptor in the pronated state (Subotnik 1985). Incorrect timing of this biomechanical change, leading to the application of abnormal forces to the leg, may result from either excessive or prolonged

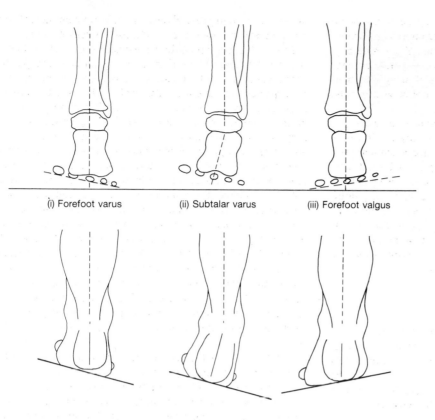

(i) Forefoot varus   (ii) Subtalar varus   (iii) Forefoot valgus

FIG. 9.23 Biomechanical abnormalities of the foot: (i) forefoot varus (inversion deformity of the head of the talus and the forefoot in relation to the calcaneus); (ii) subtalar varus (inversion deformity of the calcaneus in the neutral position); (iii) forefoot valgus (eversion deformity of the head of the talus and the forefoot in relation to the calcaneus).

pronation (Donatelli 1987). Problems may also arise when the foot remains on the running surface for too long—that is, dorsiflexing too much as a result of plantarflexor weakness or of the nature of the terrain (e.g. sand or ice). The centre of gravity then extends too far anteriorly at toe-off, creating hyperextension of the knee. Within the gait cycle (just prior to toe-off), as the heel leaves the ground, the foot should be in the neutral position. In this position, the heel is perpendicular to the ground, the subtalar joint is neither supinated nor pronated, and the plane of the metatarsal heads is at right angles to the heel. This normal position may be demonstrated in the static standing position by externally rotating the leg with the foot on the ground. When a patient is examined in this position and the articulation of the talar head with the navicular is palpated, abnormalities between the rearfoot and the forefoot, and their relationships with the leg

and the ground, may be detected. Such abnormalities may be the cause of overuse injury.

A number of variations from the norm of both forefoot and hindfoot are seen (Fig. 9.23). *Abnormal compensatory pronation at the subtalar joint (STJ)* is usually secondary to forefoot varus (Brown and Yavorsky 1987) or to ankle equinus, which is often due to tightness of the Achilles tendon. The uncompensated and compensated positions of the foot with forefoot varus are shown in Figs 9.24 and 9.25. The excessive STJ motion is necessary for the forefoot to reach the ground. The resultant excessive internal rotation of the tibia is accompanied by transmission of similar forces to the femur. Injury patterns include Achilles tendinitis, posterior tibialis tendinitis, plantar fasciitis, medial periostitis of the tibia, and the patellofemoral stress syndrome (McKenzie *et al.* 1985).

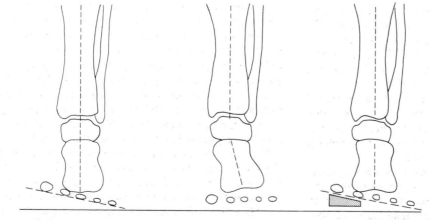

Forefoot varus   (i) Uncompensated   (ii) Compensated   (iii) Orthotic posting under first ray

FIG. 9.24 Forefoot varus: (i) uncompensated; (ii) compensated (by subtalar pronation); (iii) orthotic posting under first ray (MT 1 and medial cuneiform).

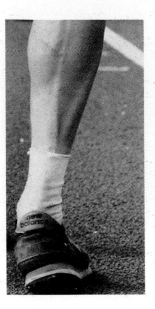

FIG 9.25 Clinical appearance of everted heel (subtalar pronation) as a compensatory mechanism for forefoot varus.

The *cavoid foot* is quite different: the dissipation of forces on heel-strike is inadequate, as unlocking of the foot does not take place owing to the relative rigidity of the subtalar and midtarsal joints. Rearfoot varus (an inverted heel) may be substantial. Supination persists through the stance phase, resulting in loss of the normal internal rotation of the lower leg: the knee retains a slight varus position, contributing to tightening of the lateral knee structures. Injury patterns include a predisposition to iliotibial tract bursitis, stress fractures, Achilles tendinitis, and lateral ankle sprains.

The positions of the STJ in neutral and of the forefoot relative to the hindfoot may be observed when the patient lies prone on the couch with his feet hanging over the edge. A weightbearing assessment is required to appreciate fully the degree of excessive pronation (in the relaxed compensated position) that is associated with a 'weak' foot due to ligamentous laxity or hypermobile first ray (MT1 and medial cuneiform). On the other hand, abnormal pronation may be due to biomechanical abnormalities associated with malalignment—for example, femoral anteversion, increased Q-angle, genu varum and valgum, and leg-length inequality. Video recordings and clinical observations on a treadmill often give valuable information on the prevailing biomechanical forces, and may be augmented by a study of the distortion and wear pattern of the running shoe.

Therapeutically, simple mechanical measures may effect adequate control. An extra insole of a few millimetres thickness inside the running shoe of a short leg may adjust the running biomechanics so as to reduce incidence of injury, even when the leg-length inequality is of the order of 1 cm or more. If the insole forces the foot too far out of the shoe, a responsible shoe manufacturer may be prevailed upon to increase the depth of the sole. An athlete may attempt to control pronation by the substitution for the running-shoe insole provided by the manufacturer by a soft arch support purchased 'off the shelf'. If this measure fails, podiatric assessment is desirable in order to diagnose the cause, whether from within the foot or from the lower limb as a whole, of any abnormal subtalar biomechanics. A soft insole or temporary posting of the hind- or forefoot may be employed. Subsequently, a hard orthotic is used if necessary. The long-term

use of orthotics to control biomechanical abnormalities appears to reduce the likelihood of further injury. Orthotics are considered further in Chapter 11, p. 197.

Training characteristics may need to be examined further and modified if necessary. Loading may need to be decreased, or crosstraining increased. Counter-clockwise sprint training around athletic tracks leads to different supinating and pronating forces on the left and right feet. For example, excessive torque on the right knee due to external rotation of the right leg during 'push off' may lead to medial symptoms. Care should be taken to achieve a well-balanced training schedule.

Inadequate footwear. The modern training shoe incorporates a number of features that assist in shock absorption and support for the foot (see Fig. 11.3, p. 186). The midsole (often made from the polyurethane compound ethylene vinyl acetate (EVA) in varying densities) and the wedge assist in shock absorption. This may be assisted further by other materials that can be incorporated into the manufacture of a running shoe in the form of an insole. The wedge also contributes to heel lift. A firm heel counter and 'arch cookie' help to control subtalar joint motion, though regrettably the flimsy arch support (cookie) is often ineffective. Pronation may be controlled by a firm heel counter, medial arch support, and a board-lasted shoe (in which the upper part of the shoe is connected to a firm fibrous innersole board). Shoes with lateral rearfoot flares should be avoided; varus wedges may help (Anthony 1987). The cavoid foot requires a board-lasted rearfoot, a lateral flare, and a firm heel counter, combined with a decent wedge and slip-lasted forefoot (in which the upper has been brought beneath the foot and stitched as a moccasin to provide greater flexibility).

It is essential for the patient with a running injury to bring in his training shoes for inspection. Inappropriate shoes (for example, casuals sold as trainers) may have been used, and it is not unusual to find over-worn footwear. Simple advice on the purchase of a suitable shoe may be all that is required for some patients. For further information on the running shoe, the reader is referred to Cavanagh (1980).

Growth characteristics. Carefully graded intensification of training schedules is obviously necessary for young athletes. It is important to recognize that, during growth spurts, increased bone-length may not always be accompanied by corresponding musculo-tendinous elasticity. Hence there is a particular need for an adequate long slow stretch programme. Youngsters are prone to heel pain if insufficient support is available from footwear. All too often, children are expected to participate in physical education programmes of all kinds, including running, in flimsy plimsolls. Physical education should include advice on warm-up, stretching, and footwear to all age groups.

Hormonal and dietary factors. Low bone density increases bone fatigue and the incidence of stress fractures as the result of repetitive loading in women (Bennell *et al.* 1996). Amenorrhoea and late menarche are recognized as risk factors.

References

Andrews, J. R. (1983). Overuse syndrome of the lower extremity. *Clin. Sports Med.*, **6**, 291–320.

Anthony, R. J. (1987). The functional anatomy of the running training shoe. *Chiropodist*, **42** (12), 451–9.

Batt, M. E. (1995). Shin splints—a review of terminology. *Clin. J. Sports Med.*, **5** (1) 53–7.

Baumgartl, F. (1964). *Das Kniegelenk*, p. 452. Springer Verlag, Berlin.

Bennell, K. L., Malcolm, S. A., Wark, J. D., and Brukner, P. D. (1996). Models for the pathogenesis of stress fractures in athletes. *Br. J. Sports Med.*, **30**, 200–4.

Brodsky, A. E. and Khalil, M. A. (1986). Talar compression syndrome. *Am. J. Sports Med* **14** (16), 472–6.

Brown, L. P. and Yavorsky, P. (1987). Locomotor biomechanics and pathomechanics: a review. *J. Orthop. Sports Phys. Ther.*, **9**, 3–10.

Cavanagh, P. R. (1980). *The running shoe book*. Anderson World, Mountain View, CA.

Donatelli, R. (1987). Abnormal biomechanics of the foot and ankle. *J. Orthop. Sports Phys. Ther.*, **9**, 11–16.

Doxey, G. E. (1987). Calcaneal pain: a review of various disorders. *J. Orthop. Sports Phys. Ther.*, **9**, 25–32.

Ficat, R. P. and Hungerford, D. S. (1977). *Disorders of the patello-femoral joint*. Williams and Wilkins, Baltimore, MD.

Goodfellow, J., Hungerford, D. S., and Zindel. M. (1976). Patello-femoral joint mechanics and pathology. *J. Bone Jt. Surg.*, **58B**, 287–90.

Hontas, M. J., Haddad, R. J., and Schlesinger, L. C. (1986). Conditions of the talus in the runner. *Am. J. Sports Med.*, **14** (6), 486–90.

Hungerford, D. S. and Barry, M. (1979). Biomechanics of the patellofemoral joint. *Clin. Orthop. Relat. Res.*, **144**, 9–15.

James, S. L., Bates, B. T., and Ostering, L. R. (1978). Injuries to runners. *Am J. Sports Med.*, **6** (2), 40–50.

Kager, H. (1939). Zur klinik und diagnostik des Achillesehnenrisses. *Chirug*, **11**, 691–5.

Kettelkamp, D. B. (1981). Current concepts review: management of patella malalignment. *J. Bone Jt Surg.*, **63A**, 1344–8.

Kilmartin, T. E. (1999). Tension night splints for the treatment of recalcitrant heel pain. *Br. J. Podiatry*, Feb 1999, 17–20.

King, J. B., Perry, D. J., Mourad, K., and Kumar, S. J. (1990). Lesions of the patellar ligament. *J. Bone Jt. Surg.*, **72B**, 46–8.

Leach, R., Jones, R., and Silva, T. (1978). Rupture of the plantar fascia in athletes. *J. Bone Jt. Surg.*, **60A**, 537–9.

Mahler, F. and Fritschy, D. (1992). Partial and complete ruptures of the Achilles tendon and local corticosteroid injections. *Br. J. Sports Med.*, **26**, 7–14.

McKenzie, D. C., Clement, D. B., and Taunton, J. E. (1985). Running shoes, orthotics and injuries. *Sports Med.*, **2**, 334–7.

McMurray, T. P. (1950). Footballer's ankle. *J. Bone Jt. Surg.*, **32B**, 68–9.

Mubarak, S. J., Gould, R. N., Lee, Y. F. *et al.* (1982). The medial tibial stress syndrome. *Am. J. Sports Med.*, **10**, 201–5.

Murphy, P. C. and Baxter, D. E. (1985). Nerve entrapment of the foot and ankle in runners. *Clin. Sports Med.*, **4** (4), 753–63.

Styf, J. (1989). Chronic exercise-induced pain in the anterior aspect of the lower leg. *Sports Med.* **7**, 331–9.

Subotnick, S. I. (1985). The biomechanics of running: implications for the prevention of foot injures. *Sports Med.*, **2**, 144–53.

Torg, J. S., Pavlov, H., and Torg, E. (1987). Overuse injuries in sport: the foot. *Clin. Sports Med.*, **6**, 291–320.

Wiberg, G. (1941). Roentgenographic and anatomic studies on the femoropatellar joint. *Acta Orthop. Scand.*, **12**, 319–410.

Wood, G. A. (1987). Biomechanical limitations to sprint running. *Med. Sport Sci.*, **25**, 58–71.

10 Investigations

M. A. HUTSON AND D. B. L. FINLAY

Non-radiological investigation

M. A. HUTSON

Clinical assessment of patients suffering from sports-related injuries combines a thorough history and a detailed musculoskeletal examination. This alone often is sufficient to establish a diagnosis. For full assessment, however, further investigative procedures may be needed. Since rheumatological conditions sometimes masquerade as sports trauma, rheumatological screening may be required. Additional information on those tissues which are deep-lying and therefore not easily inspected or palpated—for example, intervertebral discs and (intra-articular) menisci—may be gained by radiological or pathological investigation. Thus CT scans, MRI scans, and scintigraphy may complement straight radiological techniques. Biopsy of muscle or synovium occasionally may be useful.

Certain procedures—for instance, joint aspiration and epidural injection of procaine—may have both diagnostic and therapeutic applications. However, the employment of local anaesthesia as a diagnostic tool usually should be unnecessary if a satisfactory clinical examination has been conducted.

Tests for muscle function may be performed on an isokinetic dynamometer, and the results computerized in a tabulated or graphical form: they are considered further in Chapters 11 and 12.

Joint aspiration

This may be performed in either a mono- or polyarthropathy for the following reasons.

1. Detection (and therapeutic aspiration) of a haemarthrosis. The additional presence of fat globules indicates an intra-articular fracture.

2. Detection of *inflammatory cells*. Other than a haemarthrosis, an effusion may be either clear (serous) or turbid. Turbidity indicates the presence of a large number of inflammatory cells which are secondary to infection or inflammatory joint disease. High white cell counts (for example, up to 50 000 per cubic millimetre) are found in infection, and also in rheumatoid and psoriatic arthropathy.

3. Detection of *organisms*. Gram-staining identifies the presence of gonococcal, staphylococcal, and streptococcal bacteria. A Ziehl-Neelsen stain is used if the presence of *Mycobacterium tuberculosis* is suspected.

4. Detection of *crystals*. The use of a polarizing microscope is necessary to detect the presence of needle-like urate crystals in gout: strongly negative birefringence is found. Weakly positive birefringence indicates pseudogout (rhomboid or rectangular-shaped pyrophosphate crystals). Spectrophotometry is required to identify hydroxyapatite crystals, which are thought to be responsible for low-grade joint inflammation (and are present in 'calcific' tendinitis).

Haematological and serological tests

Hb, WBC and differential, and ESR. Anaemia is found in chronic inflammatory disease. White cell count is elevated in the presence of infection. ESR may of course be elevated in the presence of active disease, though it is an unreliable indicator of the presence or the progress of the various polyarthritides.

Latex and rheumatoid factor, ANF and DNA binding. The latex and rheumatoid factor tests are positive in rheumatoid arthritis and negative in osteoarthritis. ANF and DNA binding are positive in systemic lupus erythematosus.

Uric acid. Hyperuricaemia indicates a gouty tendency. Positive clinical findings or crystals are necessary to confirm the diagnosis of gout.

Tissue typing. The HLA B27 antigen test is most useful if one of the spondyloarthritides is suspected: 96 per cent of cases of ankylosing spondylitis and 50 per cent of Reiter's syndrome are positive.

Plasma proteins, calcium, phosphate, and alkaline phosphatase. These investigations are necessary to exclude metabolic and bone disease as a cause of back pain.

Creatine phosphokinase (CPK or CK). The level of this enzyme is often substantially raised in the presence of muscle damage resulting from overtraining. It is also high in polymyositis.

Biopsy

Virtually any tissue may be biopsied, should the need arise. In practice synovial biopsy is used occasionally, though its application is limited because of the non-specificity of the observed inflammatory changes. Muscle biopsy may reveal mitochondrial abnormalities, an uncommon cause of recurrent muscle dysfunction. Fibre-typing is largely a research procedure.

Urinalysis

Other than its general use in screening and in detection of certain specific diseases, there are few other indications for urinalysis in sports trauma. Haemoglobin or myoglobin may be detected in the urine after endurance activities or after gross muscle trauma.

Radiological investigations

D. B. L. FINLAY

Plain film radiography

The principal imaging technique for the diagnosis of fractures is plain film radiography. A fracture most commonly is seen on the radiograph as a line of lucency—the greater the displacement of the component parts of the fracture, the wider and more obvious is the fracture line. The visibility of this line also depends on its alignment with the X-ray beam, and if it is oblique it becomes less visible. There is a degree of obliquity at which each individual fracture line will not be seen. However, it is unusual for the fracture line not to be visible on a further radiograph obtained at right angles to the first (Fig. 10.1). These

(a)

(b)

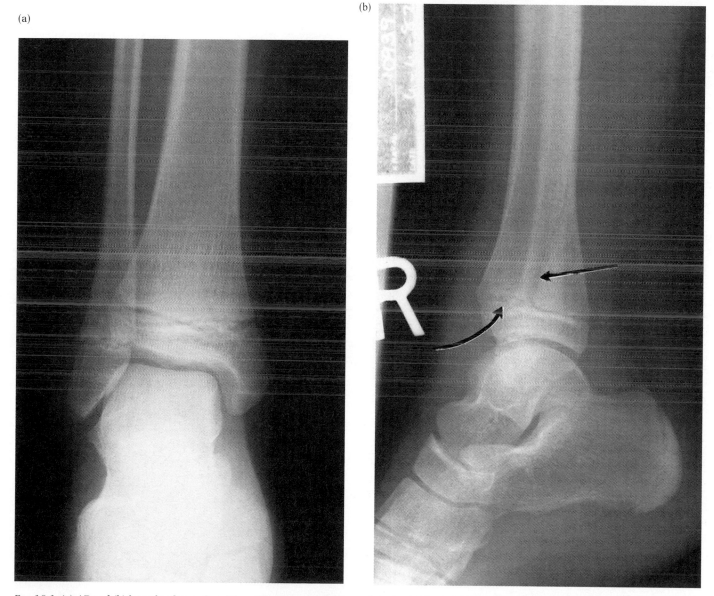

FIG. 10.1 (a) AP and (b) lateral radiographs of the ankle of a child. Fracture of the lower tibia is only visible on the lateral radiograph (arrowed). There is separation of the lower tibial epiphysis (curved arrow) (Salter II epiphyseal injury)

observations apply to fractures involving most of the circumference of a bone. However, for identification of fractures which involve only part of the circumference, in particular fractures of the end of a bone within a joint or avulsion fractures by tendons or ligaments, further radiographs may need to be obtained. To a lesser extent this is also true of fractures involving the proximal or distal shaft of a bone. *Therefore, it is important that information be given by the requesting physician about the precise location of the injury and the suspected nature.* This helps to ensure that adequate radiographs are obtained for diagnosis.

The sports physician is particularly interested in fractures inside a joint and in ligament or tendon avulsions. It is important to note abnormal alignment of one bone with another. Even

if no fracture is visible, malalignment suggests the presence of ligamentous damage, which is of particular importance in the fingers (Fig. 10.2). It is necessary to verify the articulation of individual bones in areas in which multiple joints exist in the wrist and foot.

Fractures can be seen as areas of increased density due to impaction. This is common in fractures of the femoral neck, in depressed fractures of the skull vault, and in some stress fractures (see Fig. 10.11, p. 184). In comminuted and other fractures where the alignment of fragments of bone with the X-ray beam is altered, there may be increased density. This also occurs when bones overlap, as in a dislocation.

It is important that the same rule of two radiographs, usually obtained at right angles, is remembered in examining joints. It is easy to miss a dislocation when only one view is obtained. When a long bone is fractured, the joints above and below should be included on the radiograph.

Two additional types of fracture occur in children. Incomplete fractures are commonly classed as *greenstick* fractures. One cortex may be fractured and the other bent or bowed but intact, as commonly occurs in the mid-shaft of the radius and the ulna; alternatively, they may be compression fractures, causing bulging of one or both cortices, as commonly occurs at the end of the long bones, particularly the radius and the ulna (Fig. 10.3). The second group of fractures are *epiphyseal separations.* These occur with or without an accompanying metaphyseal fragment, and are the childhood equivalent of a dislocation or ligamentous injury (Fig. 10.4).

For further information on fractures, the reader is referred to the book by Rogers (1982).

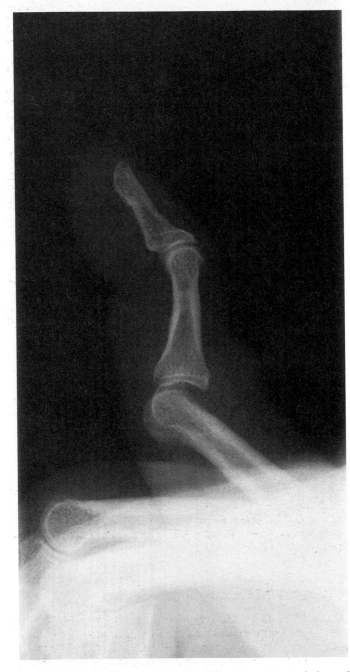

FIG. 10.2 Lateral radiograph of the finger. The proximal interphalangeal joint is hyperextended due to acute volar plate disruption.

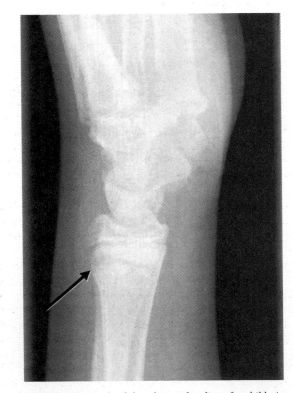

FIG. 10.3 Lateral radiograph of the ulna and radius of a child. A greenstick fracture is demonstrated. Bulging of the posterior cortex is seen (arrowed).

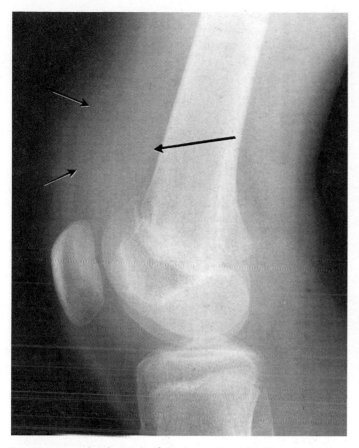

FIG. 10.4 Lateral radiograph of the knee of a child. There is anterior displacement (Salter I) of the lower femoral ephiphysis and a large effusion in the knee joint (arrowed).

Soft tissue signs

Unfortunately, radiographs do not image soft tissues well. Soft tissue swelling is a useful marker of damage and possible underlying fracture (Fig. 10.5). Although some injuries, for instance complete tears of the Achilles tendon, may be identified on the radiograph, this is of little primary value. A complete tear will be seen as a disruption of the normal convex curve of the tendon. There is normally a lucent triangle bounded by the Achilles tendon posteriorly, the deep layer of posterior tibial muscles anteriorly, and the superior margin of the tuberosity of the calcaneum inferiorly. This is obliterated when there is damage—either incomplete or complete rupture of the Achilles tendon (see Fig. 9.18, p. 167).

At the knee, infrapatellar tendon ruptures are demonstrated by superior displacement of the patella (Fig. 10.5) associated with a soft tissue mass in the region of the infrapatellar tendon. There may be avulsion fractures from the inferior pole of the patella or from the tibial tubercle. In the normal knee, the length of the infrapatellar tendon is approximately the same as the longest diameter of the patella.

When there is an effusion in the knee joint, swelling of the suprapatellar pouch above the knee can be seen (Fig. 10.4). In the normal knee this is visible only as a stripe, the width of the thickness of two layers of synovial membrane surrounded by extra-synovial fat. If there has been a fracture in the joint which

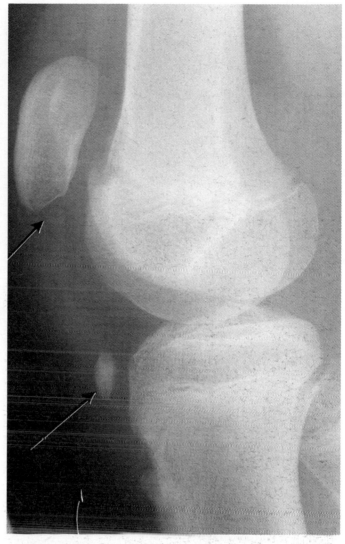

FIG. 10.5 Patellar tendon avulsion. Lateral radiograph of the knee shows that the patella lies high. (The distance from the lower pole of the patella to the tibial tuberosity should equal the longest oblique diameter of the patella.) There are fragments avulsed from the inferior pole of the patella and the anterior tibial tubercle (arrowed). Soft tissue swelling is seen in the area of the patellar tendon (curved arrow).

has released fat, this lipohaemarthrosis may be seen on a horizontal lateral radiograph as a fat fluid level within the joint.

At the elbow, a joint effusion may be identified by elevation of the anterior fat pad, as a sail-shape, away from the anterior cortex of the distal humerus (Fig. 10.6). The posterior fat pad, which is not normally in evidence behind the lower humerus, becomes visible.

Avulsion fractures

Fragments of bone are avulsed by ligaments or tendons. They may vary in size from small slivers to quite large fragments, as occurs, for instance, at the base of the fifth metatarsal owing to avulsion by the peroneus brevis (Fig. 10.7). They indicate serious damage to the soft tissues, rather than just fractures of the bone. They occur in many characteristic sites, but are partic-

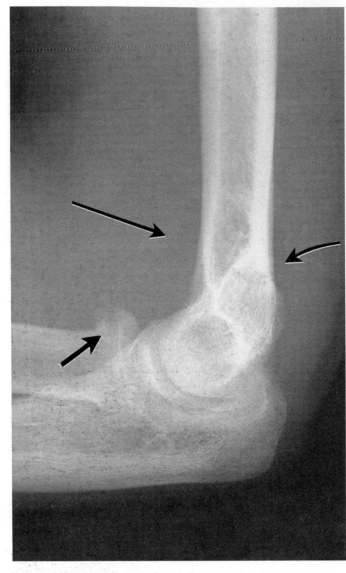

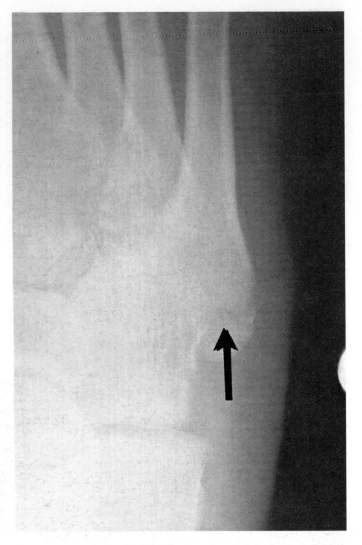

FIG. 10.7 AP radiograph of the foot. Avulsion of the base of the fifth metatarsal by the peroneus brevis has occurred (see also Fig. 9.2, p. 152).

FIG. 10.6 Lateral radiograph of the elbow. Elevation of the anterior fat pad which is sail-shaped (arrow) and the posterior fat pad (curved arrow) are demonstrated. The radial head is fractured (thick arrow).

ularly common at the ankle and foot (see Fig. 9.16, p. 165). From the malleoli of the ankle, avulsion fractures are caused by the medial and the lateral collateral ligaments; in the foot, they occur from the navicular and talus. In the pelvis, the anterior superior iliac spine is avulsed by the sartorius, the anterior inferior iliac spine by the rectus femoris, and the ischial tuberosity by the hamstrings (see Fig. 1.13, p. 13). It is important to note that avulsion of the ischial tuberosity commonly produces a large mass of bone in the healing phase, which may be misdiagnosed as a tumour. Avulsion fractures also commonly occur in the fingers—for example, avulsion of the extensor tendon at the base of the distal phalanx, of the profundus tendon on the volar surface of the base of the distal phalanx, and of the volar plate at the base of the middle phalanx. In the knee, damage to the extensor mechanism may cause avulsion of the superior and inferior patellar tendon attachments (Fig. 10.5), avulsion of the tibial tubercle, or complete fractures of the patella (Fig. 10.8).

In the foot, avulsion fractures must be distinguished from accessory ossicles and normal apophyses. The ossicles occur in characteristic sites. Examples are the os tibialis externa (Fig. 10.9(a)), which lies proximal to the medial tuberosity of the navicular, the os supranaviculare, which is related to the dorsal aspect of the navicular (Fig. 10.9(b)), and the apophysis of the base of the fifth metatarsal. These do not 'fit' the adjacent bone and have rounded corticated margins. In these sites, avulsed fragments which are larger than slivers should fit with the underlying bone, should have sharp well-defined margins, and may be associated with soft tissue swelling.

Stress fractures

Stress fractures occur in normal bone in response to the stress of repeated activity. Their sites are characteristic. They commonly occur in the distal part of the second and third metatarsal shafts (Fig. 10.10), the proximal and distal shaft of the tibia and fibula, the neck of the femur, and the pubic rami. A radiograph of the

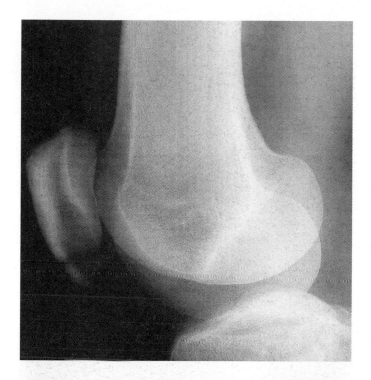

FIG. 10.8 Lateral radiograph of the knee. There is a transverse fracture of the lower pole of the patella.

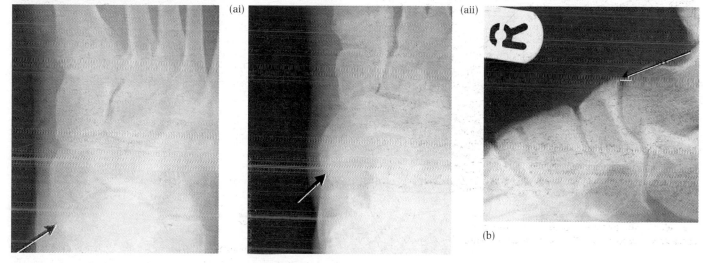

(ai)   (aii)

(b)

FIG. 10.9 (a) (i) and (ii) Dorsiplantar radiographs of the foot. An os tibialis externa is seen. Its margins are corticated and rounded, seen particularly laterally where its margin is seen in profile without the overlying navicular bone (arrowed). Importantly, this is the characteristic site of this os. (b) Lateral radiograph of the foot. An os supranaviculare with rounded margins is seen at its characteristic site.

area involved is normal at the time of injury. No evidence of a fracture will be seen for between ten days and three weeks. The fracture may first be seen as a thin translucent line, or periosteal callus may be visualized without evidence of the fracture line. Occasionally the fracture may be seen as sclerosis due to impaction, for example in the tibia or calcaneum (Fig. 10.11).

In the tibia, multiple stress fractures in the anterior cortex may produce marked thickening, with a wavy outline that is sometimes associated with multiple horizontal radiolucent defects (Fig. 10.12). This appearance represents multiple stress fractures at different stages in healing. Occasionally periosteal and endosteal thickening of the cortex may be observed without

a fracture line. If not seen in profile, a stress fracture may appear as a rounded lucency within thickened cortical bone.

There is often concern that these radiological abnormalities may be due to bone tumours. This is particularly so in lesions in the tibia, especially near the knee joint. An osteosarcoma initially may be visualized predominantly as periosteal elevation (Fig. 10.13); an osteoid osteoma normally causes sclerosis and cortical thickening. In the latter case, a well-defined area of rarefaction is commonly seen in the bone (Fig. 10.14); in an osteosarcoma, rarefaction is indiscrete. The osteoid osteoma gives a history of pain, predominantly at night, which is relieved by aspirin. Other tumours and infection do not usually cause great problems in differential diagnosis, provided that the history

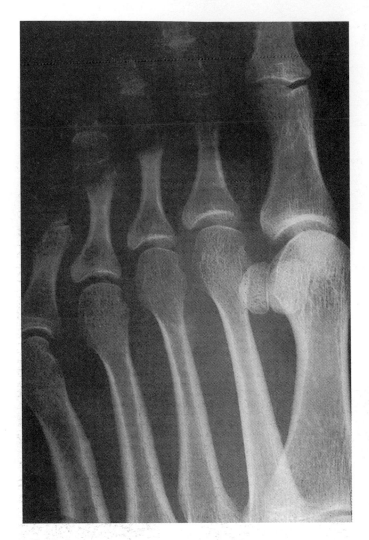

Fig. 10.10 Oblique radiograph of the foot. A stress fracture of the third metatarsal neck is identified by the presence of callus formation, without a fracture line being evident.

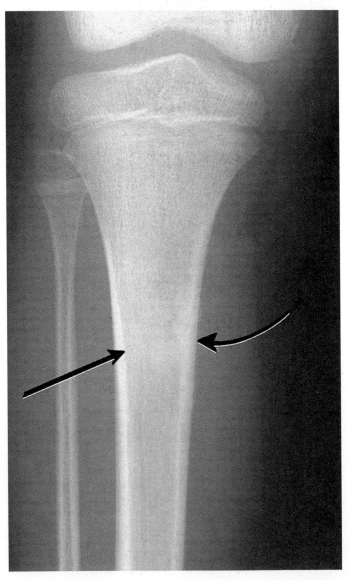

Fig. 10.11 AP radiograph of the upper tibia of a child. Sclerosis (arrowed) and periosteal elevation (curved arrow) are due to a stress fracture.

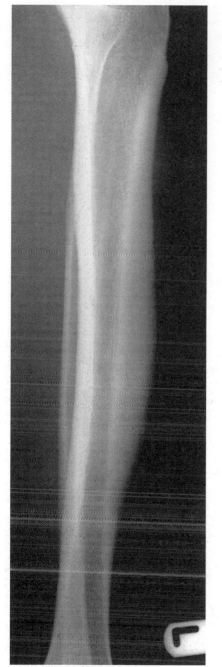

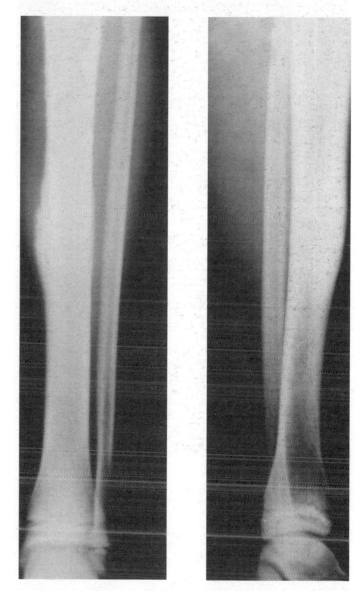

Fig. 10.12 Lateral radiograph of the tibia. Marked thickening of the anterior cortex is seen. The wavy appearance is due to multiple old stress fractures.

Fig. 10.13 (a) AP and (b) lateral radiographs of the tibia. Initially, an osteosarcoma may be visualized predominantly as periosteal elevation.

and the characteristic sites of stress fractures are remembered. Very occasionally the diagnosis can only be determined by biopsy.

Sesamoid fractures

In common with avulsion fractures, the opposing surfaces of a fractured sesamoid should appear to fit together and seem sharp and possibly jagged (Fig. 10.15). In practice, it is probably impossible to make the diagnosis in the absence of suitable clinical findings. Sesamoid fractures, when they occur, are seen most commonly in the medial and fibular sesamoids related to the big toe.

Myositis ossificans

This results from calcification arising in a post-traumatic haematoma. It occurs characteristically in the quadriceps muscle, and produces an area of calcification which is orientated longitudinally along the limb (see Fig. 1.8(b), p. 7). Initially the appearances are of a cloud of calcification within the tissues, but, with time, this becomes organized and actual bony trabeculae can be identified.

Calcification is seen occasionally in certain areas of the body after chronic trauma, for instance in the medial collateral ligament of the knee (see Fig. 9.10, p. 149), the Pellegrini–Steida lesion, and in the adductors of the thigh, as seen in horse-riders.

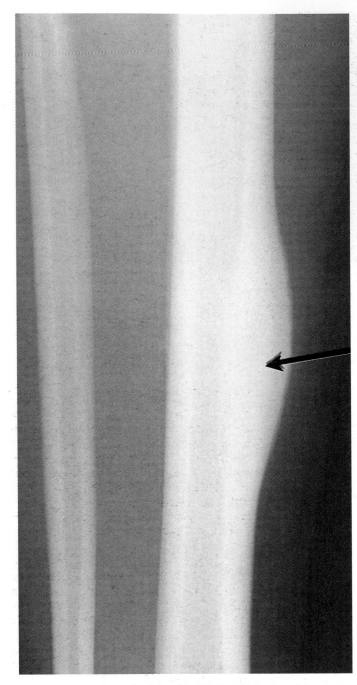

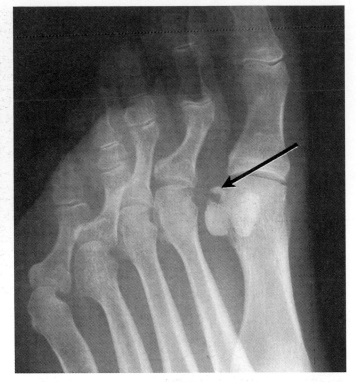

FIG. 10.15 Oblique radiograph of the big toe. A fragment is seen distally which fits 'with the rest of the sesamoid'. Its margins are not rounded— a fracture of the medial sesamoid.

FIG. 10.14 AP radiograph of the tibia. Marked thickening of the cortex with a central lucency (arrowed) is due to an osteoid osteoma.

Bands of calcification, indicative of chondrocalcinosis, may be seen in fibrocartilage such as the knee menisci.

Osteochondral and chondral fractures

Abnormal joint movements associated with subluxation or dislocation may produce fractures of one or both joint surfaces. The resulting fragment may be cartilage alone, which will not be visible on plain radiographs, or may consist of a fragment of bone and cartilage. These fractures occur in characteristic sites, and close examination of the radiograph often is neces-

sary to detect them. They are found after dislocation of the patella, and arise from the medial facet of the patella (Fig. 10.16) or the lateral femoral condyle. They are often best seen on the skyline view. Osteochondral fractures of the dome of the talus occur on both the medial and lateral aspects, and result from inversion injuries. They are usually best seen on the mortise view of the ankle joint (see Fig. 8.13, p. 148). Osteochondral fractures are also commonly observed in the capitellum and radial head.

Osteochondritis dissecans

In osteochondritis dissecans, a fragment of bone which is concave away from the joint becomes separate from contiguous bone, although the overlying articular cartilage may be intact. At its most minimal, it may be identified only by a line of lucency around it (Fig. 10.17); at its most maximal, a fragment of bone and its overlying cartilage may become free within the joint. These lesions are seen particularly in the femoral condyles, and may also be demonstrated in the talus and hip joint.

Dislocations

The need for suitable clinical information upon which the correct radiological views are taken is highlighted at the shoulder. Posterior dislocation of the shoulder joint is easily missed on the AP radiograph, as the radiographic features are subtle. The most reliable sign is that the head looks unusually oval because the upper arm is in forced internal rotation.

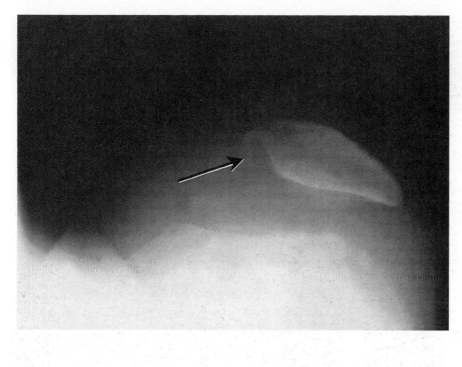

FIG. 10.16 Skyline view of the patella. Fragments of bone (arrowed) have fractured from the medial surface of the patella after dislocation.

Recurrent dislocations

These commonly occur in two sites—the patellofemoral and the glenohumeral joints. At the knee, the patella is dislocated in a lateral direction: this is associated with a low lateral femoral condyle seen on the skyline view of the patella, and a long infra-patellar tendon (patella alta). Recurrent anterior dislocation of the shoulder is associated with damage to the anterior glenoid labrum with or without the separation of a bony fragment (Bankart lesion).

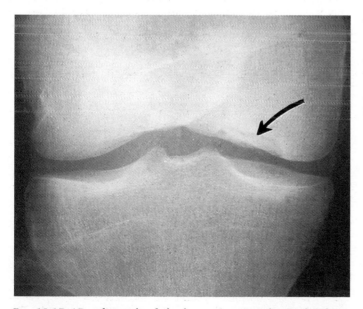

FIG. 10.17 AP radiograph of the knee. An area of osteochondritis dissecans with a line of lucency around it (curved arrow) is demonstrated.

Radioisotope bone imaging

In the diagnosis of sports injuries, radioisotope bone imaging is most commonly used to detect stress fractures. The images are obtained by a gamma camera after the intravenous injection of technetium-99m-labelled phosphate or diphosphonate. The amount of local radioactivity seen on the isotope scan correlates with the rate of mineralization of the bone; increased tracer localization or so-called 'hot spots' are seen in stress fractures. Hot spots can be seen at fracture sites as early as twenty-four hours after injury. This is well before evidence will be available on a radiograph.

In addition to facilitating early diagnosis, radioisotopic bone imaging is also of use in a patient in whom there is a history of pain, but in whom no fracture or abnormality can be detected radiologically even after a delayed period. This occurs particularly in the foot, where fractures of the navicular and cuneiforms may be difficult to see on a radiograph (see Fig. 9.22, p. 170). The detection of a hot spot on the radioisotopic scan allows a more localized search of the radiographs for a fracture; further views or CT scanning may be indicated.

Investigation of the joints

Magnetic resonance imaging (MRI) is now the modality most often used for the examination of the joints. Relying for its effect on the excitation of protons by a magnetic field and not requiring ionizing radiation, it has no known side-effects and is extremely sensitive. Although images, which highlight different structures, can be produced by different sequences, the images are known as being T_1 or T_2 weighted. Fat, marrow fat, fat pads, and fat planes between muscle are shown to good advantage on T_1 weighting. Fluid is demonstrated on T_2 weighting: effusions within joints are particularly well seen, as are cysts.

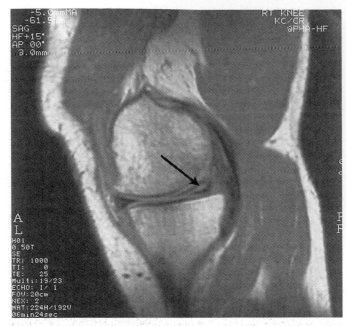

Fig. 10.18 Oblique tear (arrowed) of the posterior horn of the medial meniscus demonstrated by MRI on a T_1 weighted sagittal slice through the medial compartment of the knee.

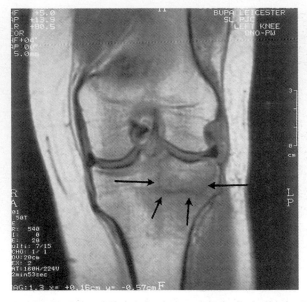

FIG. 10.20 Coronal T_1-weighted image through the knee. A line of reduced density (arrowed) is seen surrounding a minimally depressed fracture of the lateral tibial plateau. This injury occurred in a skier; the clinical diagnosis was a lateral meniscal tear. Plain films were normal.

The knee

MRI has revolutionized the investigation of traumatic knee disorders. Images are produced most commonly in the sagittal, coronal, and axial planes.

In the knee, MRI is highly accurate. A normal MRI examination almost totally excludes significant abnormality in the knee. A meniscal tear is seen as a line crossing the meniscus involving one or more articular surfaces. Oblique (Fig. 10.18), horizontal, and vertical tears can be differentiated easily. The specific features of bucket-handle tears are also well visualized. The ante-

rior cruciate ligament is normally well demonstrated; its disruption (Fig. 10.19) and site of disruption can be diagnosed in a high percentage of cases. It is, however, not possible to differentiate partial from complete ACL tears with certainty. Coronal images allow assessment of the collateral ligaments; axial images assessment of the patellofemoral joint and confirmation of the presence or absence of meniscal cysts. Minor degrees of abnormality of the patellofemoral joint, in particular chondromalacia patellae, cannot be diagnosed with certainty. However, in other patella conditions, particularly dislocation, features can be seen which confirm the diagnosis. Stress fractures of the tibial plateau (Fig. 10.20) which may present in sportsmen with pain simulating a meniscus tear are also well demonstrated.

The ankle

The ankle joint can be investigated by MRI or ankle arthrography. Ankle arthrography is used to demonstrate tears of the calcaneo-fibular ligament. When this ligament is torn, contrast is seen to fill the peroneal tendon sheath, which lies in immediate proximity to the calcaneofibular ligament. Ankle arthrography can also be used to confirm that loose bodies lie within the joint.

The arthrogram is performed by the introduction of a needle under radiographic screening into the anterior tibiotalar joint space on its anteromedial aspect. One to two millilitres of radio-opaque contrast are introduced, and the joint is then distended by the introduction of approximately 6 ml of room air. Anteroposterior and lateral and both oblique radiographs are obtained. Tomography may be necessary to confirm the presence of fragments of bone within the joint.

MRI is not as accurate at diagnosing calcaneofibular ligament disruption as is ankle arthrography. If a normal calcaneofibular ligament is demonstrated on MRI, it is intact. However, its apparent absence does not mean that it is ruptured. MRI, however, has the advantage that it is extremely good at demon-

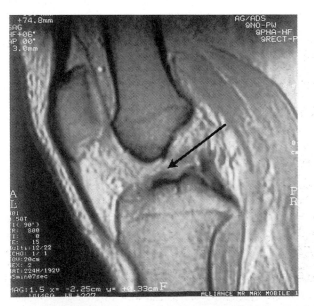

FIG. 10.19 MRI investigation of the knee. T_1-weighted sagittal image through the intercondylar fossa of the knee. The anterior cruciate ligament is torn; its inferior part only is seen (arrowed).

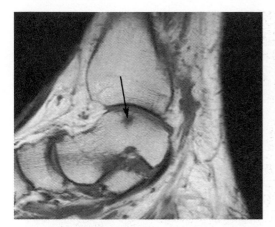

FIG. 10.21 MRI sagittal T_1 sequence through the ankle showing an osteochondral abnormality in the talar dome (arrow)

strating injuries of the talar dome (Fig. 10.21). To increase the accuracy of MRI with respect to the ligaments to the same level as arthrography, it is necessary to perform an MRI arthrogram. Gadolinium is introduced into the joint as a contrast material, which enhances the fluid signal in the joint.

The shoulder

MRI is particularly useful in the evaluation of tears of the rotator cuff. Disruption of the elements of the cuff, commonly the supraspinatus tendon, may be visualized (Fig. 10.22). Fluid in the subacromial bursa is also well demonstrated. The ability of MRI to evaluate the soft tissues and the availability of images in any plane required provide assistance to the clinician in dealing with the impingement syndrome (Fig. 10.23). The accuracy of diagnosis of rotator cuff tears in particular can be increased by the use of gadolinium.

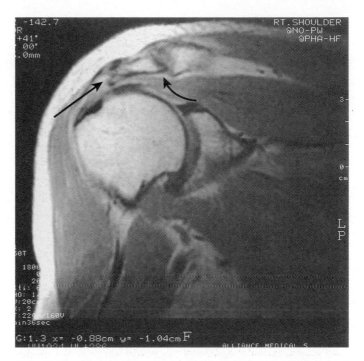

Fig. 10.23 MRI investigation of subacromial impingement. Coronal oblique T_1-weighted image of the shoulder showing an osteophyte arising from the acromion (arrow) impinging on the supraspinatus tendon; there is also an osteophyte arising from the acromioclavicular joint (curved arrow) impinging on the supraspinatus muscle.

Although defects of the glenoid labrum are readily seen on MRI (Fig. 10.24), CT shoulder arthrography is more commonly performed as part of the investigation of recurrent dislocation of the shoulder. In the case of an anterior dislocation, deformity of the anterior inferior rim of the glenoid and its overlying articular cartilage may be seen (Bankart lesion). In the case of a posterior dislocation, a defect of the posterior aspect of the labrum may be seen.

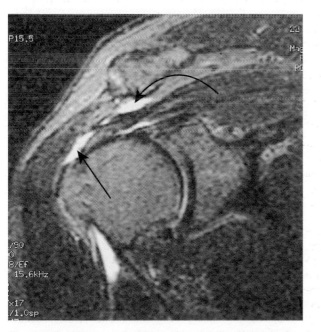

FIG. 10.22 MRI coronal oblique T_2 sequence through the shoulder showing a tear in the rotator cuff (straight arrow). Fluid is seen in the subacromial bursa (curved arrow).

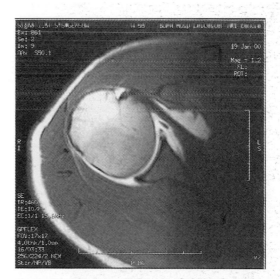

FIG. 10.24 MRI axial images in a patient with a known previous anterior dislocation. The MRI post-gadolinium enhancement shows damage to the anterior glenoid labrum (arrow) not visible on a non-enhanced MRI.

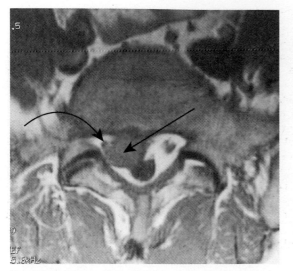

FIG. 10.25 MRI axial T_1 image at the level of L5/S1 showing a large disc prolapse (straight arrow) impinging on the right S1 nerve root (curved arrow).

The arthrogram is performed by the introduction of a needle, most commonly anteriorly, between the humeral head and the glenoid. Under radiographic screening, approximately 4 ml of radio-opaque contrast is introduced followed by 10 ml of room air. In the diagnosis of tears of the rotator cuff, contrast may be seen extending into the subacromial and subdeltoid bursae. When a frozen shoulder is present, the joint capsule is shown to be contracted; this is particularly evident in the small size of the axillary recess. It is then often useful to introduce local anaesthetic and steroid into the joint, and distend it until rupture and leakage of air from the joint capsule occurs. Active physiotherapy with maximum movement of the joint is then encouraged.

The spine

MRI is the investigation of choice for the spine. Images are commonly obtained both in the sagittal and axial planes. Disc prolapses can be demonstrated confidently and their relationship to the central neural tissue and the emerging nerve roots ascertained (Fig. 10.25).

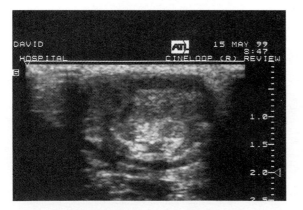

FIG. 10.26 Axial ultrasound image of a grossly abnormal, swollen Achilles tendon with heterogeneous signal. Chronic tendinopathy.

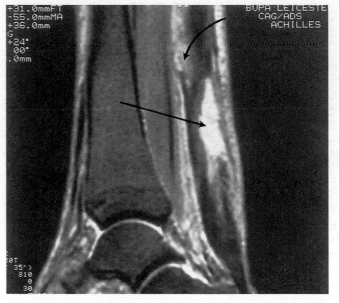

Fig. 10.27 MRI T_2-weighted sagittal image of the ankle showing haemorrhage (arrow) at the site of a tear in the Achilles tendon; haemorrhage is also seen in the soleus muscle (curved arrow).

Soft tissues

The soft tissues can be imaged both by diagnostic ultrasound and by MRI. Diagnostic ultrasound images are produced by sound of between five and ten MHz transmitted into the patient through the skin by a transducer which then receives echoes back. A coupling agent such as olive oil allows good contact between the transducer and the patient. When used in these quantities, ultrasound is harmless. It is a relatively cheap investigation, but is operator dependent. By and large, ultrasound and MRI produce similar images, but MRI has the advantage of producing a clearly understandable cross-sectional image. The Achilles tendon and its paratenon can be imaged by both, and a range of appearances in chronic tendinopathy can be demonstrated (Fig. 10.26). Complete rupture is better assessed by MRI (Fig. 10.27). Both modalities demonstrate retrocalcaneal and retroachilles bursae. Both techniques can be used to assess the patella tendon. Intramuscular haematomas can also be assessed by both techniques, but MRI allows better anatomical definition (Fig. 10.28). Other tendons, particularly in the fingers, can be demonstrated, but again MRI does allow for a more complete anatomical evaluation. Ultrasound enables the early diagnosis of stress fractures, particularly in the metatarsals, by the demonstration of soft tissue swelling around the fracture site.

Computerized tomography

Computerized tomography (CT) is at present the principal diagnostic tool in the evaluation of trauma in the brain. Both extradural and subdural haematoma (Fig. 10.29) are well visualized. An extradural haematoma produces a biconvex abnormality in relation to the skull vault. A subdural haematoma is seen as a layer outlining the surface of the brain. Both types of haematoma appear dense in the first two weeks, after which

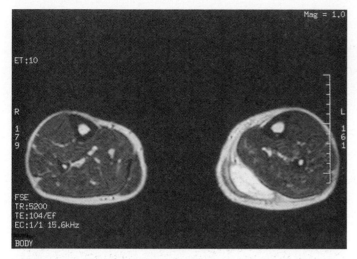

FIG. 10.28 MRI axial T_2 sequence through the calf showing a large haemorrhage in gastrocnemius (arrow).

time they reduce in density, eventually becoming less dense than the underlying brain. There is a stage at which they show the same density on the CT scan as the underlying brain tissue. Both these collections of blood cause displacement of the midline of the brain away from the haematoma and tend to obliterate the ventricular system.

Evidence of concussion to the brain may be seen either as an area of increased density due to oedema, or as increased density due to blood lying within the brain tissues. The number and size of areas of haemorrhage may vary greatly. CT scanning occa-

sionally may reveal an increase in brain volume recognizable by obliteration of the ventricles, basal cisterns, and cerebral sulci.

CT is the primary modality in the diagnosis of subarachnoid haemorrhage. Increased density due to blood may be found in the sylvian fissures and the basal cisterns, and in the ventricular system. In approximately 25 per cent of cases of subarachnoid haemorrhage, however, the CT scan is normal.

MRI is now used in the assessment of brain damage in boxers. This may reveal frontal atrophy or basal ganglia degeneration.

CT is also of use in injury to the skeleton. It is of particular benefit in the spine, where it allows the production of images in the transverse plane. This is particularly helpful to the surgeon prior to consideration of operative intervention. CT is also capable of showing fractures at levels which appear normal on plain radiographs. In the pelvis, CT assists in the assessment of traumatic conditions which require surgery, and in the identification of loose bodies present within the hip joint.

References

Fornage, B. D. (1988). Ultrasound examination of the tendons. In *Ultrasonography of the musculoskeletal system*. Radiologic Clinics of North America, W. B. Saunders, Philadelphia, PA.

Rogers, L. F. (1982). *Radiology of skeletal trauma*. Churchill Livingstone, New York.

Stoller, D. W. (1997). Magnetic resonance imaging. In *Orthopaedics and sports medicine*. Lippincott Raven, Philadelphia, New York.

Vincent, L. W. (1988). Ultrasound of soft tissue abnormalities of the extremities. In *Ultrasonography of the musculoskeletal system*. Radiologic Clinics of North America, W. B. Saunders, Philadelphia, PA.

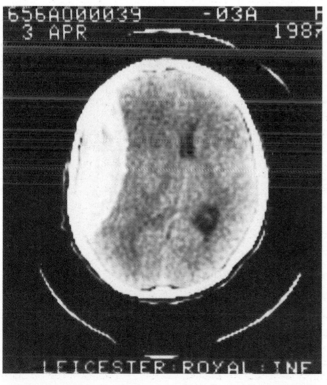

Fig. 10.29 CT slice through the skull. A dense extradural haematoma is revealed.

11 Prevention of injury

M. A. HUTSON

Responsibility of the medical profession in sports injury prevention

Members of the medical profession, in particular those involved with sports injuries (and in the broader context with sports medicine), have a responsibility to advise both sports groups and individuals on aspects of prevention of injury resulting from sport. Such advice may be offered at all levels, with the recipients ranging from sports governing bodies on the one hand to local sports clubs and individual sports participants on the other. Major strides in injury prevention have been made in certain directions, though progress is slow in others, particularly where there are financial implications and where there are possibilities of infringement of personal freedom. This advisory function should be the responsibility not only of the various associations of sports physicians on behalf of their membership, but also of individual practitioners, acting in concert with administrators, managers, and coaches in their own localities.

Protective equipment

Reduction in the incidence of injury due to direct trauma is influenced by the design of protective equipment and the obligation upon the wearer to comply with the regulations of sports associations. An obvious example is the wearing of suitable helmets by horse-riders. In horse-racing, the wearing of a skull cap of acceptable design is mandatory. In competitions under the control of the British Horse Society or the Pony Club, it is also compulsory for the riders to wear a protective helmet that conforms to the standard PAS 015 (British Standards Institute), EN 1384 (European standard), or ASTM F1163 (American standard). (Fig. 11.1). However, many competitions are not held under such control, with inevitable consequences. Even when a helmet is worn, it is important to stress the need for attachment of the chinstrap. Of course, fashion plays a part. Not long ago, Mike Brearley (an outstanding captain of English cricket in recent times) was advocating the use of head and facial protection while batting at cricket. At first, the reaction from the 'macho' element was of disbelief, but the application of protection in specific risk situations, for example batting or fielding close to the wicket, is now commonplace. In some sports, such as American football, motorcycling, cricket, and hockey (goalminders), the helmet has a visor or grille extension to reduce the incidence of maxillofacial injury (Fig. 11.1). Standards and statutory requirements vary in different sports. in some it is also necessary to comply with international regulations.

In American football, body protection has become so extensive that the sceptic is inclined to the view that the game is effectively a licence to injure. However, the incidence of head, neck, and shoulder injuries appears to be on the decline. In cricket, batsmen often protect the forearms, ribs, and thighs, as well as the genitals. In karate, the use of fist pads has been shown to reduce the severity of head injuries, which account for the majority of injuries sustained in tournaments (Johannsen and Noerregaard 1988).

(a) (b) (c)

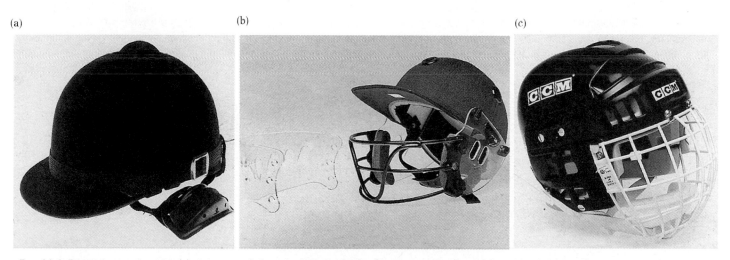

FIG. 11.1 Protective equipment: (a) equestrian helmet to BSI standards; (b) an example of a cricketer's helmet (alternative forms of visor are demonstrated); (c) ice hockey goal-minder's helmet.

Goggles are worn in a number of sports in which high speeds are encountered (see Fig. 2.5, p. 33). Special goggles made from tough polycarbonate material are available for squash. Recently a British Standard (BS 7930:1) for eye protection in squash has been published. Eye protection is now mandatory in doubles squash and in some specified SRA major junior events (see Chapter 2, Ocular injuries). However, one should not assume that the mere replacement of spectacles by contact lenses protects the eye. Increased damage to the eye may result from direct trauma to a contact lens; soft lenses are safest.

Mouth guards are compulsory in some sports, for example boxing, and their use is encouraged though not mandatory in others, such as rugby football. All contact sports participants are at risk; the highest incidences of injury to the mouth and teeth are in rugby football in the UK and American football in the USA. 'Non-contact' sports participants are not exempt, as direct trauma in these sports is not uncommon (for example, in squash and field hockey). It has been mandatory for some time for all high school and college footballers in the USA to wear mouth protectors: in the UK, progress has been somewhat slower. A suitable protector acts against trauma to the teeth, fillings, bridges, and crowns. Additionally, the likelihood of laceration of lips, mouth, and tongue from the teeth is drastically reduced, as are mandibular fractures and concussion injury which may result from the teeth being clenched together forcefully by an impact from below (Chapman 1988).

A number of different mouth guards are available. 'Off the shelf' guards are the least adequate, as they may fit badly and be displaced easily. An inexpensive guard made from a thermoplastic material, for instance a polyvinyl acetate–polyethylene polymer, and moulded by the patient usually fits better, though it may not be sufficiently extensive or resilient at points of maximal stress. A custom-made mouth guard constructed from a cast impression taken by a dental surgeon is the most satisfactory (Fig. 11.2). A number of different materials are available; however, the cost is considerably higher than in the non-custom-made types.

The design of ski boots has helped to reduce certain types of injury such as ankle fractures, though to some extent these have been replaced by boot-top tibial fractures. Modern two-mode ski-release bindings have allowed earlier release of the ski under excessive rotational stress, and thereby reduced the incidence of grade I medial collateral ligament (MCL) knee injuries, though not the more severe knee ligament disruptions (Johnson

and Ettlinger 1982). Proper care of bindings helps to reduce incidence of injury. It is also possible that further sophistication in the release system, for example from the present-day sensitivity to forward lean at the posterior attachment and twist at the toe, to a multimode system, might lower the incidence of lower-extremity injury still further.

Attention to specific clothing is important in certain sports—for example, the use of fireproof material for racing drivers, and the utilization of neoprene, reinforced by nylon, in the manufacture of water-skiing pants to prevent vaginal or rectal douches. Light-weight emergency anti-exposure clothing should be carried by hill-walkers and mountain-climbers to protect against sudden changes in the weather.

Sports arenas

Safety designs of arenas and training and competition surfaces, including pole-vaulting, high jump, and gymnastic landing areas, are important considerations. In gymnastics, the basic basemat requirement of 3 cm of padding should be augmented by mats of substantially increased thickness around the various pieces of equipment: 10 cm for the pommel horse, 20 cm for the rings, vault, bars, and high bar (men) and 12 cm for women. Suitable padding of essential props (for example, the goalposts in rugby football and ski-lift pylons) reduces the incidence of direct traumatic injury. Spring-back flagposts of non-breakable material should be used. The incidence of injuries to the thumb was higher in a fall in which the thumb is caught in the diamond-shaped gaps between the links of the older ski slopes. It seems that the incidence of this type of injury has been reduced by the introducion of the modern artificial surfaces. Indoor arenas should be designed to exclude obstacles such as radiators, which are potential sources of injury.

Rules of the game

Although body protection of different kinds may be custom-designed and, if necessary, made obligatory for sports which involve risk from extrinsic trauma, the enforcement of safety measures by the participants' adherence to rules is not always so easy. Illegal play is often dangerous. Prime examples are to be seen in rugby (union) football: both illegal collapsing of the scrum and the deliberate ploy of 'popping' the opponent upwards out of the scrum impart excessive strain on the cervical

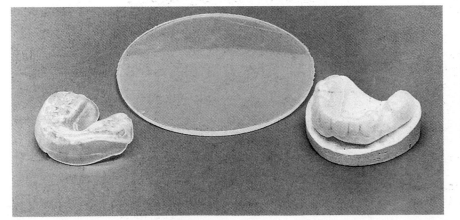

FIG.11.2 A variety of mouth guards are available. On the left an 'over the counter' gum-shaped shield is moulded by the player's teeth. On the right a 'custom made' guard is constructed from a disc of plastic (demonstrated) following a plaster impression taken by a dentist.

spine of front-row forwards (Burry and Calcinai 1988). A similar danger exists in the head-high short-arm tackle. Silver (1984) emphasized the risks to the cervical spine, and encouraged the Rugby Football Union to change certain interpretations of the laws for schools to make the game safer. The New Zealand Rugby Football Union has insisted on matching boys by weight, a sensible approach that appears to have been more difficult to enforce in the UK. Both Silver (1984) and Davies and Gibson (1978) related a percentage of rugby injuries to foul play; the collation of statistical medical information of this kind provides an example of the way in which the medical profession can be of considerable assistance to the governing bodies of sports.

Regulations regarding physical contact vary from one martial art to another; injury may result from the novice's inexperience or clumsiness, or from the expert's manipulation of the rules. Of course, lack of skill is to be expected in the beginner in any sport. In downhill snow-skiing, for instance, statistics often reveal a higher incidence of injury in the novice (Davis *et al.* 1977; Johnson *et al.* 1980). The pattern of injury may be different at the elitist level. Expert skiers tend to have a relatively higher incidence of shoulder injuries and the more severe type of knee injury. Professional soccer players accept a relatively high incidence of injury, which is more often due to the intensity of physical commitment than to dangerous play.

The control of dangerous play is in the hands of referees, umpires, and sports administrators; nevertheless, it is incumbent upon the sports physician to advise on the medical implications of unnecessary violence. Regrettably, criminal proceedings have been necessary on occasions for assault on the field of play (Grayson 1999), and it seems likely that prosecutions will become more common.

Pre-participation screening

Guidelines on individuals' fitness to compete should be established in cooperation with the relevant sports bodies. The practice of medical screening (or 'profiling') prior to participation in sport varies enormously from country to country. On the basis of prevention of illness and injury, screening makes sense. As an example, hyperextension of the knees or hypermobility in general should result in a ban from contact sports because of the risk of ligament and/or joint injury. In the UK, however, the provision of such screening services within the framework of a National Health Service that is sorely stretched in most directions is debatable. Nevertheless, a healthy debate should include the advocacy of a changing emphasis in health care towards prophylaxis against injury.

Participation in certain sports or recreational activities such as subaqua diving requires a medical examination and certification of fitness. Other sports require medical certification if the participant has reached a certain age—for example, is over 40 in parachuting. It is of some interest that people with certain medical conditions (which include giddiness and fainting) are prevented from parachuting, whereas there is no proscribed level of lower-limb musculoskeletal incompetence. Participation in the majority of sports in the UK does not require any statutory examination procedure.

A suitable pre-participation medical examination which encompasses the techniques described in individual chapters is summarized as follows.

History

Sports
Illnesses
Injuries
Surgery
Orthotics

Physical examination

Somatotype
General (body systems)

Musculoskeletal:

Spine
- Scoliosis
  Kyphosis
  Lordosis
  Pelvic tilt/leg length
  Cervical ROM ⎫
  Thoracic ROM ⎬ flexion, extension, side flexions, rotations
  Lumbar ROM ⎭
  Neural tension: upper limb (ANT)
  ⠀⠀⠀⠀⠀⠀⠀⠀⠀⠀⠀lower limb (SLR, FST)
  Reflexes: upper limb
  ⠀⠀⠀⠀⠀⠀lower limb

Shoulders
- Symmetry/deformity
  ROM: abduction
  ⠀: external rotation
  ⠀: internal rotation
  ⠀: adduction
  ⠀: flexion
- Impingement/instability signs
- Muscle power: abductors
  ⠀⠀⠀⠀⠀: external rotators
  ⠀⠀⠀⠀⠀: internal rotators

Elbows
- Cubitus valgus
- ROM: flexion
  ⠀: extension/hyperextension
- Forearm ROM: supination
  ⠀⠀⠀⠀⠀: pronation
- Muscle power: flexors
  ⠀⠀⠀⠀⠀: extensors
  ⠀⠀⠀⠀⠀: supinators
  ⠀⠀⠀⠀⠀: pronators

Wrist/hands
- ROM: wrist dorsiflexion
  ⠀: wrist palmarflexion
  ⠀: finger/thumb mobility
- Muscle power: wrist dorsiflexors
  ⠀⠀⠀⠀⠀: wrist palmarflexors
  ⠀⠀⠀⠀⠀: hand intrinsics

Hips
- Femoral anteversion (squinting patellae)
- ROM: flexion
  ⠀: extension
  ⠀: abduction
  ⠀: adduction
  ⠀: medial rotation
  ⠀: lateral rotation
- Muscle power: flexors
  ⠀⠀⠀⠀⠀: extensors

: abductors
: adductors
: medial rotators
: lateral rotators
- Flexibility: hamstrings
    : quadriceps
    : iliotibial tract

Knees
- Genu varum/valgum
- Effusion
- Q-angles
- Patella mobility/apprehension/alta
- Patella compression
- ROM: flexion/squat
    : extension/recurvatum
- Laxity: medial
    : lateral
    : anterior drawer (10° / 90°)
    : posterior drawer
    : jerk test/pivot shift
- Muscle power: flexors
        : extensors

Lower legs
- tibia vara
- Achilles stretch
- Heel deformity
- Muscle power: triceps surae (tip-toe)

Ankles
- ROM: dorsiflexion
    : plantarflexion
    : squat
- Laxity: anterior drawer
    : talar tilt
- Muscle power: foot dorsiflexors
        : foot plantarflexors
        : invertors
        : evertors

Feet
- Pes cavus/planus
- Forefoot/toe deformity

- ROM: subtalar
    : midtarsal
    : first MTP

Technical factors in overuse injury

Introduction

Reduction in incidence of overuse injury is dependent upon the prior identification of the relevant aetiological factors responsible for overload. Thus excessive or abnormal biomechanical stress, caused by poor sports technique or associated with anatomical malalignment, needs modification by appropriate means. Further stress reduction should be achieved by the choice of suitable sports shoes and equipment (such as squash and tennis rackets). Training schedules should be critically assessed in conjunction with coaches and trainers—excessive training may improve some physiological parameters, but often leads to biomechanical injury and the additional risk of overtraining syndrome.

Flexibility

Lack of flexibility in one or more joints may be found during medical examination or noted by the trainer/coach. It may be congenital—for example, the cavoid foot. Alternatively it may be due either to intrinsic joint pathology (for instance, capsular contracture or early degenerative disease) or to a lack of elasticity of the surrounding musculotendinous structures. Athletes generally may not receive appropriate advice on the relevance of stretching exercises, or may become non-compliant as a result of boredom, shortage of time, or for other reasons. It is of the utmost importance that exercise is preceded and followed by a flexibility programme for all major muscle groups to help prevent injury. Using dance as an example, considerable hip extension is required for arabesque; restriction of extension results in pelvic sway and excessive lumbar lordosis. Hamstring muscle tears (particularly in sprinters) and tendinitis are common if the hamstrings are not stretched regularly. Cyclists may also develop hamstring tendinitis, and therefore should utilize a stretching routine. Long-distance runners who have a 'shuffling' gait tend to develop limited hip movement as a result of soft tissue contracture, and are prone to pelvic stress injuries. Squash players are liable to back injury due to the combination of flexion and rotational stresses on the thoraco-lumbar spine; inadequate spinal flexibility compounds this risk. To help prevent subacromial problems in swimmers and tennis players (in whom external rotation of the shoulder may become restricted), an adequate warm-up should include a comprehensive stretching routine for the shoulders.

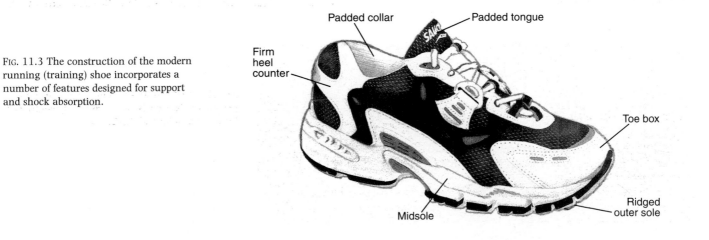

FIG. 11.3 The construction of the modern running (training) shoe incorporates a number of features designed for support and shock absorption.

Sports shoes

There has been a consistent improvement in design of running shoes over the last decade (Fig. 11.3). Excellent texts describing the construction of shoes are available (James *et al.* 1978; Cavanagh 1980; Anthony 1987), and a detailed account will not be reproduced here. However, one or two relevant general points should be made. An unsatisfactory level of support or shock absorption may be associated with the following:

(1) an inadequate shoe type, for example a casual 'trainer' or squash shoe being chosen instead of a running trainer;
(2) distortion occurring in the worn shoe;
(3) inadequate heel counter;
(4) inadequate arch support;
(5) early deterioration of the shock-absorbing properties of the midsole;
(6) disruption between the upper and the sole.

Pressure effects, giving rise to bursitis or tendinitis, may be due to the following:

(1) laces that are too tight;
(2) insufficient breadth of shoe;
(3) irritation from a heel tab;
(4) anatomical foot deformities;
(5) biomechanical abnormalities.

The overall level of medial arch support is often inadequate. The flimsy insole that is so often provided in a running shoe may be replaced by a more substantial commercially available arch support. An orthotic may be required for correction of excessive biomechanical stresses. Orthotic appliances ('orthoses') are used to realign an abnormally balanced foot by controlling either the subtalar joint or the forefoot (Fig. 11.4). A temporary 'soft' orthotic may be constructed in the surgery by the use of small pads of chiropody felt positioned on to a flexible insole: support under the medial arch and under the medial aspect of the heel is useful for overpronators. For greater sophistication, and for a long-term approach, a more rigid orthotic should be manufactured from a cast of the patient's foot made by an orthotist or podiatrist. The foot is cast in subtalar neutral; a positive mould is formed from this plaster cast by pouring in moulding plaster. (Alternatively, a foam cast may be used to replace the traditional casting method.) Suitable posting may be added to correct deformities. The orthotic is then constructed using one of a number of materials, according to the orthotist's or the manufacturer's inclination.

The most common reason for the use of orthotics is correction of compensatory overpronation of the foot associated with conditions such as forefoot varus (Subotnick 1985). Less satisfactory results are obtained with the supinated foot. Orthoses may be used to prevent injury or the recurrence of injury, or be part of the therapeutic armamentarium that is used for established conditions, such as metatarsalgia, plantar fasciitis, 'runner's knee', and iliotibial tract bursitis, when there are identifiable biomechanical foot abnormalities.

In comparison with running shoes, which have thick soles to reduce impact (and thus are unstable on change of direction), squash shoes provide greater stability, as they allow the foot to be closer to the ground.

Bicycle maintenance

Bicycles should be overhauled regularly, not only to prevent accidents resulting from major structural faults, but also to reduce the likelihood of the insidious onset of overuse injury due to abnormal biomechanical stress. In particular, emphasis should be given to the pedal–crank–bottom-bracket axle interconnections. Excessive wear or poor adjustment may result in patellofemoral pain. Further information may be gained from manuals such as *Richard's Bicycle Book* (Ballantine 1976).

Racket construction

Over the last few years, artificial materials such as graphite and boron have been used increasingly in racket construction. Although unsubstantiated at present, it may be demonstrated later that the incidence of forearm and elbow overuse injury has been altered for the worse by this trend (despite some manufacturers' claims to the contrary). Sports physicians should monitor the incidence of injury so as to be able to advise on future construction patterns in the manufacture of sports equipment.

Technique

It is apparent that inadequate technique throws abnormal biomechanical strains upon the athlete's musculoskeletal system; examples are given throughout the text in individual chapters. Vigilance is required by teachers and coaches in order to prevent injury from poor technique. The incidence of low back problems, including spondylolysis, in young dancers should be kept to a minimum by attention to posture in certain exercises. Thus care should be taken to avoid an excessive lordosis at the barre and in floor exercises (Fig. 11.5). For the older (male) dancer, a correct lifting technique is necessary to reduce lordotic stress. The founda-

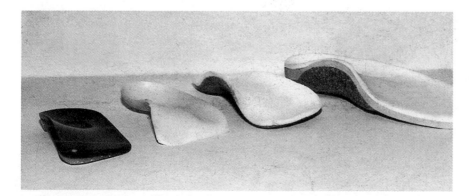

FIG. 11.4 Orthoses for the running shoe help to realign an abnormally balanced foot by controlling the subtalar joint and the forefoot.

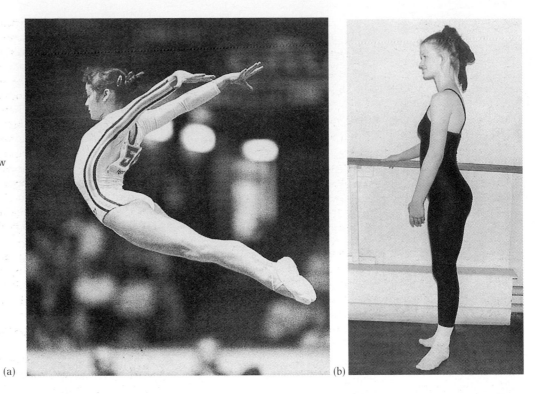

FIG. 11.5 Excessive lordosis in gymnasts and dancers may cause low back problems: (a) a stylish finish; (b) poor posture at the barre.

(a)

(b)

tion of proper dance technique is a strong well-balanced lumbar spine and pelvis. Excessive pelvic flexion or extension will undermine technique and increase the likelihood of injury.

The pivotal area of the spine, the lumbosacral junction, is also at particular risk in other sports if technique is faulty. Too much forward swing prior to powerful leg action in rowers should be corrected. Hyperflexion and hyperextension, both in the air and on water-entry, are a cause of low back injury in highboard divers. Overuse of the butterfly stroke is a further cause of low back pain in swimmers. In weight-training, injury risk may be lessened by preventing spinal flexion on attempting heavier loads.

Technique is particularly important in the various field athletics disciplines. In javelin throwing, for instance, power is maximized by rotation of the chest and body. During the throw, the knee ipsilateral to the throwing arm is brought through quickly to block forward momentum and 'square off' the body, thereby reducing the likelihood of a side-arm throw, which is more likely to incur shoulder strain. Varying degrees of upper body rotation are utilized in the different throwing styles.

In other sports, such as Alpine skiing, it is clear that technical guidance from qualified instructors may reduce the incidence of certain types of injury—for example, reduction of likelihood of injury to the first MCP joint by excluding the thumb from the leather wrist strap.

Malalignment

Femoral anteversion in young dancers increases the likelihood of lower limb injury (Fig. 11.6). Excessive internal rotation of the hips, detected most easily when a patient is examined in the prone position, is suggestive of femoral anteversion. The additional features of squinting patellae and excessive Q-angle are adverse prognostic indicators for athletes contemplating long-distance running. Both pes cavus and pes planus are associated with increased incidence of foot and lower-limb injury. Performance targets should be adjusted accordingly.

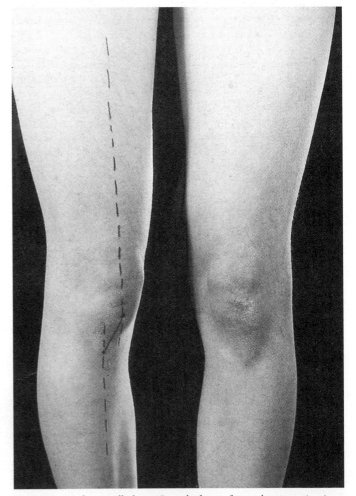

FIG. 11.6 An abnormally large Q-angle due to femoral anteversion is demonstrated in the right leg of this patient.

Biomechanics

A basic knowledge of sports mechanics is required to appreciate the factors associated with prevention of injury, aetiology of injury, and management of injury. Consideration should be given to such concepts as force, torque (force around an axis of rotation), centre of gravity, and lever arms. The axis of rotation itself has great relevance in certain joints such as the subtalar joint. In other joints, the resultant force in different positions of the surrounding levers is of greater relevance—for example, in the patellofemoral joint. Of course, muscle function depends on its physiological state of training. Its force of contraction depends on its cross-section, and its effectiveness on its position in relation to a joint. The ground-reactive forces—that is, those forces which are applied to the body by contact with the ground—depend on the magnitude of the force with which the athlete presses on the ground. Such external vertical forces amount to two and a half to three times the body-weight in running, and may increase to three or four times the body-weight in jumping, and to even higher levels on bouncing (Nigg 1988). Therefore, activities such as the more aggressive forms of 'aerobics' impose considerable repetitive strains on the legs, commonly resulting in injuries such as Achilles tendinitis and shin splints. The suitability of shock absorption, either in the training shoe or the training surface, is an important consideration in the prevention of these injuries.

The mechanics of the different types of locomotion, and the technical requirements of various sports may not be obvious in

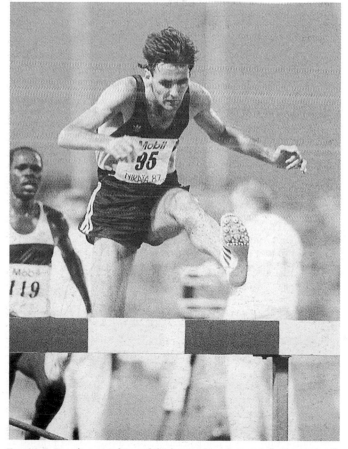

FIG. 11.7 Regular stretching of the hamstrings is especially important in hurdlers.

a particular individual without more refined study. Video recordings that allow slow-motion playback of running style on a treadmill, EMG tests, stress plate analysis, high-speed motion photography, and discussions with the trainer or coach are all ways of identifying faults. Some of the instrumentation is available principally as a research tool, though increasing use is now made of video analysis in the clinical setting. The qualified coach or trainer is familiar with kinetics (analysis of movement) and dynamics (the muscle forces required for movement), so that under his guidance suitable flexibility and strengthening regimes are included in the athlete's training programme. The sports physician should also develop a suitable baseline of knowledge of kinesiology and be able to relate this to clinical problems. For example, in sprinting, high knee action is coupled with early elevation of the heel towards the buttock as soon as the foot leaves the ground—rapid leg movement is achieved by the use of a small swing radius. Strong hip flexors and knee flexors are required. Training should concentrate on strengthening these muscles (principally the iliopsoas and the hamstrings), and creating a balance with the gluteals and the quadriceps. Routine stretching of all these muscle groups is equally important, and in hurdlers is particularly necessary for the hamstrings (Fig. 11.7).

The running style of long-distance runners (when compared with sprinters) is quite different: muscle economy is required. The running style is more of a shuffle, with little hip movement. Although powerful hamstrings are not required, nevertheless the athlete is at risk of developing hamstring contracture unless flexibility exercises are performed regularly. Poor elasticity of the hamstrings creates a risk of muscle 'pull' during bursts of activity—for example, in downhill running—that invoke greater stretch.

Further biomechanical considerations are identified by reference to the following examples, which are particularly relevant to a number of sports.

Abdominal muscle exercise

Well-developed abdominal muscles are required to stabilize the spine, acting as antagonists to the paraspinal extensors. They also reduce shear strain by their action on the dorsilumbar fascia, and unload pressure on the intervertebral discs during lifting. The extensors are rarely weak, either in athletes or in the general population, as they are postural muscles. However, the abdominals are often relatively weak: abdominal strengthening exercises are thus useful for all. A critical study of exercises which are commonly prescribed for abdominal strengthening reveals a need for differentiation between abdominal muscle contraction and hip flexor (iliopsoas) contraction. When hanging from a bar and raising the legs to the horizontal, or lying supine and raising both legs in the air, the iliopsoas contracts powerfully. There is a considerable transmission of force to the lumbar spine, increasing intradiscal pressure and increasing lordosis, thereby incurring risk of injury to the lumbar spine in those individuals who do not have established strong abdominal musculature. To offload the spine and yet exercise the abdominals instead of the hip flexors, trunk curl exercises should be performed in a specific way (Fig. 11.8(a)). In the supine position, the hips and knees are flexed as far as possible and the feet placed flat on the floor. Alternatively, both hips and knees are flexed to 90° as shown in Fig. 11.8(b). In this way, the hip flexors are disengaged. Curled trunk sit-ups ('half' sit-ups only are possible) strengthen the rectus abdominae, and angulations

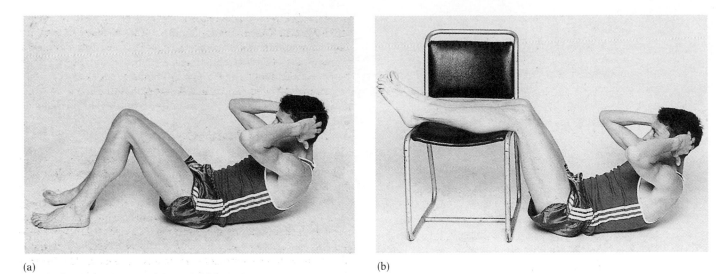

(a)   (b)

FIG. 11.8 Abdominal strengthening exercises are demonstrated (the hip flexors are disengaged and the trunk is curled).

to each side strengthen the external and internal obliques. Commonly, exercises are performed in less hip flexion, with the ankles/feet supported under a wall bar for example. Although the lumbar lordosis has been abolished to a considerable degree in this position, the iliopsoas is able to assist the abdominals (Norris 1993). The earlier part of the sit-up is by concentric abdominal contraction, and the latter half is by concentric iliopsoas contraction.

Although elitist athletes are able to perform multiple hip flexor repetitions, the relatively less fit or those recovering from injury, particularly back strain, require expert guidance in the first instance on the correct way to exercise the abdominals and paravertebral muscles that, acting in concert, stabilize the spine. Initially, motor control and recruitment of the spinal segmental stabilizers—transversus abdominis and multifidus—rather than concentration on strength and flexibility is an important part of a rehabilitation protocol (Mottram and Comerford 1998).

Quadriceps femoris exercises

The rectus femoris flexes the hip and extends the knee. The vastus lateralis and intermedius extend the knee only. The vastus medialis obliquus (VMO) stabilizes the patella by pulling it medially. Examples of exercises which strengthen the knee extensor components of the quadriceps femoris are as follows:

(a) 'sitting' against a wall with both hips and knees flexed to 90° (isometric contraction);
(b) step-ups, particularly when extra load is applied by carrying free weights;
(c) squat jumps.

The muscle force increases as knee flexion increases (the lever arm extends significantly). Patellofemoral compression also increases alarmingly at the extreme of flexion—up to as much as eight times the bodyweight. Thus it may be seen that zero force is required to maintain the extended knee, i.e. in the upright position, and the VMO is not exercised significantly in these regimes.

Following injury, however, it is necessary to develop the VMO at the outset: the likelihood of patellofemoral pain is high if iso-

tonic exercises are performed too early. Thus therapists take patients through a carefully graded sequence of straight leg raises—that is, isometric contractions in full knee extension (see Fig. 12.3, p. 218). Subsequently, progressive resistance training is performed using weights from flexion through to extension. Most gymnasia incorporate equipment that loads the knee concentrically in this way. However, when this type of exercise is undertaken, the patellofemoral joint is increasingly loaded, and the quadriceps work increasingly hard *in extension*, not flexion (see Fig. 7.8, p. 131). This is an unnatural situation for most everyday activities and sports. When 'unnatural' stress is applied, for instance when the relatively untrained or the skeletally immature engage in unsupervised exercise using gymnasium equipment that utilizes a weight-stack resistance principle, particularly the leg-press station, the risk of injury is significantly raised.

Biomechanics of running

The terms 'overpronation', 'podiatric assessment', and provision of 'orthosis' have become familiar to many competitive athletes, who may assume (not unreasonably) that functional support in the running shoe is an important factor in prevention of injury. It behoves the physician to understand the basic principles involved in a biomechanical assessment, to eschew a too theoretical approach to mechanics, and to search for the practical applications. An understanding of the biomechanics of running facilitates this strategy.

The subtalar joint (STJ) is a linchpin of the system of stress distribution. Its axis is triplanar, passing from posterior, lateral, and inferior to anterior, medial, and dorsal (see Fig. 8.1, p. 141). It is also described as being a mitred hinge joint, reflecting its association with pronation/supination in the foot and internal/external rotation in the lower leg. Rearfoot *valgus* (calcaneovalgus) is the hindfoot position when the subtalar joint is everted. When combined with abduction and dorsiflexion in the foot, pronation takes place. On the other hand, rearfoot *varus* indicates inversion of the subtalar joint that, when combined with adduction and plantarflexion, contributes to supination of the foot.

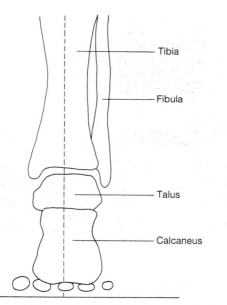

FIG. 11.9 The normal (neutral) foot (vertical calcaneus, subtalar neutral, and horizontal forefoot) observed in the midstance phase of the gait cycle.

The neutral position of the STJ (Fig. 11.9) is achieved when one-third of the movement from eversion to inversion has taken place, and is found at midstance in the gait cycle. The midtarsal (or transverse tarsal) joint comprises the talonavicular and calcaneocuboid joints, with motion occurring in all planes around longitudinal and oblique axes (see Fig. 8.2, p. 142). A full range of motion at the midtarsal joint is dependent upon the 'unlocking' of the subtalar joint in pronation. Assessment of the position of the forefoot relative to the hindfoot (with the STJ in neutral) determines any degree or forefoot varus or valgus.

The running-gait cycle includes phases of stance (heel-strike through to toe-off), float (double-limb unsupported phase), swing, and further float (Fig. 11.10). During the early stance phase, the centre of gravity passes forward over the hindfoot, requiring a relative leg shortening. The STJ everts and the foot pronates. Transmission of force and motion to the midtarsal joints, and thence to the forefoot, allows the plantar surface of the forefoot to accommodate to the ground surface. Pronation is largely a passive event without muscular control. From midstance to toe-off, supination takes place, during which both intrinsic and extrinsic foot muscles are active prior to the provision of heel-lift by the triceps surae. The limb then extends as the foot comes off the ground during acceleration.

Although the majority of long-distance runners use an initial heel-strike pattern, a small percentage (increasing as faster speeds are gained) have a midfoot strike. Sprinters usually have a forefoot strike pattern. The magnitude of the ground-reaction forces which occur during running may be measured by a force platform. Peak forces (in a biphasic fashion for rearfoot strikers, and uniphasic for midfoot strikers) of three times body-weight are seen.

Abnormal biomechanics are discussed in Chapter 9.

Training schedules

Since inappropriate training schedules are a common source of overuse injury, it is clear that this is a subject with which the physician should be familiar. Naturally, a well-balanced training schedule is sought at all times, though the athlete recovering from injury is particularly at risk of relapse or further complications, unless muscle rehabilitation has been adequate and training is undertaken at the correct pace—that is, without abnormally large incremental increases in loading. His frustration during a period of disability and subsequently impatience to increase the intensity of training combine to cause further irritation if breakdown occurs. The physician may then be criticized for his 'mis-management' of the condition: indeed, this may be a valid criticism if a suitable 'review' policy is not arranged on starting training. Particular care is required by the athlete at the beginning of a season (when he is relatively 'unfit') and towards the close of the season (when he may be 'stale'). Overtraining may led to generalized fatigue and poor competitive performance. Serum creatine phosphokinase may be significantly raised both in overtraining and in sports such as some martial arts, in which there is repetitive direct muscle trauma.

The risk of injury may be lessened by increasing muscle strength. Studies of American university footballers, for instance, have demonstrated that the frequency and severity of knee injuries are reduced by preseason total-body conditioning (Cahill and Griffith 1978). The importance of appropriate agonist–antagonist balance for a particular sport, in addition to muscle power and endurance, cannot be overemphasized. Loss of shock-absorbing capacity may occur in fatigued muscles, thus leading to increased stress and microfractures in the area of bone adjacent to their attachments. Recurrent stress (in the form of repetitive microtrauma) to musculotendinous units which are fatigued from repetitive eccentric contraction may result in tendinitis.

Regular strengthening of muscles which are not primarily involved in posture, such as the abdominals, should be performed by those who wish to undertake physical conditioning. Stretching exercises contribute to muscle warm-up, thus helping to prevent the well-recognized association of injury with 'cold' muscles. They also counteract the adaptive shortening of muscles that occurs with strength-training.

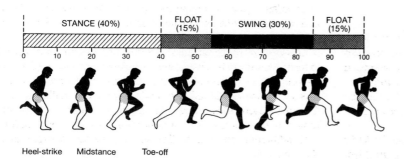

| STANCE (40%) | FLOAT (15%) | SWING (30%) | FLOAT (15%) |

Heel-strike   Midstance   Toe-off

FIG. 11.10 The running gait cycle: the phases for the right leg are shown.

Common sense

Athletes who have achieved the feeling of well-being or 'high' from the endorphin release associated with endurance exercise are not always able to adopt a logical or sensible approach when setting themselves targets or goals. The type of exercise that is chosen in the pursuit of physical fitness or conditioning may be inappropriate. It is not always appreciated by the 'prospective athlete' that endurance (aerobic) exercise is required to attain the level of 'cardiorespiratory' fitness necessary for a healthy life-style. A schedule of thirty minutes of jogging, brisk walking, cycling, or swimming three or four times a week should be the goal for those seeking recreational rather than competitive activity. For those who expand their exercise programmes, the risk is the linear association between the intensity of endurance exercise and the incidence of musculoskeletal injury.

Training characteristics

Strength training

During strength training, or recovery from disuse atrophy (for example, after immobilization), there is an increase in the number of muscle capillaries, an increase in myofibril size per cell, and an increase in mitochondria. It is possible that inter-conversion between fibre types II-A and II-B is a response to training techniques (see Chapter 1, Tissue injury—muscle, p. 6). No such interconversion appears to occur between types I and II: selective recruitment of the different type II fibres appears to be the more logical response. Generation of new fibrils occurs, and must be given time between training sessions to compensate for fibril destruction. Thus it is important to allow at least twenty-four to forty-eight hours between sessions of intensive strength training. Application of heavy work-loads is necessary in strength training (for example, 80–95 per cent of the load that may be maximally managed)—and high-intensity low-repetition regimes are used. Increases in strength of up to 70 per cent are reported as typical training effects (Thorstensson 1976). However, endurance work requires repetitive stress with loads that correspond to 20–25 per cent of maximal capacity—that is, low-intensity high-repetition regimes.

Dynamic muscle activity is often a combination of *isotonic* (dynamic or concentric) contraction when muscle shortens, and *isometric* (static) contraction when there is no change in length. Muscle may also contract *eccentrically* while lengthening. Visco-elastic energy is stored by muscle when prestretched or preloaded by eccentric contraction prior to concentric contraction. This principle is employed during a type of training known as plyometrics when various drills are used to develop power for running, jumping, and rowing. Such drills include hops, power bounds, depth jumps, and jumping with weights. Free weights, or throwing and catching a medicine ball, may be used for the upper body.

Progressive resistance training is the mainstay of the development of strength, power, and local muscle endurance. Gradually increasing overload must be applied to the musculoskeletal system as adaptation occurs. Relatively inexpensive equipment, in the form of barbells, dumb-bells, and ankle and wrist weights, relies on gravity for resistance. At no extra expense, an athlete may utilize his own body-weight for resistance, for instance in bench-stepping and press-ups, in a conventional 'circuit'. Multi-gyms usually rely on the gravity effects of stacked weights,

though at somewhat greater cost. Sets of repetitions are used, with the workload depending upon both the maximal capacity and the capability of the joint over which the muscle acts. Variation is required, as it has been observed that training by concentric contraction alone will not necessarily increase the ability to contract eccentrically.

Many health clubs and gymnasia incorporate *variable resistance*, equipment such as Nautilus or Atlanta. A series of cams and levers modifies the loading on a muscle (and therefore on a joint) at different angles of contraction. Although weight is selected in a similar way to the multi-gym, the engineering is such that ballistic movements are eliminated and heavier weights are capable of being handled. In distinction from the situation found using conventional weights, the athlete is not limited to using a weight that can be moved through the mechanically 'weakest' part of the muscle's range. The variable-resistance systems include a large number of pieces of equipment for exercising specific muscles or muscle-groups.

Isokinetic training employs a more specific 'accommodating resistance' by the use of hydraulics (Fig. 11.11). A dynamometer offers an equal resistance as soon as the preset speed is reached, thus matching the muscle contraction (Hislop and Perrine 1967). Increased muscular output produces increased resistance rather than the increased acceleration that would occur in gravity-loaded systems. Systems such as Cybex, Orthotron, and Lido include a computer linkage, so that torque in foot pounds and other measurements may be made (see Fig. 11.11(d), p. 203). Peak torque is defined as the highest point on the generated torque curve in foot pounds (1 foot pound = 1.356 newton metres). The joint angle at which peak torque occurs may be measured. A change in angular velocity affects this value: for instance, quadriceps peak torque occurs later in the range of motion with increasing speeds. Work, which is a reflection of the movement of force through an angular displacement, may be measured, and is represented by the area under the torque curve (Fig. 11.11(c)). There is substantial evidence that isokinetic exercise increases the work that a muscle can do more rapidly than isometric or isotonic exercise (Moffroid *et al.* 1969).

In comparing the mechanics of an isokinetic contraction with a dynamic one using weights as a resistance, the difference in the torque curve over the range of motion is striking (Grimby 1982). In an isokinetic exercise programme at the knee, maximal resistance may be achieved throughout a complete range of motion. However, on examination of the torque values at 0°, it may be seen that, if resistance work is required at or close to full knee extension, isometric training also should be employed.

Different sports require different muscle capabilities with respect to strength, power, and endurance. Eventually, the establishment of a database from testing protocols using isokinetic dynamometers should help to determine the function of specific muscle groups in each sport (Watkins and Harris 1993). Many sports, for instance soccer, demand a background of constant running interspersed with frequent demands for explosive power in the form of short sprints. Weight-lifters also require power—that is, strong fast contraction. Therefore, training should be appropriate (sport-specific), and include a full complement of exercise, not solely that designed for endurance. Pure endurance training reduces the strength and power of muscles. Any athlete who has experienced the difficulty in coping with the bursts of activity demanded in a game such as squash rackets after a period of long-distance running training will recognize this.

FIG. 11.11 Isokinetic training (for example, with a Lido isokinetic dynamometer) utilizes the principle of 'accommodating resistance' by the use of hydraulics. Muscle function may be assessed by computer linkage. (a) Knee flexors/extensors. (b) Shoulder abductors/adductors. (c) Typical torque curves are displayed for repetitions of knee flexion/extension at 90°/sec (the curves are emphasized for clarity). The positions of the joint ('joint angle') are also illustrated. (d) A typical print-out of Lido isokinetic results: bar graphs indicate average peak torque (if an injury is present, this side is shaded); the remaining parameters are expressed digitally.

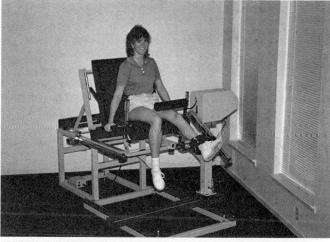

(a)

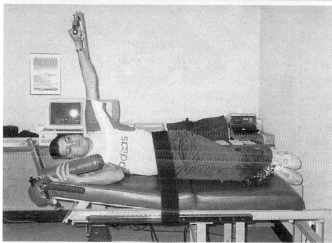

(b)

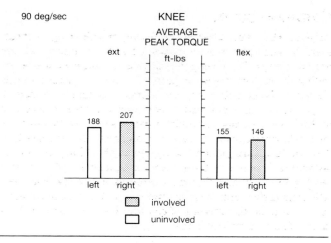

90 deg/sec KNEE AVERAGE PEAK TORQUE

ext ft-lbs flex

188 207 | 155 146

left right | left right

▨ involved
☐ uninvolved

STRENGTH

	Repetitions	5 LEFT	5 RIGHT	INV/UNIV %
PEAK TORQUE (ft-lbs)				
ext		198	210	106 %
flex		161	149	93 %
WORK PER REPETITION (ft-lbs)				
ext		162	153	94 %
flex		146	114	78 %
TORQUE RATIO (%)				
flex/ext		81 %	71 %	
PEAK TORQUE TO BODY WEIGHT RATIO (%)				
ext		104 %	111 %	
flex		85 %	78 %	
JOINT ANGLE AT PEAK TORQUE (degrees)				
ext		60	60	
flex		58	45	
RANGE OF MOTION (degrees)				
ext		98	86	
flex		99	86	

ENDURANCE

	LEFT	RIGHT	INV/UNIV %
TOTAL WORK DONE (ft-lbs)			
ext	811	765	94 %
flex	732	571	78 %

	LEFT	RIGHT	INV/UNIV %
FATIGUE INDEX (%)			
ext	90 %	92 %	102 %
flex	92 %	104 %	113 %

(d)

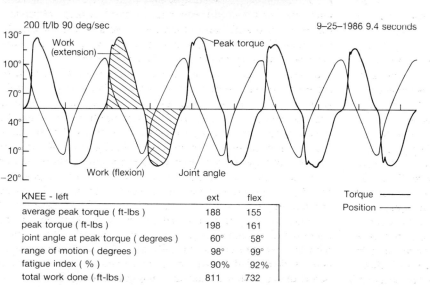

200 ft/lb 90 deg/sec 9-25-1986 9.4 seconds

Work (extension) — Peak torque

Work (flexion) — Joint angle

Torque ———
Position ———

KNEE - left	ext	flex
average peak torque (ft-lbs)	188	155
peak torque (ft-lbs)	198	161
joint angle at peak torque (degrees)	60°	58°
range of motion (degrees)	98°	99°
fatigue index (%)	90%	92%
total work done (ft-lbs)	811	732

(c)

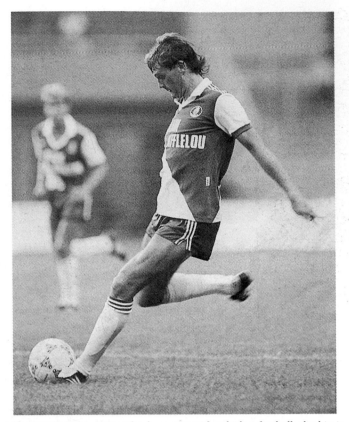

FIG. 11.12 To maximize the force required to kick a football, the hip is extended, thereby creating viscoelastic energy in the rectus femoris which subsequently is required as a powerful knee extensor.

Flexibility training

Adequate flexibility is essential for normal biomechanical function in sport. Performance may be compromised if flexibility is inadequate.

(i)   Sports techniques are difficult, if not impossible, to achieve.
(ii) Other training characteristics—for example, strength-training—may be impeded.
(iii) Excessive muscle activity is required, leading to premature fatigue.

Of the factors affecting flexibility, there are some which impose unyielding limitations—for instance, bone to bone, or bone to soft tissue impingement. However, other factors, such as the following, may be influenced by flexibility exercises:

(i) the contractile (musculotendinous) structures that span joints; and
(ii) the non-contractile (capsular/ligamentous) structures that are an integral part of joints.

The term *laxity* refers to the degree of passive distraction or shear of a joint in a specific direction: it results from ligamentous insufficiency, for instance medial laxity at the knee after MCL rupture. If mobility in a wide spectrum of joints is excessive, the term *hypermobility* is applied (see Chapter 1). Neither situation is desirable.

Muscles which are used repetitively yet remain unstretched, or muscles which are trained for strength only, become shorter.

However, viscoelastic forces allow muscles to achieve maximum force when initially stretched to approximately 120 per cent of their resting length. Thus to maximize the force required to kick a football, the hip is initially extended, thereby stretching the rectus femoris, which subsequently is required as a power knee extensor (Fig. 11.12). In throwing the javelin or discus, the trunk is rotated maximally, thereby stretching the pectoralis major (among other muscle groups), which contracts powerfully in the forward acceleration phase.

Flexibility training develops this capacity for viscoelastic energy storage by overload. *Long slow (passive) stretching* is required. Passive stretching is often reinforced with the aid of external forces, thereby creating passive 'assisted' stretching—for example, resting the heel of the outstretched leg on a plinth to stretch the hamstrings. *Ballistic* stretching, on the other hand, should not be considered to be anything other than a form of 'toning up' for muscles. It stimulates the stretch reflex and, if performed too vigorously when the athlete has warmed up inadequately, may provoke muscle pulls. De Vries (1962) found that flexibility may be improved significantly (and equally) by both static and ballistic methods. *Post-contraction relaxation* is another technique that is utilized in both training and therapeutic contexts. Muscle may lengthen further after isometric contraction at the extreme of range—therapists use this principle in the technique of PNF (proprioceptive neuromuscular facilitation).

In summary, flexibility exercises are used:

(i)   in rehabilitation to re-establish normal joint function;
(ii) prophylactically to prevent injury;
(iii) in training to achieve a maximally efficient biomechanical framework for specific sports techniques.

Examples of flexibility exercises are demonstrated in Fig. 11.14, pp. 208–10.

Fitness assessment

A number of identifiable factors are involved in the preparation of an individual or a collection of players in team sports to a level of maximal effectiveness. Some factors, such as motor skills, tactics, and team selection are clearly the responsibility of coaches, trainers, and managers. In other areas, such as the development of improved materials used in the manufacture of running shoes, and the reduction of drag in speed sports such as yacht-racing, car-racing, sprinting, and sprint cycling by streamlining including the use of wind suits, the bio-engineer plays his part. Other factors which are within the domain of the sports physician, psychologist, and physiologist are the provision of sports medical services, psychological training, and fitness assessment. A large contribution to fitness assessment may be made by the physiologist, although a 'team approach' in which the physician plays a leading role is desirable. A thorough medical examination (see previous section on 'Pre-participation screening') should precede the more dynamic (physiological) aspects of fitness evaluation.

Physiological assessment

The physiological components which contribute to athletic performance may be outlined as follows.

1. *Physique*. Whilst somatotyping individuals into ectomorphs, endomorphs, and the typically athletic mesomorph is interesting,

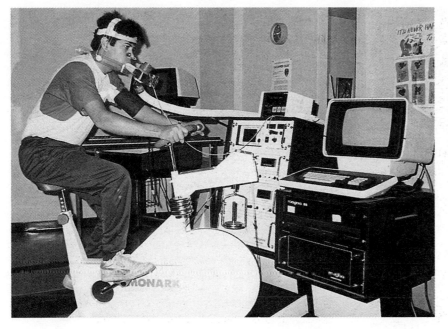

FIG. 11.13 Max. VO_2 may be measured using a recording of heart rate and expired air analysis (this test is being performed at the Sports and Fitness Assessment unit at the London Bridge Clinic). Cardiac function may be assessed simultaneously using a Marquette ECG.

it is of little practical benefit. In sports such as American football, it is quite clear that size is as important as explosive power. On the other hand, the variation in body size of 800 metre runners is quite extensive. Evaluation of body-fat per unit body-weight is of more relevance, and may be calculated by the use of skin-calipers. Reference is made to conversion tables once average values are recorded from the four skin-sites, i.e. those overlying triceps and biceps in the upper arm, at the inferior angle of the scapula, and finally over the iliac crest. Alternatively, lean body-weight may be measured by electrical impedance.

2. *Flexibility*. Although an initial evaluation should be made during medical examination, the physiologist performs his own tests. The assessment of flexibility should not be confined to an isolated test for combined trunk flexion and hamstring elasticity (touching the toes), despite its relative importance. All the major joints are examined. Specific stretch tests for muscles which span two joints are performed. At very mobile joints, the range of motion in the position of function is recorded—for example, external rotation in 90° abduction of the shoulder in tennis players. Hypermobility should be recorded if present: it should be looked for routinely in dancers and gymnasts (see Chapter 1).

3. *Aerobic fitness*. The capacity of the cardiovascular system to deliver appropriate quantities of oxygen to working muscle is conventionally assessed by measurement of maximal O_2 intake (max. VO_2). The Astrand method, depending on the use of conversion factors from a knowledge of heart rate and work performed, has been used for some time. A more accurate method requires expired air analysis (Fig. 11.13), though increased costs may be restrictive. A sport-specific ergometer should be chosen if available—for example, bicycle, treadmill, rowing ergometer, or swimming flume. Gradually increasing effort to exhaustion is required of the athlete.

Max. VO_2 should be measured in athletes whose sports involve over two minutes of continuous vigorous activity. Aerobic capacity depends on the ability of muscles to cope with the available oxygen. Muscular endurance as well as cardiovascular efficiency is improved by training. Max. VO_2 in the rela-

tively unfit may improve by up to 25 per cent following suitable training. Typical figures in athletes who depend on high aerobic capacity are 65–80 ml per kg body-weight.

4. *Anaerobic threshold (AT)*. At a given submaximal exercise intensity, muscle relies largely on anaerobic metabolism to deliver energy. Much greater amounts are available, although for limited periods of time; the accumulation of chemicals such as lactic acid causes increasing discomfort. The anaerobic threshold depends on the body's capacity to metabolize lactic acid. Therefore, determination of the AT yields information on the capacity to *sustain* high levels of aerobic work. When used to test endurance capacity, it correlates better than max. VO_2.

Its physiological basis has not been agreed universally. The onset of blood lactate accumulation (OBLA) often is measured; other parameters are associated with the sudden relative reduction of VO_2. Endurance training causes the AT to increase significantly compared with max. VO_2. The running speed at the AT correlates well with the maximal running speed over middle and long distances.

5. *Anaerobic fitness*. Explosive bursts of energy are required in a number of sports, and are provided by the creatine phosphate energy store and anaerobic glycolysis. An anaerobic test measures the quantities of work that a muscle group can produce maximally, in addition to its ability to recover. A typical example is the Wingate test using a cycle ergometer. Calculated values for the total work done and mean power output are measured for short bursts of maximal exercise, and reflect the subject's work capacity. A *recovery index* may be calculated by noting the relevant recorded data on repeated tests after short rest intervals. Alternatively, an isokinetic dynamometer may be used: the time taken for torque to drop to 50 per cent of its initial value, or the torque level after 30 contractions at a high angular velocity, for example, 300° per second, are recorded. A *fatigue index* is established by this means.

6. *Muscle strength and power*. Sheer 'strength' (which may be measured in a number of ways because it has no inherent

definition) plays its part in a number of sports. It is usually required for limited periods—for example, in rugby scrummaging. The fast delivery of force—that is, *power* which is measured In foot pounds or newton metres per second—is often much more relevant. Conventionally, when measured by an isokinetic dynamometer, the faster speeds—for example, 240° or 300° per second—are used, as it is thought that these reflect function more accurately. However, Rothstein *et al.* (1987) point out that no evidence exists to suggest that different speeds of movement test different muscular characteristics. Field tests such as sergeant jumps, short sprints, and throwing the shot in different ways offer a cruder indication of power in different muscle groups.

The Lido isokinetic dynamometer (Fig. 11.11) used by the author at the Sports and Fitness Assessment Unit at the London Bridge Clinic has a number of practical applications in assessment and rehabilitation, summarized as follows:

(1) calculation of fatigue index—an anaerobic test of local muscle endurance;
(2) establishment of a database of muscle function for fit individuals or team members;
(3) detection of muscle imbalance—as an assessment procedure or in established injury, for example by comparison of torque ratios of agonists and antagonists;
(4) rehabilitation after injury;
(5) isokinetic training.

Psychological assessment

Psychological factors have a significant effect on an athlete's capacity for (or perseverance in) training, and motivation for competition or increased intensity of effort (Yaffé, 1983). Factors which generally are believed to influence sports performance include anxiety, aggression, motivation, concentration, self-confidence, pain tolerance, and emotional state. Psychometric evaluation of abilities, aptitudes, and skills by objective measurement and techniques may be performed by the sports psychologist.

Yaffé (personal communication 1988) used Nideffer's Test of Attention and Interpersonal Style (Nideffer 1981) to assess the capacity of talented young tennis players to cope with stress, and Eysenck's Personality Questionnaire to gauge sociability, impulsiveness, emotionality, and toughmindedness. Response to specific training and competitive situations is assessed by a structured interview.

Sports psychologists now have an established role, both in the realization of potential and in reducing the incidence of injury, physical and mental, in competitive athletics and team sports.

Community fitness

The need for an increased emphasis upon disease prevention within the framework of the National Health Service in the UK has been appreciated for some time. Various arguments, not least those involving financial implications, have apparently prevented its more extensive development. Debate still continues over the relative importance of the aetiological factors implicated in the health scourge of affluent Western civilization—coronary artery atherosclerosis. There is general agreement over the adverse effects of smoking and hypertension and the association with socio-economic deprivation, though the subsidiary roles of

obesity, stress, diet, and a sedentary existence seem less clear. Hypercholesterolaemia appears to be involved, with the result that fat-reducing diets are widely available.

Studies (e.g. Kavanagh *et al.* 1979) have purported to show the usefulness of regular exercise in the prevention of progressive coronary artery disease after a first myocardial infarct. A logical extension of this argument is that exercise may prevent the initial onset of coronary artery disease in the asymptomatic subject, possibly by assisting in maintenance of serum cholesterol and weight within accepted norms. Although studies such as that by Morris *et al.* (1953) on London busmen and Paffenbarger and Hale (1975) on San Franciscan longshoremen have shown an association between active jobs and reduction in ischaemic heart disease, a causal relationship is not established. Furthermore, comparison of the apparent beneficial effects of work activity and leisure pursuits is difficult. Nevertheless, it is generally accepted that exercise reduces the likelihood of developing coronary heart disease. Morris *et al.* (1980) have shown that the important aspect of this cardio-protective effect is repeated bouts of vigorous exercise, rather than overall energy expenditure. Other benefits to health from exercise are as follows:

(i)   prevention of osteoporosis;
(ii) facilitation of management of chronic disease such as diabetes;
(iii) increase in physical working capacity;
(iv) improvement of mood.

Evaluation of risk factors is available at screening centres within the private medical sphere in the UK. The more dynamic aspects of health and fitness, with particular reference to the role of exercise, may be evaluated by appropriate tests at a smaller number of dedicated clinics. A suggested protocol of dynamic assessment comprises the following.

1. Medical examination evaluates the musculoskeletal system as well as other body systems. Flexibility is assessed. The resting blood pressure is measured.

2. Anthropometric measurements include height and weight.

3. Body-fat percentage is calculated from skin-caliper measurements.

4. Lung function is evaluated by spirometry.

5. Cardiac function is assessed by a stress ECG using a 12-channel 12-lead Marquette machine or equivalent while the subject exercises on a treadmill or bicycle.

6. Aerobic fitness is measured by expired air analysis. Maximal exercise testing (to exhaustion) using one of several protocols on a treadmill or bicycle ergometer is performed on subjects who take regular vigorous exercise. Max. VO_2 and anaerobic thresholds are calculated, where possible, and assessment made by comparison with age-related tables. Submaximal tests are used for subjects who do not take regular exercise or who are recovering from cardiac disorders or bypass surgery: nevertheless max. VO_2 may be computed from tabulated oxygen consumption. The test is concluded when the subject's heart rate rises to the target heart rate adjusted for age.

7. Muscle power and endurance (of the quadriceps and hamstrings) are assessed on a Lido (or equivalent) isokinetic dynamometer.

8. Urinalysis and haematological screening, including cholesterol and triglycerides, are undertaken.

9. Finally, a 'prescription' is issued with suggestions for a healthier life-style, including a suitable exercise regime. The subject's inclinations, musculoskeletal capabilities, and cardiovascular tolerance are taken into account in the formulation of the prescription.

Exercise prescription

Three components should be included.

1. Warm-up. During this five-minute phase, exercises to stretch large muscle-groups are performed, preparing them for sustained activity. The combination of long slow stretch and muscle-toning in the form of jogging on the spot or hopping increases muscle blood-flow.

2. Endurance or aerobic. During this phase, lasting fifteen to thirty minutes, intensity should be tailored, depending upon the baseline of fitness, to increase aerobic capacity. Although different formulae are used, a rule of thumb guide is for a target heart rate of approximately 75 per cent of maximal safe heart rate to be achieved and maintained. Maximal heart rate is usually considered to be 220 minus age. For example, for a forty-year-old 220 − 40 = 180 beats per minute; thus target heart rate in this case would be 135 beats per minute. Clearly the type of aerobic activity will depend upon a number of factors already outlined: fast walking, swimming, cycling, and jogging are commonly prescribed.

3. Cool down. During this phase body metabolism is allowed to return to normal gradually by the inclusion of a reduced level of muscle activity. Callisthenic exercises, which have the added desirable effect of improving anaerobic fitness, may be added to walking or a slow jog.

Injury prevention in children

An understanding of the pattern of musculoskeletal injury in children is required prior to a consideration of injury prevention. The patterns of injury reflect the difference in the relative strength of the structural components (bone, tendon, muscle, and ligament) in the child compared with the adult. Thus indirect stress applied to the articular framework in children is more likely to result in epiphyseal fracture than in ligament disruption. Salter and Harris (1963) classified fractures involving the epiphysis into grades I–V depending upon the extent of the involvement of the metaphysis or diaphysis. When faced with apparent joint injury in the child, radiological assessment of the epiphyses should be undertaken, and orthopaedic surgical opinion should be sought if abnormalities are detected. Joint instability tends to be caused by avulsion of a bony fragment attached to a ligament, rather than to an intraligamentous tear. The equivalent of the anterior cruciate ligament (ACL) tear in the adult is avulsion fracture of the inferior attachment of the ACL at the intercondylar area of the tibia. Surgical management by re-attachment of the bony fragment is advisable. In general, a satisfactory outcome may be expected following such fracture management.

Traction forces which result in muscle tear or tendon rupture in the adult tend to cause fracture separation of the apophysis in the child. Examples of acute avulsion fractures are found in the pelvic girdle (see Fig. 6.14, p. 122). The affected apophyses are located at:

- iliac crest—origin of gluteus medius and insertion of external oblique
- anterior superior iliac spine—origin of sartorius
- anterior inferior iliac spine—origin of rectus femoris
- ischial tuberosity—origin of hamstrings
- lesser trochanter—insertion of iliopsoas.

Fragmentation of an apophysis that results from chronic repetitive stress is referred to as a traction osteochondrosis. Examples of stress injuries to the apophyses in the upper limb are found at the coracoid process (origin of coracobrachialis and the short head of biceps brachii) and in the lower limb at the tibial tubercle (Osgood–Schlatter's disease) and the posterior calcaneal tubercle (Sever's apophysitis). The acute injuries should be treated in the same way as muscle tears—that is, with a full stretching and strengthening programme during rehabilitation. The stress injuries require reduction of load; relative rest for two to three months may be sufficient.

Overuse injury patterns are similar to those in the adult. Stress fractures are common, though they may occur at the epiphyseal growth plate as well as the diaphysis. In the upper limb, stress fractures of the proximal humeral epiphysis in Little Leaguers (baseball pitchers) and of the distal radial epiphysis in gymnasts (see Fig. 4.7, p. 66) have been recorded. X-rays often show widening of the epiphysis: bone scans may confirm the diagnosis, though interpretation is sometimes difficult as there is increased uptake in the normal epiphysis. Stress fractures in the lower limbs conform to a similar pattern to those found in adults. Stress fractures in the partes interarticulares of the lower lumbar vertebrae (spondylolyses) are largely confined to children under twelve, when they are often relatively (or completely) painless, and to adolescents (aged thirteen to seventeen), when they are usually painful (see Fig. 5.7, p. 93). Repetitive microtrauma may lead to compression fracture of the anterior margins of the vertebral bodies in the thoracic and thoracolumbar regions, giving rise to the clinical syndrome of Scheuermann's disease (see Fig. 5.5, p. 91). A tight lumbodorsal fascia associated with an increased lordosis are thought to be contributory factors (Micheli 1983).

Disorders of the articular cartilage may also occur during growth spurts. Osteochondritis dissecans of the capitellum is seen in gymnasts (see Fig. 4.4, p. 62). Osteochondritis dissecans of the knee occurs in juniors as well as in adolescents (see Fig. 10.17, p. 187). Although the aetiological factors remain unproven, recurrent microtrauma is suspected.

In the evaluation of the aetiological factors in overuse injury, abnormalities of technique, malalignment, and abnormal biomechanics should be considered as for the adult. In some sports, such as swimming, the peak of potential may be realized while the child is still in the mid-teens. Miles of swimming training may be performed each day, causing overuse strains at the shoulder, in particular, and to other anatomical areas, of which the most notorious is breast-stroker's knee (see p. 156). Other sports, including gymnastics and dance in its various forms, require training from an early age. Extreme flexibility is required in many joints. Injury patterns may be associated with lack of flexibility in crucial areas—for instance, inadequate hip mobility leading to low back injury in ballet dancers.

In some youngsters in their early teens, recurrent injury may be associated with relative tightness of the musculotendinous structures. Growth spurts involve axial lengthening of the long bones. Unless flexibility exercises (Fig. 11.14) for the contractile

FIG. 11.14 Flexibility exercises demonstrated by Jack Buckner.

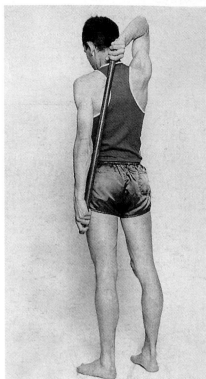

(a) External rotation of the (right) shoulder using a stick

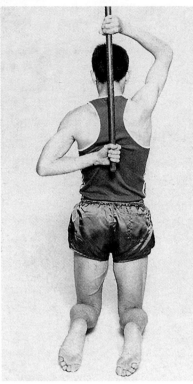

(b) Internal rotation of the (left) shoulder using a stick

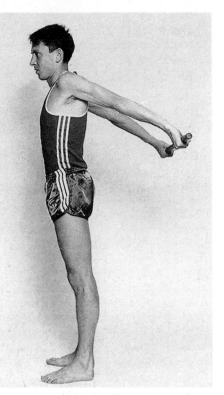

(c) Extension of the shoulders using a stick

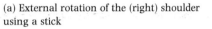
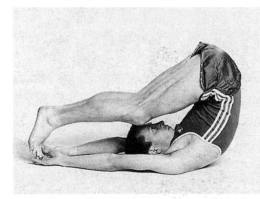

(d) Backward roll for trunk flexion

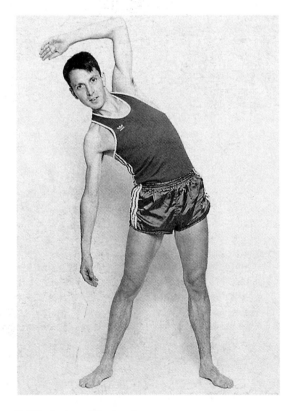

(f) Side flexion of the trunk

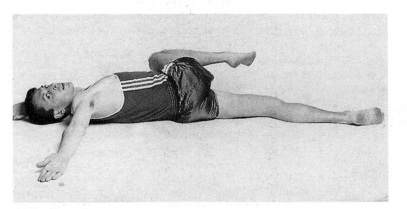

(e) Trunk rotation

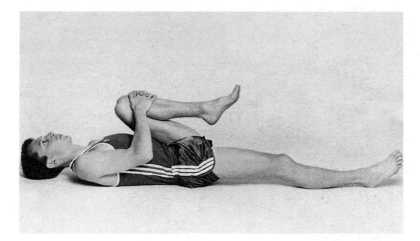

(g) Flexion of the hip

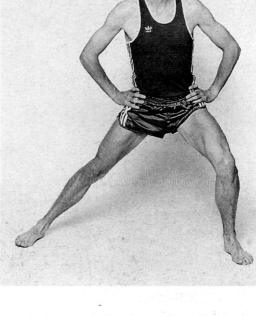

(i) Abduction of the (right) hip, standing (adductor stretch)

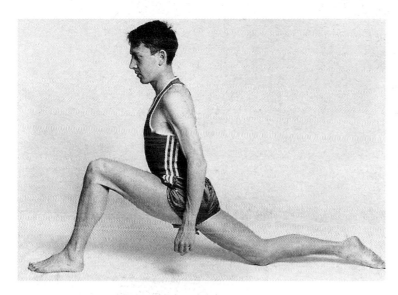

(h) Extention of the right hip (psoas stretch)

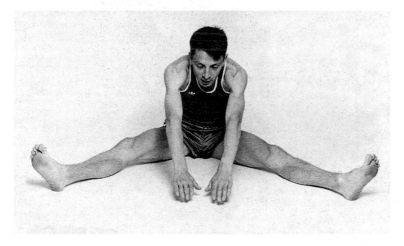

(j) Abduction of the hips, sitting (adductor stretch)

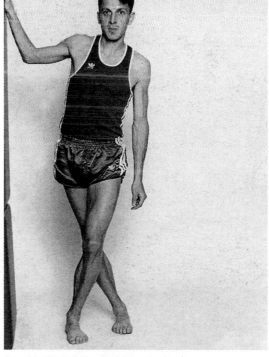

(k) Adduction of the right hip (iliotibial tract stretch)

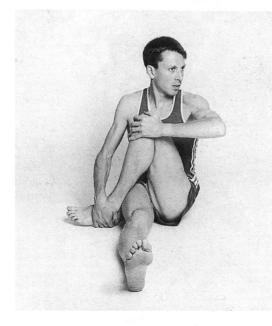

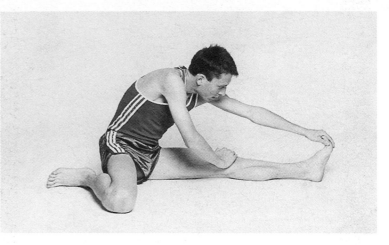

(l) External rotation of the flexed adducted hip (glutei stretch)

(m) Internal rotation of the (right) hip combined with contralateral hamstring stretch

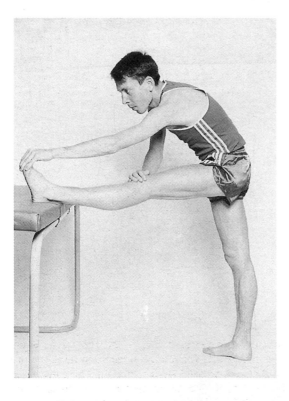

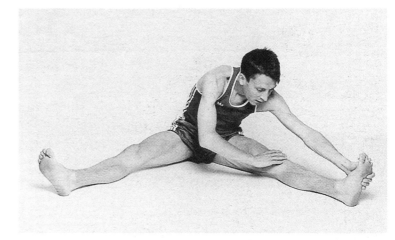

(n), (o) Hamstring stretching

tissues are undertaken at this time, recurrent muscle pulls may be sustained. Usually the child is no more inclined than the average adult to perform regular stretching exercises, and therefore must be suitably encouraged.

The possibility of long-term skeletal problems resulting from repetitive intensive exercise from an early age is conjectural. Since it is accepted that a delay in sexual maturity associated with delayed puberty may occur in girls as a result of intensive and prolonged sporting activity, it is of some concern that skeletal maturation may also be affected. Murray and Duncan (1971) and Stulberg et al. (1975) have suggested that repetitive stress to the capital femoral epiphysis in childhood could be an aetiological factor in the causation of adult osteoarthritis of the hip. It is possible that a reactive hypertrophy of the

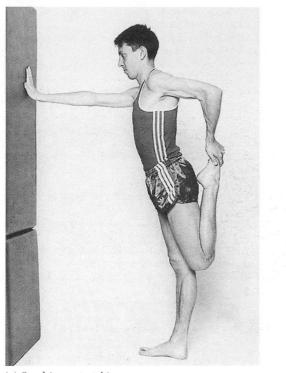

(p) Quadriceps stretching

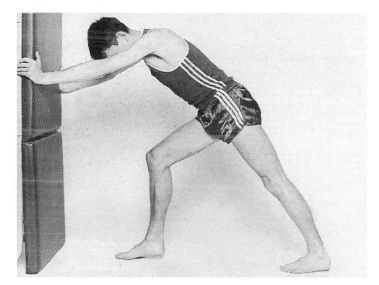

(r) Gastrocnemius stretching

(q) Soleus stretching

humeral head, secondary to the repeated stress of throwing in childhood, may cause impingement syndromes in the adult (F. Jobe in a personal communication to L. Micheli). Further research is required in these directions before definite conclusions may be drawn.

In the protection of children from inappropriate levels of stress, responsibility should be shouldered by the relevant contact groups: parents, teachers, coaches, trainers, sports clubs, and sports associations. Parents, in particular, may need suitable counselling when their child has considerable athletic potential. Sports associations have a special responsibility for grouping children by weight, as well as height and age, in contact sports such as rugby football. In New Zealand, children have been graded by weight for some time; as yet there is no statutory requirement in the United Kingdom. By definition, children are immature, and therefore need advice. Very often, however, a child, if left alone to decide for himself how much sport he wishes to play, will formulate an appropriate judgement. In this respect, he may be more mature than his advisers.

References

Anthony, R. J. (1987). The functional anatomy of the running training shoe. *Chiropodist*, **42** (12), 451–9.
Ballantine, R. (1976). *Richard's bicycle book* (revised edn). Pan Books, London.

Barry, H. C. and Calcinai, C. J. (1988). The need to make rugby safer. *Br. Med. J.*, **296** (6616), 149–50.

Cahill, B. R. and Griffith, E. H. (1987). Effect of preseason conditioning on the incidence and severity of high school football knee injuries. *Am. J. Sports Med.*, **6**, 180–84.

Cavanagh, P. R. (1980). *The running shoe book.* Anderson World, Mountain View, CA.

Chapman, P. J. (1988). The pattern of use of mouthguards in rugby league (a study of the 1986 Australian rugby league touring team). *Br. J. Sports Med.*, **22** (3), 98–100.

Davies, J. E. and Gibson, T. (1978). Injuries in rugby union football. *Br. Med. J.*, **6154**, 1759–61.

Davis, M. W., Litman, T., Drill, E., and Mueller, J. K. (1977). Ski injuries. *J. Trauma*, **17**, 802–8.

De Vries, H. A. (1962). Evaluation of static stretching procedures for improvement of flexibility. *Res. Q.*, **33**, 222–9.

Grayson, E. (1999). *Ethics, injuries and the law in sports medicine*, pp 50–54, Butterworth Heinemann, Oxford.

Grimby, G. (1982). Isokinetic training. *Int. J. Sports Med.*, **3**, 61–4.

Hislop, H. J. and Perrine, J. J. (1967). The isokinetic concept of exercise. *J. Am. Phys. Ther. Assoc.*, **47**, 114–7.

James, S. L., Bates, B. T., and Osternig, L. R. (1978). Injuries to runners. *Am. J. Sports Med.*, **6** (2), 40–50.

Johannsen, H. V. and Noerregaard, F. O. H. (1988). Prevention of injury in karate. *Br. J. Sports Med.*, **22** (3), 113–15.

Johnson, R. J. and Ettlinger, C. F. (1982). Alpine ski injuries: changes through the years. *Clin. Sport Med.*, **1** (2), 181–97.

Johnson, R. J., Ettlinger, C. F., Campbell, R. J., and Pope, M. H. (1980). Trends in skiing injuries. *Am. J. Sports Med.*, **8** (2), 106–13.

Kavanagh, T., Shephard, R. J., Chisholm, A. W., Qureshi, S., and Kennedy, J. (1979). Prognostic indices for patients with ischaemic heart disease enrolled in an exercise-centered rehabilitation program. *Am. J. Cardiol.*, **44**, 1230–40.

Micheli, L. J. (1983). Overuse injuries in children's sports: the growth factor. *Orthop. Clin. North Am.*, **14** (2), 337–60.

Moffroid, M., Whipple, R., Hofkosh, J., *et al.* (1969). A study of isokinetic exercise. *Phys Ther.*, **49**, 735–47.

Morris, J. N. *et al.* (1953). Coronary heart disease and physical activity at work. *Lancet*, **2**, 1053–7, 1111–20.

Morris, J. N. *et al.* (1980). Vigorous exercise in leisure time: protection against coronary heart disease. *Lancet*, **2**, 1207–10.

Mottram, S. and Comerford, M. (1998). Stability dysfunction and low back pain. *J. Orthop. Med.*, **20** (12), 13–8.

Murray, R. O. and Duncan, C. (1971). Athletic activity in adolescence as an aetiological factor in degenerative hip disease. *J. Bone Jt. Surg.*, **53B**, 406–19.

Nideffer, R. (1981). *The ethics and practice of applied sport psychology.* Mouvement Publications, Ithaca, NY.

Nigg, B. M. (1988). The assessment of loads acting on the locomotor system in running and other sport activities. *Semin. Orthop.*, **4** (3), 197–206.

Norris, C. M. (1993). Abdominal muscle training in sport. *Br. J. Sports Med.*, **27** (1), 19–27.

Paffenbarger, R. S. and Hale, W. E. (1975). Work activity and coronary heart mortality. *N. Engl. J. Med.*, **292**, 545–50.

Rothstein, J. M., Lamb, R. L., and Mayhew, T. P. (1987). Clinical uses of isokinetic measurements. *Phys. Ther.*, **67** (12), 1840–44.

Salter, R. B. and Harris, R. (1963). Injuries involving the epiphyseal plate. *J. Bone Jt. Surg.*, **45A**, 587–622.

Silver, J. R. (1984). Injuries of the spine sustained in rugby. *Br. Med. J.*, **288**, 37–43.

Stulberg, S. D., Cordell, L. D., Harris, W. H., *et al.* (1975). Unrecognised childhood hip disease: a main cause of idiopathic osteoarthritis of the hip. In *The Hip: Proceedings of the Third Open Scientific Meeting of the Hip Society*, Vol. 3, pp. 212–8. Mosby, St Louis, MO.

Subotnick, S. I. (1985). The biomechanics of running: implications for the prevention of foot injuries. *Sports Med.*, **2**, 144–53.

Thorstensson, A. (1976). Muscle strength, fibre types and enzyme activities in man. *Acta Phys. Scand. Suppl.* **443**, 1–45.

Watkins, M. P. and Harris, B. A. (1983). Evaluation of isokinetic muscle performance, *Clin. Sports Med.*, **2** (1), 37–53.

Yaffé, M. (1983). Sports injuries: psychological aspects. *Br. J. Hosp. Med.*, **29** (3), 224–33.

12 Treatment and rehabilitation

M. A. HUTSON

General concepts

It is useful at the outset to define terminology; that this is more than pure semantics should become obvious in the text. 'Treatment' usually refers to those therapeutic measures that are used in healing injured tissue. 'Rehabilitation', on the other hand, literally means restoration of a normal state of health or well-being, and is a more all-embracing term. Total rehabilitation transcends the anti-inflammatory phase (involving treatment by specific modalities, physical or otherwise) by incorporating recovery of musculoskeletal functions that existed before the injury. Furthermore, it may involve realignment of any pre-existing weakness or imbalance that precipitated the breakdown process. In many instances, the psychological aspect of rehabilitation is just as or more important than the physiological. Therefore, rehabilitation may be instituted from the first day of injury, and should invoke in the clinician's mind the need for maintenance of general body fitness, as well as the more specific aspect of tissue healing.

The extent of rehabilitation depends on a number of factors, including the severity and type of injury sustained, and the requirements of the specific sport. A cricketer with a fractured finger will be more severely handicapped than a long distance runner with the same injury, though he will be able to maintain general body fitness to a large degree. Conversely, a runner with shin splints may need to modify his training substantially compared with the cricketer, who might continue to practise technical skills such as batting even though he may not be able to bowl. The timing of the re-introduction of specific training schedules is dependent upon the exact demands made by each sport. It is erroneous to pursue a narrow-minded approach of first 'treatment', then 'rehabilitation'. Muscle-strengthening and flexibility exercises may be performed concurrently with anti-inflammatory therapy, albeit in a restricted fashion.

Rehabilitation programmes should include the following stages:

   (i) healing of injured tissue such as muscle, tendon, joint capsule, and ligament;
   (ii) a pain-free active range of movement;
   (iii) restoration of full flexibility of joints and contractile structures;
   (iv) recovery of muscle strength and endurance;
   (v) recovery of skill and cardiovascular fitness.

Although the final determinants of recovery (factor (v)) are often pursued by the patient after discharge to his own training schedules or to his coach, advice on timing and appropriate amendments to his schedule are required of the clinician.

Expansion of the principles of rehabilitation

Rest

The normal tissue response to injury, namely inflammation, takes at least five days, and may last for two or three weeks. During this time, some degree of reduction of applied stress is necessary. Many conditions require relative rather than absolute rest of the injured part, and numerous instances have been cited in the relevant chapters. Absolute rest by immobilization may be prescribed for complicated or unstable fractures, grade III medial collateral ligament tears of the knee, Achilles tendon ruptures, and severe muscle contusions (when the development of myositis ossificans is to be avoided). Alternatively, surgical management may be undertaken for some fractures, and ligament and tendon ruptures. Following surgery, a period of immobilization is usually indicated, though cast-bracing rather than casting may be appropriate.

For most soft tissue problems, however, the period of complete rest should be as short as possible—of the order of a few days only—and immobilization by external splintage should be eschewed whenever possible. Immobilization affects the proprioceptive mechanism adversely, as well as causing capsular stiffness by contracture, muscle wasting, loss of tensile strength of all connective tissues (Akeson et al. 1967; Viidik 1967; Laros et al. 1971), and impaired nutrition of articular cartilage (Finsterbush and Friedman 1973).

Cast-bracing

The use of cast-bracing techniques for lower limb fractures has been accepted by orthopaedic surgeons for some time. Mooney (1974) summarized his own practice as follows:

> The ambulatory care of lower extremity fractures is based on two concepts: 1) Progressive weight-bearing, with its associated muscle and joint function, improved fracture-site fluid-flow, and gradually increasing skeletal stresses—these are positive factors to achieve efficient fracture healing and early limb rehabilitation; 2) prolonged recumbency is a negative factor. The improved general body metabolism associated with ambulatory activity is good for primate organ function, including the 'psyche'.

Experience with a cast-brace for patients with knee trauma, utilizing a modified single-axis joint in which the arc of motion was restricted to 30°–90°, was described by Bassett et al. (1980). Both non-operative and post-operative management were included. Rehabilitation times were considerably shortened and stability was not compromised, even with moderately severe ligamentous injuries.

The author subsequently has utilized a cast-brace for management of both acute ankle ligament injuries (Hutson and Jackson 1982) and acute knee ligament injuries to good effect. At the ankle, the usual requirement is for lateral support following inversion injury: the provision of a plastic heel-cup and stirrups allows a limited amount of plantarflexion in addition to dorsiflexion (see Fig. 8.10, p. 146). At the knee, protected motion in the sagittal plane is limited to 10°–90°: valgus and varus stresses are controlled by the medial and lateral (adjustable) knee hinges, and rotational strain may be reduced by the application of an additional ankle brace (Fig. 12.1).

The protection afforded by such a brace invites an alternative strategy to the surgical management of substantial tears of the collateral and anterior cruciate ligaments, and of peripheral meniscal tears.

Haggmark and Eriksson (1979) have also reported the satisfactory use of a similar cast-brace (which included an ankle attachment) for control of rotation in the post-operative period after anterior cruciate ligament reconstruction. By comparison with the use of a standard cylinder cast, the rehabilitation time was much reduced. Alternatively, a knee brace, such as the Masterhinge rehabilitation brace, may be used during the rehabilitative phase after surgical ligamentous reconstruction (Fig. 12.2(a)). For established instability, the Lenox Hill derotation brace offers resistance to rotatory, AP, and medial–lateral stresses (Fig. 12.2(b)).

Therapeutic modalities

Non-steroidal anti-inflammatory drugs (NSAIDs)
The increased interest in sports and fitness in recent years, allied to the development of sports medicine, has been paralleled by the introduction of NSAIDs for the management of musculoskeletal disorders. Although the emphasis in this text is on the application of physical modes of treatment to sports injuries, a few comments on the use of NSAIDs are of relevance.

NSAIDs and salicylates have analgesic, anti-inflammatory, and antipyretic properties. Low doses produce analgesic effects, while higher doses reduce inflammation (Calabrese and Rooney 1986). The mechanism of their action appears, in part, to be due to reduction of prostaglandins by inhibition of prostaglandin synthetase. Nevertheless, the inflammatory phase of healing is essential, and the role of the prostaglandins is important (see p. 4).

Several studies have demonstrated the usefulness of NSAIDs in the management of acute sports injuries, for example in knee ligament sprains (Hutson 1986). There is less agreement on their efficacy in overuse injuries; in the author's experience their ability to hasten recovery in these conditions is disappointing. In the presence of degenerative joint disease the prescribing physician has an ethical problem to consider with respect to the possible masking of further joint deterioration resulting from exercise. A further consideration of their use is the significant incidence of dyspepsia and gastro-intestinal bleeding.

Cryotherapy
The use of ice, or at least cold applications, has been established for many years (Sloan et al. 1989). Its vasoconstrictive activity, leading to decreased blood flow and decreased capillary permeability, has a useful effect on the control of bleeding and oedema. Of equal, or greater, importance in the immediate management of acute injury is the reduction of tissue metabolism by cooling. Often this anti-inflammatory action is combined with elevation and compression (ICE) in the early stages of tissue healing. Subsequently it may be used throughout the subacute

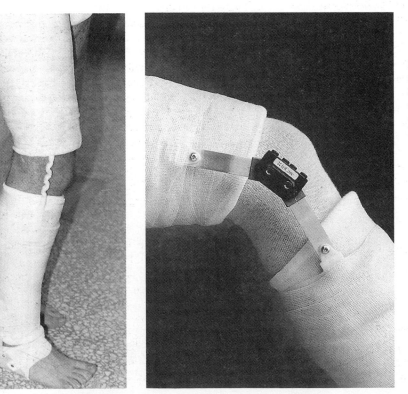

FIG. 12.1 An ambulatory cast-brace for management of knee ligament injuries includes both knee and ankle hinges to control varus, valgus, and rotational stress: (a) using a polycentric hinge; (b) using a Masterhinge (InCare Orthopaedics).

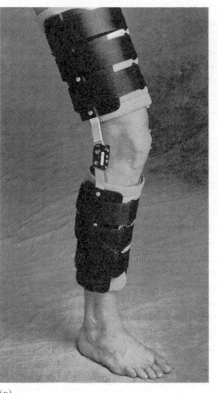

(a)

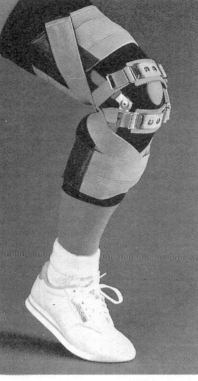

(b)

FIG. 12.2 (a) A knee brace may be used during rehabilitation after surgical ligamentous reconstruction: a Masterhinge rehabilitative knee brace is demonstrated. (b) The Lenox Hill derotation brace offers resistance to rotary, AP, and medial–lateral stresses for established instability.

stage during the institution of a graded exercise programme. Muscle spasm and pain are minimized, thus allowing earlier resumption of mobilizing exercises.

Cold applications or ice may be applied in a number of ways. Crushed ice wrapped inside a suitable bag or wet towel has the advantage of being moulded around the affected area to some extent. Ice that has been produced inside a polystyrene container in a freezer may be used by snipping off the top of the container, thus facilitating the technique of ice massage. The extremities may be immersed in iced water, though this does not allow the concomitant use of elevation. Finally, numerous commercial cold packs which are re-usable are available. Ice applications or cold packs should be used for ten to twenty minutes, and reapplied every two hours or so from the time of the injury for forty-eight hours.

Although cryotherapy is used almost universally, it is not without its dangers. Ice itself should not be allowed to stay in direct contact with the skin, as iceburns may result: motion or massage should be employed. Frostbite has been reported. Nerve palsy has also been documented (Drez *et al.* 1981) when ice is applied over areas in which an underlying nerve lies superficially.

Heat

Heat may be employed in a variety of ways, and is dependent upon the following therapeutic properties:

increased metabolism;

increased blood flow (vasodilatation);

increased threshold of sensory nerve endings.

Shortwave diathermy. A high-frequency current (frequency 27.12 MHz) generated in a machine circuit and coupled to a patient's circuit is used to treat the patient with as deep a form of heat as any available to the therapist. The method of application is either via electrodes or by insulated cable. It is particularly valuable for deep-seated conditions—for example, at the hip joint—and for relief of muscle spasm prior to active exercises. Like other forms of heat, it is not used immediately after injury, particularly after haemorrhage.

Ultrasound therapy

Ultrasound therapy employs frequencies well beyond the range of hearing: 1 MHz (for deep-seated lesions such as joint capsules) to 3 MHz (for more superficial lesions). A high-frequency current is converted via a crystal into an ultrasound beam transmitted through a treatment head. Intensity is variable, though most therapeutic ultrasound is used in the range 0.25–1.0 Watts/cm^2. Continuous wave and pulsed wave outputs are available—pulsing lowers the overall intensity. A coupling medium is required to transmit the waves. Physiological, psychological, and physical mechanisms are involved in the therapeutic effect on tissues (Dyson 1987). The principal effects are acceleration of repair and reduction of pain.

A *physiological* response within twenty-four hours of injury may be due to stimulation of the release of histamine and chemotactic agents by mast cells, thereby attracting polymorphs and monocytes to the injured site. This process involves a change in permeability of the cell membrane, thereby increasing the transport of calcium ions into the mast cells. As the inflammatory phase proceeds to the proliferative phase, fibroblasts may also be stimulated by diffusion of calcium ions, facilitated by ultrasound, resulting in increased collagen synthesis. Increased endothelial activity occurs with the formation of new capillaries. Therefore, the overall physiological effect of ultrasound is to accelerate both the inflammatory phase and the proliferative phases of tissue repair (Dyson and Pond 1970). During the subsequent remodelling, the strength of the scar is greater if ultrasound has been used early on.

One of the *physical* properties of ultrasound is the production of heat, which may be minimized by the use of pulsed waves; it is not usually desired immediately after acute injury. At a later stage, the thermal effect may be used to increase the extensibility of collagen, and to reduce pain and muscle spasm. Among the non-thermal physical effects is a micromassage that occurs at cellular level, facilitating the reduction of oedema that is associated with both acute and chronic conditions. Acoustic streaming, a unidirectional flow of tissue fluid, affects cellular permeability, thereby increasing protein synthesis and reducing pain (possibly by stimulation of mechanoreceptors, or by a direct effect on nerves). A potential hazard is transient ('unstable') cavitation, in which cells may be damaged by the implosion of small gas bubbles: the risk is reduced by continued mobility of the transducer, and the use of a low intensity (0.1–0.2 Watts/cm^2).

The *psychological* (placebo) effect is associated with alteration of plasma endorphin levels: patients often find therapy to be soothing.

A major advantage of ultrasound lies in the fact that it may be used in acute traumatic conditions, when reduction of oedema and adhesions are required. Although there is controversy over dosage schedules, perhaps the most practical guide is to rely on the personal experience of the therapist. Absorption of hydrocortisone cream is facilitated by ultrasound energy (phonophoresis). A further therapeutic use of ultrasound depends on its softening effect on established scar tissue at both an early and a later stage following injury.

Interferential therapy

Interferential therapy is so called as a result of the use of the 'interference' between two medium-frequency currents to produce the desired low-frequency current. The resultant frequency of between 0 and 250 Hz is produced in the crossover area between two applied circuits. Interferential stimulation is a form of transcutaneous electrical nerve stimulation (the classical pain-relieving form of which is better known as TENS). The electrodes are applied diagonally across the treatment site. Claimed clinical benefits are as follows:

(1) reduction of inflammation—for example, in shoulder-joint synovitis;
(2) muscle re-education—for example, foot muscle exercises, pelvic floor exercises;
(3) pain relief (150–250 Hz).

Lasers (*light amplification by stimulated emission of radiation*)

Cold or soft lasers produce a flow of photons at a specific wavelength. For treatment of soft tissue lesions, the energy is released in a pulsed mode, which reduces the average intensity to safe levels. This energy 'helps reinstate normal conditions by overcoming tissue resistance that occurs with trauma. Healing is enhanced in this manner by the resumption of normal cellular metabolism ... Various researchers have disclosed the following results from studies involving cold lasers; (1) elevated ATP production; (2) enhanced DNA replication; (3) reduction of prostaglandin production; (4) oedema reduction, especially in the acute phase of injury; (5) increased collagen production and vascularization; and (6) increased tensile strength of collagen.' (Gieck and Saliba 1987).

Massage

Massage may take many forms, and may be used for a multitude of soft tissue problems. Although at one time it fell into some disrepute, as a result of its association with 'massage parlours', therapeutic massage is now being employed to its rightful extent. Undoubtedly it has physiological effects. Depending upon the type used, these effects include relaxation, neural stimulation, increased lymphatic drainage, increased local blood-flow, and possibly an effect on muscles whereby recovery from post-exercise muscle soreness is accelerated. However, the indications should be clear to the clinician and therapist, and it is important that the correct type of massage is used. Types of massage which may be of therapeutic value are detailed below.

Effleurage helps to relieve congestion, particularly the unwanted presence of oedema around joints and in traumatic periostitis. Repeated upward stroking movements are employed. The massage is repeated daily and followed by application of a double Tubigrip support.

Deep friction. This technique, developed by Cyriax, helps to maintain or restore mobility to those (often deeply seated) lesions that are prone to develop adhesions or scarring. Its application is principally to muscles, tendons, and ligaments. Accurate localization of the lesion is imperative; thus the technique may not be employed until oedema has been reduced by *effleurage*. Its action is to promote mobility of the healing or scarred area and create hyperaemia, which results in analgesia, and to increase mechanoreceptor stimulation, which further reduces pain by blocking afferent sensory stimuli. It is imperative that it is used properly by transverse movements across the line of the fibres in their relaxed position, and by the abolition of any movement between the therapist's finger and the patient's skin, so that finger and skin move as one across the underlying tissues. Although it is painful initially, subsequently there is a numbing effect.

When used for muscle lesions, its effect is to reduce adhesions between individual fibres, and to allow natural broadening upon contraction. For ligamentous lesions, the purpose is to reproduce the normal mobility of the ligament over the underlying bone and to reduce fibrotic attachments, thereby improving joint mobility. Examples of its use are in lesions of the femoral attachment of the medial collateral ligament of the knee, of the coronary ligaments of the knee, and of the dorsal ligaments of the wrist. In tendinous lesions, it may help to reduce intratendinous scarring and thus facilitate stretching. It may have an excellent effect on tenosynovitis (though steroid injections have an even quicker effect) by mobilizing the sheath around the tendon.

Other types of massage include kneading and vibration massage using commercially available vibrators; probably these assist by their pleasurable effects and by increased local blood flow.

Mobilization exercises

The benefits of mobilization are the reverse of the adverse effects of immobilization: the primary considerations are the maintenance and subsequent improvement of muscle tone, reduction of joint stiffness, and increased tensile strength of connective tissue, particularly ligaments. Although conventional orthopaedic teaching in the past has suggested that six weeks is required for healing of a ligament tear by immobilization (for example, in a POP cast), it is probable that this healing time is less when a joint is mobilized, if necessary with an appropriate degree of functional support. Collagen deposition is more 'orderly' with respect to the laying down of fibres in parallel during this phase when under the influence of controlled exercise. The constraints to early mobilization of connective tissues should be the presence of oedema or effusion, the patient's complaint of discomfort or pain, and the minimum amount of time taken for tissues to progress to the repair stage of healing. However, such constraints should not result in an all-or-nothing situation. Sound healing of a muscle tear may take three or four weeks (and indeed many months for full maturity of the scar), though graded stretching exercises should take place well before then. The diagnosis of 'microscopic' rather than 'macroscopic' damage in ligament injury—that is, a stable joint—should lead to commencement of both active and passive mobilization exercises as soon as pain and oedema allow. The use of a cast-brace for ligament rupture allows earlier introduction of a restricted range of joint mobility.

Prolonged tissue oedema may have devastating effects on local musculoskeletal function, and is influenced considerably by the judicious use of graded mobilization. In the lower limb, a distinction should be made between the adverse effects of prolonged standing and abnormal gait on the one hand (in the mistaken belief that any form of ambulation is correct), and the usefulness of deliberate careful, though biomechanically correct, gait on the other.

The acute phase. Both active and passive range of motion exercises may begin early after joint injury. They have a similar effect on joint mobility, though only active exercises maintain some degree of muscle tone. The therapist may need to encourage joint motion initially, to a point at which slight discomfort is appreciated by the patient, followed by active exercises within the same range. A skilled therapist is able to gain the patient's cooperation, and proceed through a gradually increasing range of movements on a daily basis. In many instances, the patient may be taught to perform these exercises himself.

When treating muscle injury, movement of the affected muscle should be maintained passively within the limit of pain. Passive stretching should not be instituted too early, for fear of disrupting healing scar tissue, though it will begin gently after a week or so. Faradic stimulation may be considered in the early stages, when little active contraction is possible otherwise. Dynamic muscle exercise may be instituted in the recovery phase.

Recovery phase. Forced passive movements are sometimes necessary to break down adhesions or to stretch capsules. Adhesions form at the knee and ankle joints, particularly after immobilization or surgery. Capsular contracture is a common accompaniment to immobilization of any joint, whatever the pathology of the preceding injury. It is often profound at the shoulder in post-traumatic capsulitis (and in the second phase of adhesive capsulitis), and may require stretching exercises for several months (see Fig. 11.14, p. 208). The elbow joint warrants special mention, as it often responds adversely to passive mobilization or stretching. Whether secondary to dislocation, fracture, or severe contusion, stiffness of the elbow may be profound, resolving slowly over many months. Attempts at forceful extension exercises create further loss of mobility. Overvigorous exercises may cause myositis ossificans in the surrounding muscles.

\ Flexibility exercises should be undertaken, gently at first and more vigorously later, to restore full mobility at the affected joint and full elasticity of an affected muscle or tendon. The principle of the two Ss—full *stretch* and *strength*—cannot be overemphasized in muscle rehabilitation, as so often they are overlooked. Strengthening exercises are considered further, while the reader is referred to Chapter 11 for an account of flexibility exercises.

Strengthening exercises

Whatever the nature of the injury sustained, a well-designed management plan includes rehabilitation of weakened muscle. Muscle function may be stimulated in a number of different ways.

Isometric exercise. The phenomenon of active muscle contraction with constant length is utilized during the early stages of recovery from joint injury. In some situations, for instance disorders of the patellofemoral mechanism, it may be the only effective way of maintaining or developing muscle tone during the early stages of rehabilitation. The therapist may need to demonstrate and subsequently monitor contractions, and in certain circumstances be required to provide manual resistance. However, most isometric exercise may be performed by the patient without assistance. Examples have been provided throughout the text. Further consideration is now given to two regions that require careful monitoring: the knee and the shoulder.

Early loss of quadriceps tone and bulk are easily measured (by a tape measure) and demonstrated to the patient. During recovery from either ligament or meniscus injury, it is usually possible to proceed rapidly to dynamic isotonic or isokinetic exercise once the ability to straight leg raise has been demonstrated (see Fig. 7.8, p. 131). However, recovery from injury to the extensor mechanism, particularly the variety of problems associated with the patellofemoral syndrome, is hindered by the risk of exacerbation of symptoms if muscle conditioning is attempted from a significant degree of knee flexion.

Isometric contraction drills in extension are prescribed to build up the vastus medialis and thereby maintain patellar stability (Fig. 12.3). Isometric exercise is undertaken initially in a supine or sitting position, though subsequently it may be performed on standing. A maximal contraction is maintained for as long as possible (that is, up to ten seconds), followed by two to three seconds relaxation, and then by a further similar contraction. This sequence is continued to muscle exhaustion, usually involving up to ten repetitions. The set of contractions is repeated several times a day.

Just as the vastus medialis contributes largely to patellar stability, so the rotator cuff is primarily responsible for stability of the mobile glenohumeral joint. Once tendinitis resolves, a schedule of isometric exercise for each of the elements of the cuff in turn should be instituted. Initially the therapist manually resists movement, subsequently instructing the patient in other forms of isometric exercise which may be performed at home. Particular attention is paid to contraction of the abductors (with the arm in the dependent position) and the external and internal rotators. Graded introduction of isotonic exercise follows, using surgical tubing or hand-held weights (see Figs 3.25 and 3.26, pp. 52 and 53).

Isotonic exercise. Concentric contraction occurs when muscle shortens during contraction. Resistance may be provided by a variety of methods that are available to the therapist and patient. Exercise with cliniband, surgical tubing, weighted boots, and free weights may be undertaken in the treatment room (Fig. 12.4(a)). More sophisticated equipment—for example, multi-

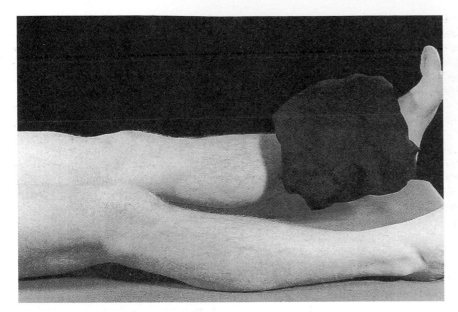

FIG.12.3 Isometric exercise in extension for the knee extensors may be augmented by loading—for example, with a weight attached to the ankle.

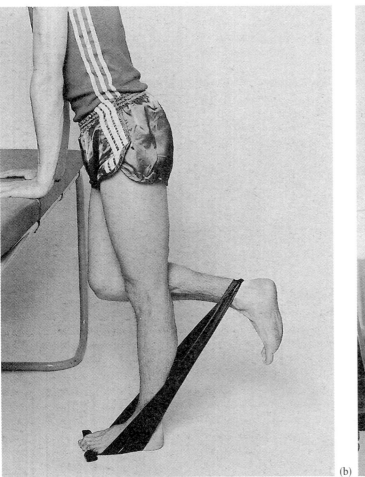

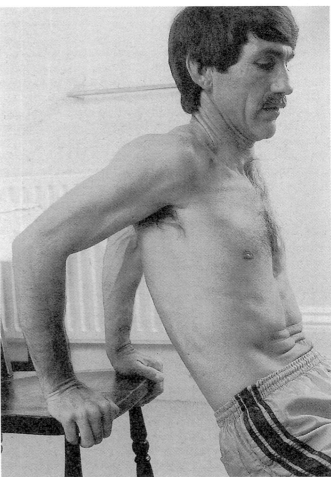

(a)   (b)

FIG.12.4 (a) Cliniband (made from pure latex) is a suitable material for use in remedial exercise. (b) The patient's own body-weight is often utilized in circuit-training exercises.

gym stations—may be available in a gymnasium. The patient's own body-weight is often utilized in circuit-training exercise. Strict monitoring is required to establish and expand a suitable programme of exercises.

Eccentric exercise. Eccentric contraction takes place when muscle contracts during lengthening—for example, triceps contraction during controlled elbow flexion using body-weight as a resistance (Fig. 12.4(b)). Mennell (1960) emphasizes the importance of this aspect of management by stating that 'when a long muscle becomes weakened by shortening through any cause it can only be strengthened once more by the use of lengthening, eccentric decelerating exercises rather than by concentric, shortening accelerating exercises which are more commonly used in a routine manner by most therapists.' The author considers that a sensible balance is advisable.

At a relatively advanced stage of rehabilitation, plyometric drills are particularly useful. These depend on a powerful concentric response to eccentric loading, and go a considerable way towards reproducing the physiological characteristics inherent in sporting activity.

Isokinetic exercise. Isokinetic contraction is dynamic muscle activity performed at a constant angular velocity. The speed of motion is preselected and controlled by an isokinetic dynamometer, in which internal resistance is created to accommodate to the force applied. As soon as the preset angular velocity is reached (which takes a few degrees of movement) the resistance offered by the machine is determined by the effort of the patient, and may be measured as torque (in foot-pounds). Grimby *et al.* (1980) have described the usefulness of isokinetic rehabilitation after knee ligament surgery. There are now numerous reports on rehabilitative isokinetic exercise involving the quadriceps and hamstrings. Most recorded work has been performed on the Cybex, originally developed by Perrini in 1969, although there are other machines such as the Orthotron and the Lido (see Fig. 11.11, p. 203).

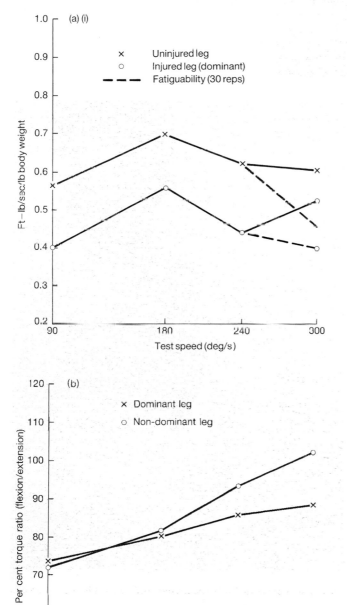

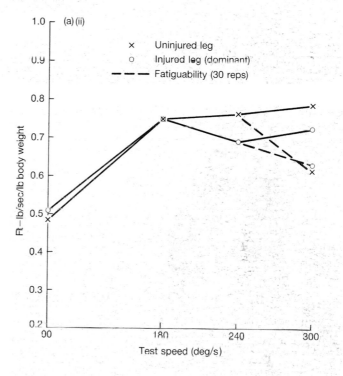

Fig. 12.5 (a) Comparison of power output of the combined knee flexors and extensors per pound body weight (i) shortly after injury to the knee and (ii) after three weeks' rehabilitation on a Lido isokinetic dynamometer. (b) % Torque ratio (knee flexion/extension) vs. test speed in tennis players.

Isokinetic exercise differs from dynamic exercise using externally applied weights by allowing muscle to work maximally throughout the full arc of motion. In addition, an athlete's training or rehabilitation programme may be adapted by selection of exercise speeds varying from 0° to 300° per second, to simulate the type of muscular contraction employed in a particular sport. A major advantage is safety: in recovery from injury a joint may not tolerate the compression, traction, or torsion effects of external weights, though it may be perfectly safe when responding to the inbuilt accommodative effects of the dynamometer, particularly at the higher speeds.

From the author's experience in isokinetic rehabilitation following knee or thigh muscle injury, two parameters have been found to be useful:

(i) power per pound body-weight of both the knee flexors and the knee extensors at different angular velocities—additionally, fatiguability is assessed at the higher speeds;
(ii) hamstring-to-quadriceps torque ratios at different speeds.

Rehabilitative exercise concentrates on normalizing deficiencies or imbalances by reference to the normal leg and the type of sport played (Fig. 12.5). Allowances are made for the dominant and non-dominant legs. Isokinetic training is described further in Chapter 11.

Whatever the arguments for or against the use of certain types of exercise such as isokinetics in rehabilitation, it should be recognized that muscle activity of this type is *not physiological*, and that the graded reintroduction of specific sports training at an appropriate stage is an important step in rehabilitation.

Manipulation

Manipulative techniques are used in a variety of circumstances, though some old-established concepts require critical reassessment. Normal joint mobility is lost in the majority of acute injuries. The mobilization techniques already described may be successful in restoring mobility, though specific indications exist for the use of procedures which utilize a greater degree of thrust.

Peripheral joints. Manipulation may readjust the position of an intra-articular fragment, namely a loose body or a meniscal tear. The techniques involve a combination of distraction and rotational movements of the affected joint. The reader may learn the techniques of manipulation of the knee and elbow, for instance, by reference to Cyriax's *Textbook of orthopaedic medicine*. A joint may be 'unlocked' by a manipulative procedure, though, since the offending loose or torn fragment is still present in the joint, the ultimate management is referral for surgical removal. A patient may learn the knack of self-releasing a locked joint, in which case the history alone provides the physician with a sus-

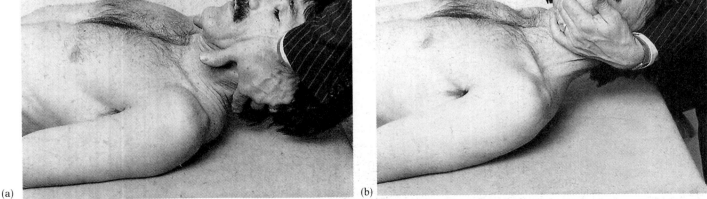

(a)   (b)

Fig. 12.6 (a) The position of the patient and physician are demonstrated in assessment of joint-play in the cervical spine. (b) A commonly used position of facet locking prior to manipulation is demonstrated.

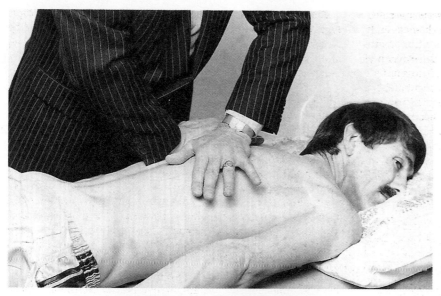

(a)

FIG. 12.7 The position of the patient and physician are demonstrated for
(a) thoracic joint manipulation and
(b) segmental manipulation of the lumbar spinal joints.

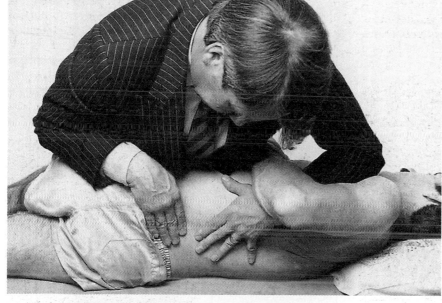

(b)

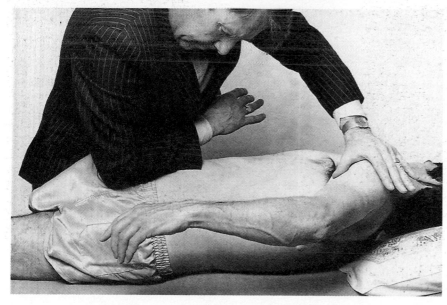

FIG.12.8 The position of the patient and physician are demonstrated for manipulation of the sacroiliac joint.

picion of intra-articular derangement. Other manipulative techniques used for mobilizing joints which are 'dysfunctional'—that is, have lost their normal range of motion due to neurophysiological disturbance or capsular contracture—are described by Mennell (1960) and Maitland (1986).

Spinal manipulation. There is much debate over the nature of the spinal lesion that is responsive to manipulation. The author's belief is that sacroiliac dysfunction and facet (apophyseal) joint dysfunction in the cervical, thoracic, and lumbar spine are the manipulable lesions. In any event, as long as appropriate criteria of suitability for treatment by manipulation have been established (see Chapter 5) the standard manipulative procedures (Figs 12.6–12.8) are safe and effective, if only on empirical grounds. Since a variety of techniques are available, the reader is advised to pursue his interest by attending courses and symposia run by the British Institute of Musculoskeletal Medicine, the Society of Orthopaedic Medicine, or the London College of Osteopathic Medicine. Referral of a patient to a suitably qualified physiotherapist or osteopath is the alternative approach.

Relative contraindications to manipulation in the cervical and lumbar spines are nuclear disc protrusions. They may be suspected by the presence of radicular symptoms (root pain, paraesthesiae, and numbness), dural signs, and articular signs. Positive neurological signs (motor weakness or altered reflexes) are confirmatory evidence. Under these circumstances, sustained daily traction or (in the case of sciatica) epidural or root block injections should be employed. A suspicion of vertebrobasilar insufficiency is a contraindication to the use of cervical manipulation by the inexperienced manipulator. An absolute contraindication is the inability to diagnose a benign mechanical lesion.

A suitable manipulation schedule is to review the patient every two to three days, reassess, and remanipulate until resolution of the signs—that is, until establishment of normal joint mobility. Once mobility is restored, a suitable range of exercises is prescribed to strengthen the abdominal and pelvic muscles in lumbar or sacroiliac disorders, and the neck muscles in cervical disorders. This is particularly important when the patient intends to return to vigorous exercise, such as rugby football.

Spinal traction. The indication for spinal traction is the diagnosis of nuclear disc protrusion (HNP). There is radiological evidence from epidurographic studies that the size of a disc protrusion is reduced by a suitable distracting force in the long axis of the spine. Daily sustained traction is applied using one of a number of commercially available traction couches (see Fig. 5.16, p. 90). A skilled therapist adjusts the level of traction according to the site of the lesion and the weight of the patient. It may be applied for between fifteen and thirty minutes to a maximum of 25 lb to the neck, and 140 lb (for a well-built male) to the lumbar region. Daily reassessment of symptoms and signs is made, though improvement may not be detected until half-way through an average course of ten treatments. However, treatment should be continued until the signs have resolved or until no further benefit is gained (fifteen sessions may be required).

Dry needling

Acupuncture and intramuscular stimulation (IMF) rely on needle stimulation without drugs. Myofascial pain syndromes are characterized by shortened tender hypertonic muscle—a consequence of neural dysfunction at the spinal level (Gunn 1996). During treatment by IMF, muscle relaxation occurs

within a few minutes following penetration of the hypertonic segment by an acupuncture needle. Manual twisting of the needle for a second or two facilitates this process.

Injection techniques

The indications for and techniques of localized injections, usually for the purpose of infiltration of steroids and/or local anaesthetic, must be understood by the practising sports physician. The indications may be as follows.

1. **Diagnostic** using local anaesthetic—for example, infiltration of the subacromial space for the detection of subacromial bursitis, or epidural anaesthesia with 0.5 per cent procaine to diagnose lumbar nerve-root irritation in a patient with posterior thigh pain of undetermined origin. With increasing experience, it becomes less necessary to confirm diagnosis by these methods. The addition of local anaesthetic to a steroid suspension during treatment is largely to demonstrate to the patient that immediate improvement reflects accurate localization.

2. **Therapeutic**. The rationale is the accurate introduction of anti-inflammatory drugs into inflamed tissues.

(i) *Local anaesthetic* alone occasionally is effective, although the desired effect is often enhanced by the addition of steroid. Lignocaine 1 per cent, for instance, may be used in injection of trigger points which are secondary to spinal joint dysfunction. The effect of the injection may be due as much to the needling of the tissues as to the chemical effect of the lignocaine. It may have a similar effect to that of the vapocoolant spray developed by Travell (Travell and Simons 1983), or the use of subcutaneous salicylate injections developed by Fox (1981). Reflex inhibition of the pain impulse may occur. Melzack and Wall (1965) consider this and other concepts in their 'gate theory' of pain control.

(ii) *Steroid injections*. The advantages and disadvantages of the use of injectable steroids should be fully appreciated. Unfortunately, the general public have become suspicious of their use, for a number of reasons. First, they are often assumed to be in the same mould as anabolic steroids, known universally to be involved in drug abuse in sport. Many patients are acquainted with the fact that high dosage of steroids—for example, used for collagen diseases or for cerebral oedema—causes side-effects including 'moon face'. Lastly, patients sometimes believe, often quite rightly if steroids are used indiscriminately in the absence of an appropriate rehabilitation programme, that an injection may simply ameliorate the symptoms without establishing a cure.

The advantage of a localized injection of steroid is the rapid anti-inflammatory response that is gained: in some instances, it may be quite dramatic. Conditions such as medial coronary ligament sprain of the knee, even if present for several months, resolve within a few days of treatment by injection. Other conditions such as subacromial bursitis are difficult to treat by other means because of their anatomical position.

The disadvantages are the side-effects which may occur with overdosage. The effect on collagen is such that subcutaneous seepage may give rise to the typical mauve-coloured discoloration and thinning of the skin overlying a lesion. This is cosmetically undesirable, and often indicates poor technique and/or overdosage. Repeated injections rarely give rise to systemic side-effects, such as weight gain or peptic ulceration, though a metabolic effect may be seen in diabetics, in whom there can be a temporary increase in insulin requirement. There may be a disturbance of the menstrual cycle in susceptible females in the form of intermenstrual bleeding. Flushing occasionally occurs. To a large extent, the likelihood of such side-effects is reduced by using the minimum dosage of triamcinolone hexacetonide (or equivalent) according to the following guidelines.

Soft tissue, for example ligament or teno-osseous junction	10 mg
Intra-articular	10–20 mg depending upon size of joint—for example, 20 mg for shoulder or knee joint, 10 mg for acromioclavicular joint
Epidural	20–40 mg

Normally 10 mg of triamcinolone or methyl prednisolone is all that is required—this is one-quarter the dose that may be commercially available in a 1 ml ampoule. Injections that need to be repeated should preferably be of the lower dosages. One further major disadvantage of injectible steroid is the weakening effect on collagen, particularly tendons. There is **no indication for injecting into a weightbearing tendon**—for example, the Achilles tendon. Although there is controversy over whether rupture may be caused by intratendinous injection, the argument should become a theoretical one: the sheath or paratenon only should be injected. The minimal pressure needed to inject into a tendon sheath is quite different from the force required to inject into the tendon.

A summary of the indications is as follows.

1. *Intrabursal*—for example, for subacromial bursitis, postcalcaneal bursitis, and anserine bursitis. A dramatic response may be expected in acute conditions, and early relief from months of discomfort in chronic conditions in which adhesions and fibrosis are features.

2. *Intrasynovial* (a) When used in tenosynovitis—for example, de Quervain's tenosynovitis or tenosynovitis of the foot dorsiflexors—the response may be dramatic. When used for primary Achilles paratendinitis, the response is equally dramatic: when paratendinitis is secondary to significant pathology of the tendon, additional therapeutic modalities are needed.

(b) Intra-articular (IA) injections have tended to fall into some disrepute as a result of the concern over the possible degradative effect on articular cartilage. Although discretion is advocated in the use of IA injection of the weightbearing joints of the lower limb, nevertheless a 'one-off' injection may be extremely useful. There should be evidence of the persistence of synovitis (for example, discomfort, dysfunction, synovial thickening, and restriction of joint movements in the capsular pattern) beyond what may reasonably be expected after trauma. Chondral or osteochondral injury should be excluded. Synovitis of the elbow, after jarring or overuse, may require two or three injections. Interphalangeal joint injuries may give rise to prolonged discomfort and stiffness, which are often helped by one IA injection. There is hardly a synovial joint in the body that does not occasionally merit IA injection: numerous examples are given in the text. The shoulder joint is worthy of further consideration: both adhesive capsulitis and post-

traumatic capsulitis respond to IA injections, which should be repeated at one- to three-weekly intervals until the pain settles (at least until the patient is comfortable at night). Graded stretching exercises may then be instituted on resolution of the inflammatory phase.

3. *Intraligamentous.* Some ligament sprains, for example, coronary ligament sprains of the knee, respond dramatically. Without localized injection or friction massage they may linger for months. Degenerative joints are more prone to ligament sprain. The knee is one example; the acromioclavicular joint is another. A localized intraligamentous injection at the acromioclavicular joint may be combined with an IA injection.

Discomfort that persists for an inordinate length of time after partial ligamentous disruption, for example at the femoral attachment of the MCL of the knee and the lateral collateral ligament of the ankle, may be helped by localized infiltration.

4. *Intratendinous.* As previously indicated, injections into the substance of tendons, particularly weightbearing tendons, are eschewed. No indication exists, and there is a risk of steroid-induced rupture. However, lesions at teno-osseous junctions (enthesopathies) may be injected. Examples of such conditions are lateral and medial epicondylitis, patella apicitis, chronic adductor tendon strain in the groin, and insertional tendinitis of the supraspinatus tendon. Care is taken to rehabilitate the involved musculature, and sufficient time is allowed after the injection to establish sound healing. Steroid injections should not be given purely for pain relief to allow competitive sport to be undertaken.

Precautions

(i) An aseptic technique using disposable syringes and needles should be used at all times. An injection is withheld in the presence of local skin sepsis.

(ii) Single-dose ampoules of steroid and local anaesthetic are preferable.

(iii) Skin preparation with chlorhexidine in 5 per cent spirit or a Mediswab is satisfactory. If a 'marker' is required, the use of a pen or the impression made by a thumb-nail prior to swabbing is ideal.

(iv) The minimum dosage of steroid is used.

(v) Patients are warned that occasionally, particularly in the treatment of enthesopathies, pain may be exacerbated for up to forty-eight hours.

(vi) Care should be taken to explain to patients the nature of the treatment and the need to rest the injury for a week or so after the injection.

The more common injection techniques are now outlined.

The shoulder

The *shoulder joint* is entered most easily and with most certainty posteriorly: there is no preferred indication for an anterior or lateral approach. The patient lies prone (or sits if this position is too painful) with the affected arm internally rotated across the abdomen. The index finger of the examiner's non-dominant hand palpates the coracoid process, and the thumb the spine of the scapula as it angulates forwards by 90° to become the acromion. The needle pierces the skin 1 cm inferior to the thumb and is directed anteriorly towards the index finger (Fig. 12.9). After penetrating the infraspinatus, the resistance of the capsule is felt, and then a loss of resistance as the joint cavity is entered; impingement against bone or articular cartilage is felt.

FIG. 12.9 (a) Injection of the left glenohumeral joint by the posterior approach is demonstrated. (b) The posterior aspect of the shoulder. The examiner's thumb palpates the spine of the scapula as it angulates forwards to become the acromion.

(b)

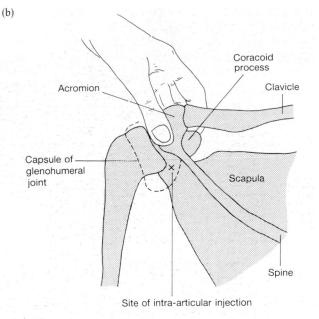

(a)

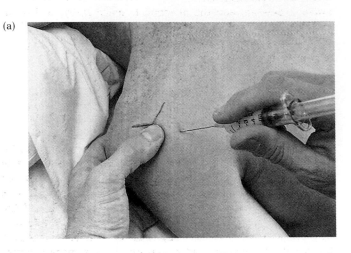

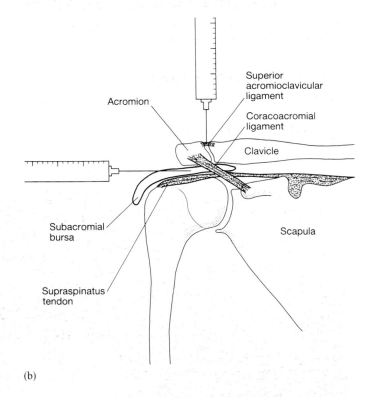

(b)

FIG. 12.10 (a) The subacrominal bursa may be injected via a postero-lateral approach. (b) Injection techniques for the acromoclavicular joint and subacromial bursa.

(a)

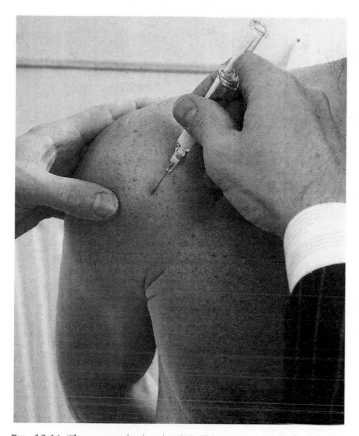

FIG. 12.11 The supraspinatus tendon insertion is injected with the patient sitting with arm internally rotated.

The following materials are required:

5 ml syringe
2 inch 21 G needle
20 mg of triamcinolone hexacetonide in 1 ml
4 ml of 1 per cent lignocaine.

The *subacromial bursa* is approached most easily in the sitting patient from the posterolateral aspect of the shoulder. The needle pierces the skin immediately posterior to the head of the humerus and inferior to the acromion (Fig. 12.10) and is directed anteromedially. A loss of resistance is felt when the bursa is entered, and the injection is made easily. If 5 ml or more is injected bulging is noted over the anterior aspect of the subacromial space.

The following materials are required:

5–10 ml syringe
1½ inch 21 G needle
20 mg of triamcinolone hexacetonide in 1 ml
4–9 ml of 1 per cent lignocaine.

The *supraspinatus insertion* is approached from the anterior aspect of the shoulder. The patient is seated with his arm medially rotated behind his back (Fig. 12.11) so that the greater tuberosity is rotated anteriorly. The supraspinatus tendon may be palpated through the deltoid muscle and the tenderness (of insertional tendinitis) identified. The injection may be made either at right angles to the skin, or by inclining the needle downwards and backwards from a more superior approach.

The following materials are required:

2 ml syringe
1 inch 23 G needle
10 mg of triamcinolone hexacetonide in 1 ml
1 ml of 1 per cent lignocaine.

The *infraspinatus tendon* is approached from the posterior aspect of the shoulder when the patient lies prone, resting on his elbows with the forearms externally rotated (Fig. 12.12). The infraspinatus may be palpated immediately inferior to the posterior margin of the acromion. It is usually this site—the musculotendinous junction—that is affected in infraspinatus tendinitis. A direct approach at right angles to the skin is made.

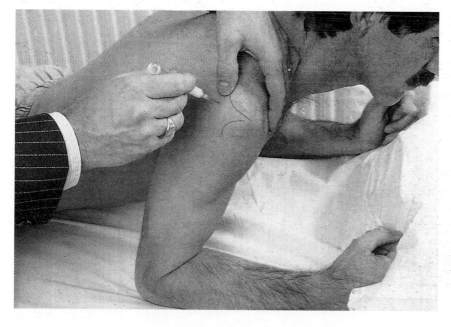

FIG. 12.12 The position of the patient is demonstrated for injection of the infraspinatus (at the musculotendinous junction).

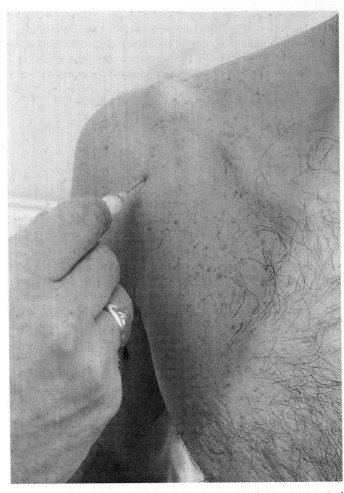

FIG. 12.13 The patient sits with his arm by his side during injection of the subscapularis tendon.

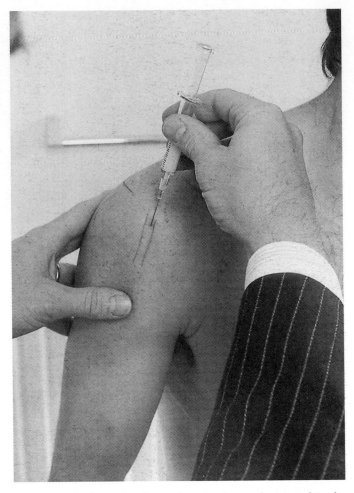

FIG. 12.14 The biceps brachii tendon sheath may be injected in the bicipital groove.

The following materials are required:

2 ml syringe
1 inch 23 G needle
10 mg of triamcinolone hexacetonide in 1 ml
1 ml of 1 per cent lignocaine.

The *subscapularis tendon* is approached from the anteromedial aspect of the shoulder when the patient is seated with his arm hanging loosely by his side (Fig. 12.13). In the presence of subscapularis tendinitis, the affected tendinous insertion into the lesser tuberosity is found to be tender, and may be injected from a direct anterior approach.

The following materials are required:

2 ml syringe
1 inch 23 G (or $1\frac{1}{2}$ inch 21 G) needle
10 mg of triamcinolone hexacetonide in 1 ml
1 ml of 1 per cent lignocaine.

The *biceps brachii tendon* may be palpated in the bicipital groove when the patient's arm hangs loosely by his side, or when the arm is supported in external rotation. The injection is made (Fig. 12.14) almost parallel to the tendon—that is, into the tendon sheath—and the resistance to the injection is minimal.

The following materials are required:

2 ml syringe
1 inch 23 G needle
10 mg of triamcinolone hexacetonide in 1 ml
1 ml of 1 per cent lignocaine.

The *acromioclavicular joint* may be injected from a superior approach. If identification of the joint is difficult, the joint surfaces may be palpated when stress is applied concomitantly to sublux the joint by applying a distracting force to the upper arm. The superior acromioclavicular ligament is infiltrated and then penetrated for intra-articular injection. The direction of the needle is downwards, and slightly forwards and medially, to accommodate the contiguous joint surfaces which are often disposed obliquely (Figs 12.10 and 12.15).

The following materials are required:

2 ml syringe
1 inch 23 G needle
10 mg of triamcinolone hexacetonide in 1 ml
1 ml of 1 per cent lignocaine

The elbow, forearm, and wrist

The *common extensor* and *common flexor* origins from the relevant epicondyles are identified by digital palpation in the treat-

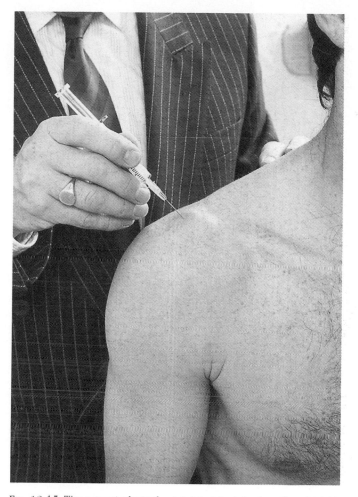

FIG. 12.15 The acromioclavicular joint is injected when the physician stands behind the patient

ment of epicondylitis. From one puncture site droplets are infiltrated into the teno-osseous junction (Fig. 12.16). In the treatment of enthesopathies, injections are made into the tendinous attachment down to the underlying bone. The patient rests his elbow in a comfortable position on the examination couch.

The following materials are required:

2 ml syringe
1 inch 23 G needle
10 mg of triamcinolone hexacetonide in 1 ml
1 ml of 1 per cent lignocaine

The *elbow joint* is approached most easily from the posterolateral aspect (between the radial head and the lateral epicondyle). The patient lies prone with the affected forearm fully supinated. The gap between the radial head (inferiorly) and the posterior margin of the lateral epicondyle (superiorly) is palpated. The needle is inserted (Fig. 12.17) in an anteromedial direction into the joint cavity. If an effusion is present, this should be aspirated initially using a syringe of larger capacity.

The following materials are required:

2 ml syringe
1 inch 23 G needle
20 mg of triamcinolone hexacetonide in 1 ml
1 ml of 1 per cent lignocaine

Tenosynovitis of the tendons of the short extensor and long abductor of the thumb may occur in the distal forearm (as intersection syndrome) or overlying the radial styloid (as de Quervain's tenovaginitis) (Fig. 12.18). In the forearm, a 21 G needle is introduced into the swollen tendon sheath at an angle that is close to parallel. A 23 G needle is used at the radial styloid with a similar technique.

The following materials are required:

2 ml syringe
1 inch 23 G or $1\frac{1}{2}$ inch 21 G needle
10 mg of triamcinolone hexacetonide in 1 ml
1 ml of 1 per cent lignocaine

The *carpal tunnel* is approached at an angle of 45° to the skin. The needle is inserted at the distal wrist crease midway between the pisiform (medially) and the scaphoid tubercle (laterally) (Fig. 12.19). If the palmaris longus tendon is present, the injection should be made on its ulnar side. A loss of resistance is felt after needle penetration to a depth of between 1.0 and 1.5 cm.

The following materials are required:

2 ml syringe
1 inch 23 G needle
10 mg of triamcinolone hexacetonide in 1 ml
1 ml of 1 per cent lignocaine.

The hip

The *hip joint*. An injection (or aspiration) occasionally may be required for which the anterior route is entirely safe. Needle entry is made from a point 3 cm lateral to the femoral artery and 2–3 cm inferior to the inguinal ligament (Fig. 12.20). The approach is anterior–posterior. Alternatively a lateral route may be used, when the needle penetrates in a medial, and slightly superior and anterior, direction from a point adjacent to the superior margin of the greater trochanter.

The following materials are required:

5 ml syringe
2 inch 21 G needle (or $3\frac{1}{2}$ inch 20 G spinal needle for lateral approach)
20 mg of triamcinolone hexacetonide in 1 ml
4 ml of 1 per cent lignocaine.

Trochanteric bursitis is identified by tenderness that is localized to the superolateral aspect of the greater trochanter. A direct approach is used and the injection is made over an area of approximately 2 cm².

The following materials are required:

10 ml syringe
2 inch 21 G needle
10 mg of triamcinolone hexacetonide in 1 ml
9 ml of 1 per cent lignocaine.

The knee

Iliotibial tract bursitis is identified by tenderness that is localized to the lateral epicondyle of the femur or the portion of the iliotibial tract that is immediately adjacent to this (see Fig. 7.3, p. 126). Infiltration is made down to the underlying periosteum.

The following materials are required:

2 ml syringe
1 inch 23 G needle
10 mg of triamcinolone hexacetonide in 1 ml
1 ml of 1 per cent lignocaine.

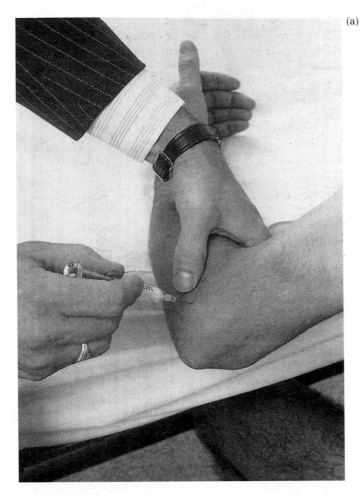

(a)

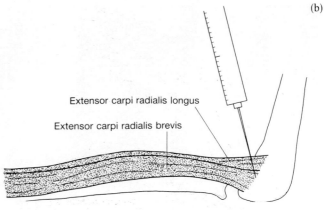

(b)

Extensor carpi radialis longus

Extensor carpi radialis brevis

FIG. 12.16 (a) The patient sits with his elbow supported in 90° flexion prior to injection of lateral epicondylitis. (b) Injection of lateral epicondylitis ('tennis elbow').

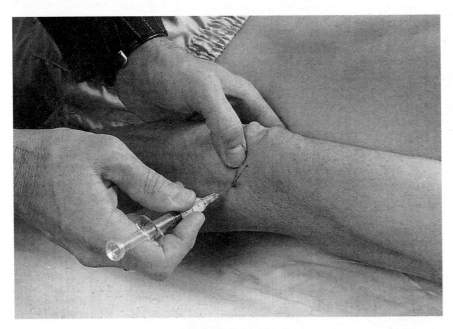

FIG. 12.17 The elbow joint may be injected from a posterolateral approach when the patient lies prone with his forearm supinated.

The *knee joint* may be approached superiorly, inferiorly, medially, or laterally, though it is recommended that one approach is used regularly to gain experience. The author favours the medial approach. With the patient supine and the patella stabilized by digital pressure to its lateral border, the needle is inserted in the gap between the patella (at its medial midpoint) and the femur (Fig. 12.21). The direction of penetration is horizontally and posteriorly; loss of resistance indicates that the joint cavity has been entered. An effusion should be aspirated (using a 20–50 ml syringe) prior to steroid injection.

The following materials are required:

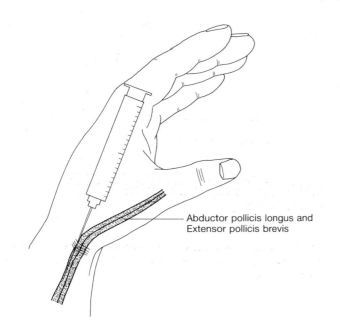

FIG. 12.18 The injection site for de Quervain's tenosynovitis of the long abductor and short extensor of the thumb is shown.

Abductor pollicis longus and Extensor pollicis brevis

5 ml syringe (50 ml for aspiration)
2 inch 21 G needle (20 G for aspiration)
20 mg of triamcinolone hexacetonide in 1 ml
4 ml of 1 per cent lignocaine.

Coronary (meniscotibial) ligament sprains are identified by localized tenderness and induration. Needle penetration is tangential to the joint line and the injection is made (using firm pressure) over approximately 2 cm (Fig. 12.22).

The following materials are required:

2 ml syringe
1 inch 23 G needle
10 mg of triamcinolone hexacetonide in 1 ml
1 ml of 1 per cent lignocaine.

The ankle region

The *ankle joint* is approached anteriorly with the patient lying supine. The skin is pierced between the tendons of tibialis anterior (medially) and extensor hallucis longus laterally (Fig. 12.23). The needle is directed posteriorly and superiorly (to accommodate the convex articular surface of the talus). An effusion should be aspirated initially.

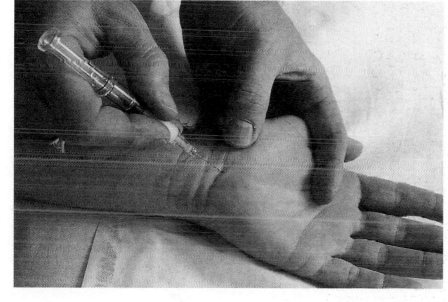

FIG. 12.19 The injection site (at the level of the distal wrist crease) for the carpal tunnel is demonstrated.

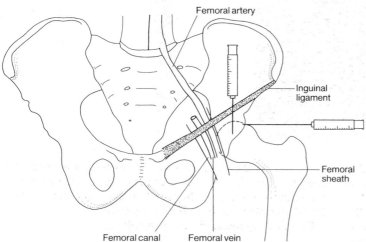

FIG. 12.20 The injection sites for the hip joint are demonstrated.

Femoral artery

Inguinal ligament

Femoral sheath

Femoral canal   Femoral vein

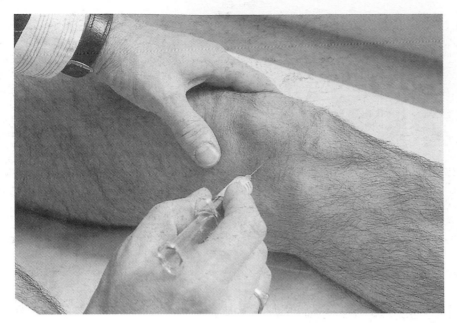

FIG. 12.21 The medial approach for intra-articular injection of the knee joint is demonstrated.

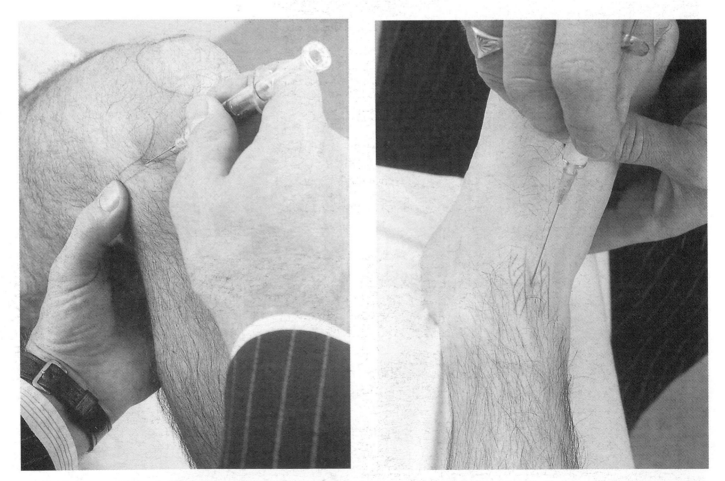

FIG. 12.22 An approach tangential to the joint line is made for injection of a medial coronary ligament sprain of the knee.

FIG. 12.23 An anterior approach for intra-articular injection of the ankle joint is demonstrated.

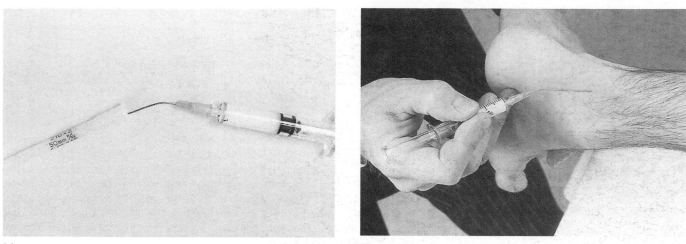

(a)   (b)

FIG. 12.24 (a) A bent needle is useful to inject the Achilles paratenon. (b) Injection of the Achilles paratenon.

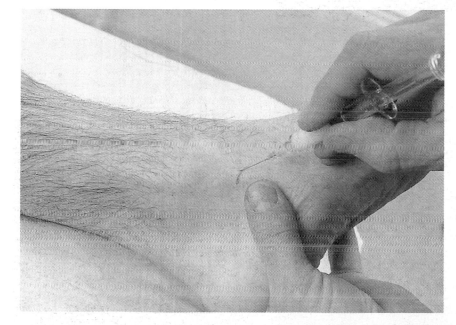

FIG. 12.25 The subtalar joint may be injected from a medial approach above the sustentaculum tali.

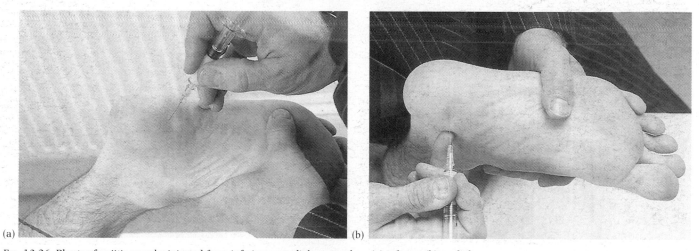

(a)   (b)

FIG. 12.26 Plantar fasciitis may be injected from inferior or medial approaches: (a) inferior; (b) medial.

The following materials are required:

5 ml syringe
$1\frac{1}{2}$ inch 21 G needle
20 mg of triamcinolone hexacetonide in 1 ml
4 ml of 1 per cent lignocaine.

The *Achilles paratenon* is approached posteriorly with the patient lying prone. Injections are made parallel to the tendon, both medially and laterally. Once attached to the syringe, the needle inside its guard may be bent to 20° close to its base (Fig. 12.24) to facilitate the direction of penetration.

The following materials are required:

5 ml syringe
2×2 inch 21 G needle
10 mg of triamcinolone hexacetonide in 1 ml
4 ml of 1 per cent lignocaine.

The *subtalar joint* may be approached most easily from the medial side. The sustentaculum tali is identified below the medial malleolus and the needle is inserted above its superior margin and directed laterally (Fig. 12.25). Alternatively, the sinus tarsi may be approached laterally via the hollow that is felt antero-inferior to the lateral malleolus, or the posterior subtalar joint penetrated from a posterolateral approach.

The following materials are required:

2 ml syringe
1 inch 23 G needle
10 mg of triamcinolone hexacetonide in 1 ml
1 ml of 1 per cent lignocaine.

Plantar fasciitis is identified by localized tenderness over the medial tubercle of the calcaneus: the patient lies prone for ease of access. The injection may be made either by penetration of the needle at right angles to the lesion or from a more medial approach (Fig. 12.26). Infiltration is made at the fibro-osseous junction: firm pressure is required.

The following materials are required:

2 ml syringe
1 inch 23 G needle
10 mg of triamcinolone hexacetonide in 1 ml
1 ml of 1 per cent lignocaine.

The spine

A *caudal epidural* injection (for back pain and/or sciatica) is given via the sacral hiatus (Fig. 12.27). The patient lies prone and the sacral hiatus is identified by palpation of the depression between the sacral cornua. Local anaesthesia to the skin and subcutaneous tissues as far as the hiatus is induced initially. The epidural needle pierces the skin at an angle of approximately 45° and penetrates the ligament overlying the hiatus, whereupon a loss of resistance is felt. Attempted aspiration excludes the penetration of an epidural vein or the dura mater (which normally terminates at the level of S2). The injection is given slowly over ten minutes, taking account of the severity of any reproduction of the patient's symptoms. A period of recumbency of ten to thirty minutes following the procedure allows early lightheadedness, when resuming the upright position, to dissipate rapidly.

Rarely, the patient reacts 'adversely' to a caudal epidural approach if the above precautions are taken. Nevertheless, the procedure should be carried out with adequate nursing help and with resuscitation facilities available, in view of the occasional reported case of hypersensitivity to local anaesthetic.

The following materials are required:

2 ml syringe, 23 G needle, and 2 ml of 1 per cent lignocaine for skin anaesthesia
24–50 ml syringe
2 inch 21 G needle (or $3\frac{1}{2}$ inch 20 G needle for obese patients)
20–50 ml of 0.5 per cent procaine HCl
± 20–40 mg of triamcinolone hexacetonide.

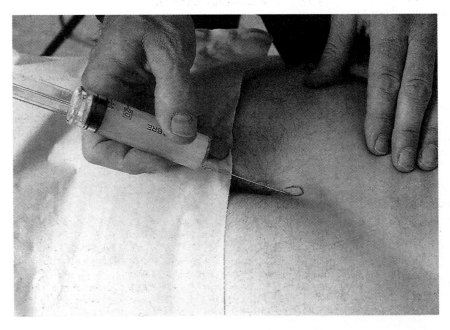

FIG. 12.27 A caudal epidural injection is given via the sacral hiatus.

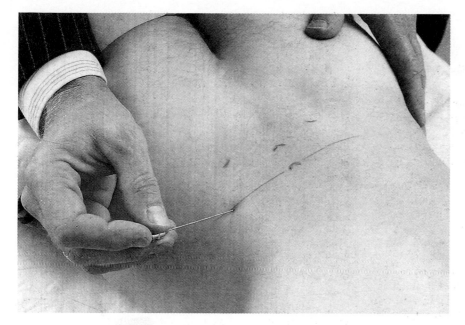

Fig. 12.28 The oblique approach for the right L4/5 facet (posterior apophyseal) joint is demonstrated. A similar approach, in a slightly more caudal direction, may be used for L4/5 or L5/S1 sinuvertebral (foraminal) nerve-block injections.

The *lumbar facet (apophyseal) joints* which are most commonly injected are L4/5 and L5/S1. The patient lies prone and the relevant facet joint position is identified by dropping an imaginary line down (anteriorly) from the level of the relevant spinous process (for example, L4 spinous process for the L4/5 facet joint) 3 cm from the midline. When the typical resistance offered by capsule and ligament to the needle is met, the injection is given with only moderate pressure. Infiltration of the posterior aspect(s) of the joint(s) is made. Commonly, bilateral injections are required.

Alternatively, an oblique approach (from a skin position approximately 6 cm from the midline, as demonstrated in Fig. 12.28) may be used. Certainty of entry into the facet joint capsule is only possible with fluoroscopic screening and contrast media. Such screening greatly facilitates accurate injection, though in the author's experience it is often unnecessary for therapeutic efficacy in facet joint syndromes. The oblique approach, in a slightly more caudal direction, is used for L4/5 or L5/S1 sinuvertebral (foraminal) nerve-block injections.

The following materials are required:

5 ml syringe
2 inch 21 G needle
20 mg of triamcinolone hexacetonide in 1ml
4 ml of 1 per cent lignocaine
(for oblique approach: $3\frac{1}{2}$ inch 20 G (spinal) needle + 2 ml syringe, 23 G needle, and 2 ml of 1 per cent lignocaine for skin anaesthesia).

The *sacroiliac joint* is approached from the midline (or within 1–2 cm of the midline) at the level of the L4/5 interspinous ligament. The direction of the needle is anteriorly, inferiorly, and laterally. The correct angle is essential, and the full length of a 3 inch needle is often required.

The following materials are required:

2 ml syringe, 23 G needle, and 2 ml of 1 per cent lignocaine (for skin anaesthesia)
5 ml syringe

$3\frac{1}{2}$ inch 20 G (spinal) needle
20 mg of triamcinolone hexacetonide in 1 ml
4 ml of 1 per cent lignocaine.

Sclerosant injections are given to the low lumbar and sacroiliac ligaments in patients with lumbar and/or sacroiliac instability. Prior sedation, for example with intravenous midazolam, is recommended. From one puncture site between the L4 and L5 spinous processes, the following ligaments are injected at their ligamento-osseous junction:

L4/5 supraspinous and interspinous ligaments
L5/S1 interspinous ligaments
L4/5 capsular ligaments
L5/S1 capsular ligaments
iliolumbar ligaments
sacroiliac interosseous ligaments
posterior sacroiliac ligaments
sacrotuberous ligaments

The following materials are required:

2 ml syringe, 23 G needle, 23 G butterfly IV set, and 2 ml of midazolam
10 ml syringe
$3\frac{1}{2}$ inch 20 G (spinal) needle
5.0 ml of P2G (Boots plc)
5.0 ml of 2 per cent lignocaine.

References

Akeson, W. H., Amiel, D., and LaViolette, D. (1967). Connective tissue response to immobility. *Clin. Orthop.*, **51**, 183–97.

Bassett, F. H., Beck, J. L., and Weiker, G. (1980). A modified cast brace: its use in nonoperative and postoperative management of serious knee ligament injuries. *Am. J. Sports Med.*, **8** (2), 63–7.

Calabrese, L. H. and Rooney, T. W. (1986). The use of non-steroidal anti-inflammatory drugs in sports. *Physician Sportsmed.*, **14** (2), 89–97.

Cyriax, J. and Russell, G. (1984). *Textbook of orthopaedic medicine*, Vol. 2, *Treatment* (11th edn). Baillière Tindall, London.

Drez, D., Faust, D. C., and Evans, J. P. (1981). Cryotherapy and nerve palsy. *Am J. Sports Med.*, **9** (4), 256–7.

Dyson, M. and Pond, J. B. (1970). The effects of pulsed ultrasound on tissue regeneration. *Physiotherapy*, **59**, 284–7.

Dyson, M. (1987). Mechanisms involved in therapeutic ultrasound. *Physiotheraphy*, **73**, 116–20.

Finsterbush, A. and Friedman, B. (1973). Early changes in an immobilised rabbit knee joint. *Clin. Orthop*, **92**, 305–19.

Fox, W. W. (1981). *Arthritis: is your suffering really necessary*. Sheldon Press, London.

Gieck, J. H. and Saliba, E. N. (1987). Application of modalities in overuse syndromes. *Clin. Sports Med.*, **6** (2), 459–61.

Grimby, J., Gustafsson, E., Petersen, L., and Renstrøm, P. (1980). Quadriceps function and training after knee ligament surgery. *Med. Sci. Sports*, **12**, 70–5.

Gunn, C. C. (1996). *Treatment of chronic pain: intramuscular stimulation for myofascial pain of radiculopathic origin* (2nd edn.) Churchill Livingstone, New York.

Haggmark, T. and Eriksson, E. (1979). Cylinder or mobile cast brace after knee ligament surgery. *Am. J. Sports Med.*, **7** (1), 48–56.

Hutson, M. A. (1986). A double-blind study comparing ibuprofen 1800 mg or 2400 mg daily and placebo in sports injuries. *J. Int. Med. Res.*, **14** (3), 142–7.

Hutson, M. A. and Jackson, J. P. (1982). Injuries to the lateral ligament of the ankle: assessment and treatment. *Br. J. Sports Med.*, **16** (4), 245–9.

Laros, G. S., Tipton, C. M., and Cooper, R. R. (1971). Influence of physical activity on ligament insertions in knees of dogs. *J. Bone Jt. Surg.*, **53A**, 275 86.

Lewit, K. (1985). *Manipulative therapy in rehabilitation of the motor system*. Butterworth, London.

Maitland, G. D. (1986). *Vertebral manipulation* (5th edn). Butterworth, London.

Melzack, R. and Wall, P. D. (1965). Pain mechanisms: a new theory. *Science*, **150**, 971–9.

Mennell, J. McM. (1960). *Back pain*. Little, Brown, Boston, MA.

Mooney, V. (1974). Cast bracing. *Clin. Orthop.*, **102**, 159–66.

Mooney, V. and Ferguson, A. B. (1966). The influence of immobilisation and motion on the formation of fibrocartilage in the repair granuloma after joint resection in the rabbit. *J. Bone Jt. Surg.*, **48A**, 1145–55.

Sloan, J. P., Hain, R., and Pownall, R. (1989). Clinical benefits of early cold therapy in accident and emergency following ankle sprain. *Arch. Emerg. Med.*, **6**, 1–6.

Stoddard, A. (1980). *Manual of osteopathic technique* (3rd edn). Hutchinson, London.

Travell, J. and Simons, D. G. (1983). *Myofascial pain and dysfunction—trigger points manual*. Williams and Wilkins, Baltimore, MD.

Viidik, A. (1967). Effect of training on the tensile strength of isolated rabbit tendons. *Scand. J. Plast. Reconstr. Surg.*, **1**, 141–7.

Zohn, D. A. and Mennell, J. McM. (1976). *Diagnosis and physical treatment of musculoskeletal pain*. Little, Brown, Boston, MA.

13 Emergency medicine in sport

J. SLOAN

Any sports physician needs to have the competencies to treat a whole range of emergencies. The presentations of disease that might occur are so widely variable that few would become expert. Nonetheless, an understanding of some basic principles could be life saving.

In addition, the sports physician will often be prevailed upon to lecture to groups of paramedics, first-aiders, trainers, and coaches on the initial management of acute injury in sport. As far as is practically convenient, it should be considered an obligation to accept the teaching responsibilities, inherent in the physician's role as medical adviser, to sports groups and associations. These responsibilities should also extend to the provision of advice to sports clubs on the adequacy of first-aid facilities which are available to sports participants (and in the case of large stadia, to spectators also). The reader is referred to the First Aid Manual prepared by the St John Ambulance Association for a comprehensive guide to the first-aiders management of injury. It is a useful reference work for the physician when faced with the need to structure a series of lectures on this topic.

Principles of emergency care in sport

Whether treating emergencies, or equipping first-aiders, there are certain overarching principles that are always vital. Whatever the injury or emergency, three aspects of care must be quickly dealt with, always in this order:

A Ensure a patent *airway*
B Ensure that *breathing* is occurring
C Ensure that the *circulation* of blood is not compromised.

These 'ABCs' are the central pillar to any care given to an emergency. Furthermore, anyone engaging in care must have sufficient practical experience to reduce the likelihood of further injury and to promote recovery

These actions are dependent upon the recognition of the nature of the injury (at least as far as is possible by non-qualified personnel). The potential for harm must be recognized and, in this regard, there is no substitute for practical training in Basic Life Support (BLS). In addition, doctors who wish to gain broad competencies should consider both Advanced Life Support (ALS) and Advanced Trauma Life Support (ATLS) courses, and undertaking a six-month post in Accident and Emergency Medicine.

Neck protection

If spinal cord injury is suspected (for example, if the victim has sustained a fall, has been struck on the head or neck, has injured the neck in a rugby scrum collapse, or has been rescued

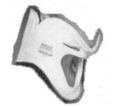

FIG. 13.1 A hard cervical collar used to support the neck in cases where spinal cord injuries is suspected.

after diving into shallow water), particular care must be taken during handling and resuscitation to maintain alignment of the head, neck, and chest in the neutral position. A hard cervical collar, similar to that shown in Fig. 13.1, should be applied. In addition, the head should be taped to the stretcher, with sand bags, or similar, supporting each side of the head. A spinal board should be used if available.

Collapse and severe trauma

A patient who collapses spontaneously, or following trauma, may require resuscitation. Excellent updated guidelines are available at the Resuscitation Council web site (http://www.resus.org.uk), from where Adult and Paediatric Life Support guidelines can be accessed.

In all such cases, as listed above, the main priorities are ABC—that is *Airway, breathing* and *circulation*. In trauma, it is important to maintain a focus on these and not be distracted by less pressing (though visually shocking) injuries. So, it follows that clearing the airway of vomit, dentures, or food takes precedence over controlling external bleeding, and that the control of external bleeding (always by direct pressure) takes precedence over management of a fracture.

If spinal cord injury is suspected, care should be taken to maintain the patient in a horizontal position during rescue as hypotension often accompanies such injuries. The patient should not be moved until an appropriate number of trained helpers is available. As detailed above, appropriate neck immobilization should be provided. One assistant supports the head and neck while the body is moved without change of position. The technique of log-roll, in which the spine is kept perfectly straight, should be familiar to the sports physician.

To obtain a satisfactory airway, the degree of head tilt should be the minimum that allows unobstructed ventilation. Jaw thrust rather than chin lift is preferable. During resuscitation, help from others may be required to maintain head, back, and chest alignment if adequate splinting is not available. Remember that successful resuscitation that results in paralysis is a tragedy, but failure to carry out adequate ventilation in cases of respiratory arrest will result in death.

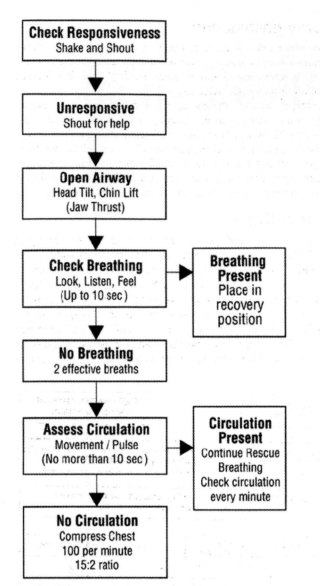

Check Responsiveness
Shake and Shout

↓

Unresponsive
Shout for help

↓

Open Airway
Head Tilt, Chin Lift
(Jaw Thrust)

↓

Check Breathing
Look, Listen, Feel
(Up to 10 sec) → **Breathing Present**
Place in recovery position

↓

No Breathing
2 effective breaths

↓

Assess Circulation
Movement / Pulse
(No more than 10 sec) → **Circulation Present**
Continue Rescue Breathing
Check circulation every minute

↓

No Circulation
Compress Chest
100 per minute
15:2 ratio

FIG. 13.2 Adult basic life support.

The correct sequence of actions is as follows:

1. Ensure the safety of rescuer and victim.
2. Check the victim and see if he responds: ask loudly: 'Are you all right?'
3. If he responds by answering or moving, leave him in the position in which you find him (provided he is not in further danger), check his condition, get help, and reassess him regularly.
4. If he does not respond, shout for help. Open his airway by tilting his head and lifting his chin: if possible, with the victim in the position in which you find him, place your hand on his forehead and gently tilt his head back keeping your thumb and index finger free to close his nose if rescue breathing is required. At the same time, with your finger-tip(s) under the point of the victim's chin, lift the chin to open the airway. If you have any difficulty, turn the victim on to his back and then open the airway as described. Try to avoid head tilt if traumatic injury to the neck is suspected.
5. Keeping the airway open, look, listen, and feel for breathing (more than an occasional gasp): look for chest movements

and listen at the victim's mouth for breath sounds. Feel for air on your cheek. Do this for up to 10 seconds before deciding that breathing is absent.

6. If he is breathing (other than an occasional gasp), turn him into the recovery position (see below; Fig. 13.3) and check for continued breathing. Send someone for help, or, if you are on your own, leave the victim and go for help.
7. If he is not breathing, send someone for help or, if you are on your own, leave the victim and go for help. As soon as possible, return and turn the victim onto his back if he is not already in this position. Remove any visible obstruction from the victim's mouth, including dislodged dentures, but leave well-fitting dentures in place. Ensure head tilt and chin lift. Pinch the soft part of his nose closed with the index finger and thumb of your hand on his forehead. Open his mouth a little, but maintain chin lift. Take a breath and place your lips around his mouth, making sure that you have a good seal. Blow steadily into his mouth over about $1^1/_2$–2 seconds, watching for his chest to rise. Maintaining head tilt and chin lift, take your mouth away from the victim and watch for his chest to fall as air comes out. Take another breath and repeat the sequence as above to give two effective breaths, each of which makes the chest rise and fall. If you have difficulty achieving an effective breath, re-check the victim's mouth and remove any obstruction. Re-check that there is adequate head tilt and chin lift. Make up to five attempts in all to achieve two effective breaths. Even if unsuccessful, move on to assessment of circulation.
8. Assess the victim for signs of a circulation. Look for any movement, including swallowing or breathing (more than an occasional gasp). Check the carotid pulse. Take no more than 10 seconds to do this.
9. If you are confident that you can detect signs of a circulation within 10 seconds, continue rescue breathing, if necessary, until the victim starts breathing on his own. About every minute, re-check for signs of a circulation; take no more than 10 seconds each time. If the victim starts to breathe on his own but remains unconscious, turn him into the recovery position (Fig. 13.3). Check his condition and be ready to turn him onto his back and restart rescue breathing if he stops breathing.
10. If there are no signs of a circulation, or you are at all unsure, start chest compression. Locate the lower half of the sternum (breastbone): using your index and middle fingers, identify the lower rib margins. Keeping your fingers together, slide them upwards to the point where the ribs join the sternum. With your middle finger on this point, place your index finger on the sternum. Slide the heel of your other hand down the sternum until it reaches your index finger; this should be the middle of the lower half of

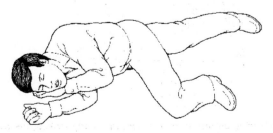

FIG. 13.3 The recovery position.

the sternum. Place the heel of one hand there, with the other hand on top of the first. Interlock the fingers of both hands and lift them to ensure that pressure is not applied over the victim's ribs. Do not apply any pressure over the upper abdomen or bottom tip of the sternum. Position yourself vertically above the victim's chest and, with your arms straight, press down on the sternum to depress it 4–5 cm ($1^1/_2$–2 inches). Release the pressure, then repeat at a rate of about 100 times a minute (a little less than two compressions a second). Compression and release should take an equal amount of time. Combine rescue breathing and compression: after fifteen compressions, tilt the head, lift the chin, and give two effective breaths. Return your hands immediately to the correct position on the sternum and give a fifteen further compressions, continuing compressions and breaths in a ratio of 15:2.

11. Continue resuscitation until the victim shows signs of life, or qualified help arrives to assist, or you become exhausted.

The recovery position

If the patient appears to be breathing, use the recovery position as follows:

- Remove the victim's spectacles
- Kneel beside the victim and make sure that both his legs are straight
- Open the airway by tilting the head and lifting the chin
- Place the arm nearest to you out at right angles to his body, elbow bent with the hand palm uppermost
- Bring his far arm across the chest, and hold the back of the hand against the victim's nearest cheek
- With your other hand, grasp the far leg just above the knee and pull it up, keeping the foot on the ground
- Keeping his hand pressed against his cheek, pull on the leg to roll the victim towards you onto his side
- Adjust the upper leg so that both the hip and knee are bent at right angles
- Tilt the head back to make sure the airway remains open
- Adjust the hand under the cheek, if necessary, to keep the head tilted
- Check breathing regularly

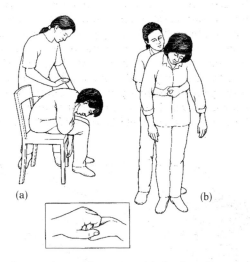

FIG. 13.4 Clearing an airway obstruction. (a) Gently striking the back. (b) The Heimlich manoeuvre, with the position of the hands shown.

Airway obstruction

Airway obstruction is more common in children than in adults. The commonest causes are external compression (the paediatric trachea is compressed much more readily), inhaled foreign bodies, and pharyngeal swelling.

Treatment should always be designed to restore a patent airway as a matter of extreme priority. Inhaled foreign bodies are best dealt with by gently striking the back and, if this fails, by the Heimlich manoeuvre, as shown in Fig. 13.4. A small foreign body may pass beyond the vicinity of the larynx and into the lungs. Patients with such foreign bodies tend to have a monophonic wheeze, and subsequent X-ray will show segmental collapse.

Acute asthma

Asthma still kills 2000 people per annum in the UK. Many of these deaths are due to the fact that the severity of asthma has been misunderstood. Severity is best judged by an assessment of peak flow rate, together with tachycardia. Exercise-induced asthma is very common, and it is therefore useful for a sports physician to acquire a small peak flow meter. Young, fit adults would be expected to have flows in excess of 350–400 (women) and 450–500 (men). More precise nomograms are available to calculate a patient's expected peak flow. Certainly any patient

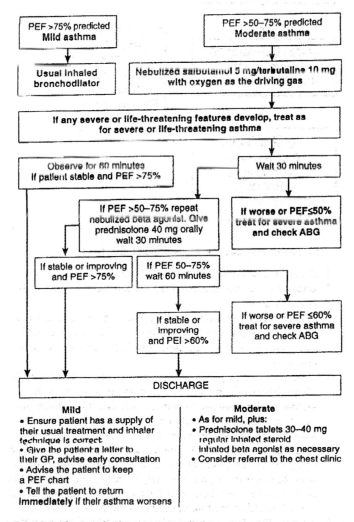

FIG. 13.5 The British Thoracic Society advice on treatment of asthma.

with a peak expiratory flow rate of less than 75 per cent of predicted should receive bronchodilator therapy. More severe restrictions of peak flow that should be treated according to Fig. 13.5, which represents advice given by the British Thoracic Society.

Anaphylaxis

Anaphylaxis is a pathophysiological condition resulting from a type 1 hypersensitivity reaction. As a result of previous sensitization, mast cells degranulate, histamine is released, and this is followed rapidly by a massive release of other mediators of inflammation.

Circulatory collapse, laryngeal swelling, broncho-spasm, urticarial skin rash, and gastrointestinal symptoms frequently occur. The situation may develop extremely rapidly and the reaction may, on occasions, prove fatal. Treatment should consist of management of the collapsed patient, together with administration of adrenaline. Classically, the adrenaline was recommended to be given subcutaneously, but most emergency physicians would agree that it should be diluted, 1 mg in 10 ml, and given by slow intravenous titration against the response.

There is little evidence to support the effectiveness of other drugs such as steroids and antihistamines.

Heat illness

Heat illness is a range of syndromes, all associated with excess body heat. Heat syncope is not unusual, especially in lengthy exertion in hot surroundings (for example, summer marathons). Heat exhaustion and heat stroke are much less common.

Heat syncope

Heat syncope results from dehydration and hypotension, usually from peripheral vasodilatation. Thermoregulation is not affected, and the condition responds to cooling by simple removal of clothing and fluid support.

Heat exhaustion

Again, thermoregulation remains intact, but the patient's temperature may rise into the range 38–41°C. The general cause is environmental excessive heat with resulting dehydration and electrolyte depletion. Patients are usually not confused but look unwell and may require intravenous fluids. Electrolyte imbalance may occur and occasionally rhabdomyolysis (that is, muscle cell breakdown), and cardiac damage may result.

Heat stroke

In this much more serious condition, there is a breakdown of normal thermoregulation, and cerebral damage may result as the core temperature rises above 41°C. Central nervous system symptoms such as convulsions and coma may occur. Management obviously consists of cooling from the environmental point of view together with circulatory support. Heat stroke will always require hospital treatment. In the event of the need for anaesthesia, patients should never be given suxamethonium, as this worsens the hyperkalaemia and hyperthermia. Always bear in mind that Ecstasy may be behind an unexplained hyperpyrexia, and was probably the commonest cause of hyperpyrexia in the late 1990s.

Seizures and status epilepticus

Most patients who have seizures are known to have epileptic fits. Occasionally, patients present with a single first fit. The most useful thing that can be done for such patients is to document the fit very accurately. Such patients should be assessed within a hospital environment, as there are diverse causes.

In status epilepticus, continuous seizures lasting over 10 minutes occur, or there are recurrent seizures without full recovery between episodes. This is a much more serious problem as there is a risk of permanent cerebral damage and such fits should be brought under control as soon as possible. Care should be designed to maintain the airway, breathing, and circulation. An intravenous benzodiazepine is the most effective way to stop fitting. It can be difficult to achieve intravenous access, and rectal administration is also very effective.

No sportsman or woman should be allowed to compete shortly after an unexplained fit. The Brazilian footballer, Ronaldo, was the focus of a great deal of attention in the World Cup of 1998 in France. At the last minute, he was included in the team for the final match against France, apparently hours after a possible first fit, only to perform very poorly.

Near drowning

Patients who drown are subject to multiple problems. Often the most significant within the UK is the hypothermia that is associated with drowning (see section below on Hypothermia). Salt-water drowning presents much less pathophysiological challenge to the body than fresh-water drowning. Successful resuscitation can occur after several minutes of immersion in salt water, particularly in younger patients and particularly when the temperature is low. Fresh-water drowning results in a great deal of water intoxication and haemolysis. Consequently, the serum potassium level serves as a marker of the likely effectiveness of resuscitation. Emergency treatment should be designed to restore the airway, breathing, and circulation, while re-warming as quickly as possible.

Following rescue, patients may regain consciousness, only to suffer significant pulmonary oedema, and this should be guarded against by avoiding large fluid boluses, and by sitting the patient upright if possible. They should always be treated in a hospital environment.

Hypothermia

Hypothermia occurs when the temperature of the body core falls below 35°C. Overall, the most common cause is urban hypothermia in the elderly. However, exposure and immersion hypothermia in younger patients is associated with various sports, especially climbing, off-piste skiing, heli-skiing, caving, sailing, and windsurfing. Many ramblers have become victims of hypothermia following trivial ankle injuries.

When a serious injury has been sustained, particularly out of doors in the winter months, an adequate body temperature should be maintained. Blankets or extra clothes should be made available. The use of modern heat-retaining blankets and 'space suits' has become commonplace in endurance events, when sudden reduction in muscle activity may give rise to hypothermia. They are of limited use alone.

As the temperature drops into the realm of mild hypothermia, (33–34°C), amnesia, ataxia, and dilated pupils are seen. Once the temperature drops to 32°C and below, the conscious level becomes depressed and bradycardia begins to develop. Increased muscle rigidity and ventricular fibrillation may develop from 28°C and below. Eventually, as the temperature drops lower, asystole occurs with absent reflexes. In view of this, the cardinal rule is that no patient should be declared dead until they have been warmed to normal body temperature. Following rescue, rapid re-warming may cause peripheral vasodilatation, with a drop in the core temperature and consequent circulatory collapse. In addition, ventricular fibrillation may occur, particularly from insertion of tubes into the oesophagus. For these reasons, care must be provided in an expert hospital setting.

Lightning injury

Only a handful of people are killed every year by lightning in the UK, but many more are injured. Golfers and walkers are most vulnerable.

Lightning strike may cause many injuries, ranging from cardiac arrest through burns, to musculoskeletal trauma from sudden muscular contractions. Blunt trauma may occur if a victim is thrown by the lightning strike. Deep muscle damage may occur from conduction through muscle compartments. Patients may remain confused or amnesic for days.

Perhaps the most merciful injury is the 'flash over' effect, causing a fern-like pattern on the skin. These lesions often resolve within a number of days. All lightning strike patients should be admitted to hospital for 24 hours observation and continuous ECG monitoring.

Hypoglycaemia

Hypoglycaemia in sporting patients is not uncommon and is not confined to those known to be suffering from diabetes. Young adults will often push themselves beyond reasonable limits, missing meals, and dropping their blood glucose below 2.5 millimoles per litre, at which point many patients begin to be symptomatic. If a patient is still conscious, he or she can be given glucose orally with safety. Once they lose consciousness, however, this route should not be used. Glucagon intramuscularly is a useful way of elevating the glucose and is much less aggressive to the body's biochemistry (and the veins) than intravenous glucose. Diabetics who become hypoglycaemic usually can manage their own sugar levels once they are alert and orientated, but they should be advised to consult their supervising nurse or doctor for further advice as soon as possible.

Musculoskeletal injury

Of course, musculoskeletal injury is the commonest emergency sustained by sports men and women. Management depends on the initial assessment, which should be made by looking, feeling, and moving the injured part.

A fracture should be suspected when there is:

(i)   pain
(ii) swelling
(iii) deformity
(iv) dysfunction.

The more experienced will be able to distinguish between the temporary 'numbing' effect of direct trauma to exposed bone (for example, the shin), which causes periosteal bruising, and the disabling effect of the tibial fracture. Pain and soft tissue swelling are often poor guides to diagnosis when compared with the resultant dysfunction. Once a general appraisal of the situation has been made, an evaluation of whether the injured player is able to move the limb is the most important step. If voluntary movement has become completely inhibited, there is a significant risk of substantial structural injury. Patients with a fracture do not squirm or roll around in apparent agony—they will lie still. This is an indication for the most careful degree of handling, more particularly if spinal injury is suspected.

A joint dislocation gives rise to distortion and dysfunction. The pain is different from that a fracture in that it is often more severe, and not eased by keeping still. The site of deformity will give an additional clue that a dislocation has occurred. Pain relief, splinting, and an early X-ray are required.

It is necessary to stress the importance of neurovascular assessment—for example, the subject's comments on skin sensation, and the observation of abnormal skin colour or absent arterial pulsation distal to the injury. The supracondylar elbow fracture is one of the best known fractures to result in arterial injury.

A ligament sprain or tear may be suspected by the nature of the stress or wrench applied to a joint. Thus medial knee pain in a rugby player following a valgus force during a tackle is likely to be due to injury to the medial collateral ligament. Pain may be substantial, and early swelling is a possibility. Dysfunction following a ligament injury is usually less profound than with a fracture, even in the presence of substantial ligament tears. For instance, following knee injury, players involved in team sports may attempt to carry on playing for a while, and indeed may be encouraged to do so by an unsuspecting trainer if the initial assessment has failed to establish the true nature of the injury. Within five or ten minutes, however, it becomes obvious to the player, his attendants, and his manager that all is not well, so that a further careful examination in the treatment room is required. A rapidly developing joint effusion is usually present by this stage.

Experienced sports physicians should be able to detect instability by stress-tests on examination of the limb at the time of injury. All too often, it is apparent to the medical officer observing from a distance that a trainer's only assessment of knee function following an injury on the pitch is the range of passive flexion and extension (which offers very limited information on injury to the soft tissues, though it may give some confidence to both the player and his examiner).

A tear or rupture of a muscle/tendon may be suspected when there is a history of sudden pain and dysfunction in a limb when there is no evidence of direct trauma. There is often little in the way of alternative diagnosis—for example, in acute hamstring tears in sprinters.

Although life threatening contusional injuries to the soft tissues or vital organs are uncommon in sport, nevertheless a medical officer may be required to assist in the management of severe injuries sustained by victims of spectator tragedies (for instance, in the case of crush injuries at Hillsborough and at the

Heysel Stadium, and the severe burns resulting from the fire at the Bradford City Football Club). In less serious incidents, in which direct trauma is involved, the treating individual may not appreciate that muscle, as well as skin and subcutaneous tissues, may be contused—for example, in the charley horse injury to the quadriceps femoris. When muscle is torn, movement is usually hampered and strength impaired, though there is rarely any initial evidence of swelling. In the case of a quadriceps haematoma developing, immediate cessation of play and the application of ice packs will reduce later impairment.

Continuation of play and promotion of recovery

An ill or injured player should not be allowed to continue unless the examiner is satisfied that the condition is relatively minor. The determined attempts of a player to continue to participate in a game when clearly he is unfit to do so, for instance with a locked knee or flail arm, or when concussed, should be met with equal resistance. The senseless approach of a small minority that a player should continue to play in pain should be discouraged.

If the physician is satisfied that an injury is relatively minor, a coolant spray may be applied to the skin overlying soft tissue trauma. Although of temporary benefit only, the reassurance that is implied in this 'therapeutic' action may have great effect. Dowsing of the head and the back of the neck with cold water is time-honoured, and appears to have a stimulant effect! If a player is able to continue, review of the injury on the completion of the game should be made in a well-lit treatment or first-aid room.

The principles of the early stages of treatment of soft tissue injuries are incorporated in 'RICE':

R—rest
I—ice
C—compression
E—elevation.

This phase of first-aid management merges with the inflammatory phase of healing. It is important to stress that during the first 48 hours after injury, the priority, other than for a thorough assessment, is for a period of rest in which there is minimal activity of the injured area.

Bleeding, whether internal or external, should be controlled in preparation for the subsequent physiological vasodilation of the healing phase. The use of elevation, by a sling for the upper limb and by recumbency with limb elevation for the lower limb, is important for comfort, reduction of further bleeding, and reduction of tissue pressure from oedema. This is especially relevant to injuries below the knee, when gravitational oedema and bruis-

ing may cause prolonged or severe inflammatory responses. Suitable strapping techniques help to control both periarticular and intra-articular swelling. For added protection, the use of wool and crepe is time-honoured, particularly in the form of the Robert Jones bandage for knee joint injuries. The use of strapping should not be a substitute for an adequate period of rest. In particular, players injured in those team sports which traditionally are associated with after-match drinking should be discouraged from persuing these social activities by standing 'propped up' at the bar.

The use of ice or one of the proprietary cold applications which are universally available is hardly ever contraindicated once the casualty has been assessed and stabilized in the relatively comfortable surroundings of the treatment or first-aid room. Twenty minutes of ice application, repeated every three hours or so, is considered to be helpful by most authorities. Care should be taken to avoid ice-burns by wrapping ice in a thin damp cloth or plastic bag, or by the application of massage techniques. In view of the occasional reports of nerve damage, ice compression should be avoided over exposed nerves, such as the common peroneal nerve at the head of the fibula.

Conclusion

Facilities for early diagnosis and first-aid management at sports clubs and arenas vary widely. A treatment room should be available, and equipped with a refrigerator for ice or cold compresses, and an adequate supply of bandages and gauze swabs. A stretcher in good working order should be readily available. For the equipment to be used with maximum effectiveness, it is necessary for as many club members as possible to have attended a first-aid course, augmented by training in management of sports injuries. A baseline of knowledge of those injuries that tend to be encountered frequently in individual sports should be provided.

Posters demonstrating BLS techniques should be displayed prominently. From time to time, BLS drills should be organized by the medical officer: if necessary, the help of certified teachers from the St John Ambulance Association should be enlisted. Suitable equipment such as a Brook airway and Ambu bag should be maintained in an easily accessible area.

References

First Aid Manual (1982) The authorised manual of the St John Ambulance Association and Brigade. St Andrews Ambulance Association, and the British Red Cross Society. Dorling Kindersley, London.

Epilogue: whither sports injury services?

M. A. HUTSON

Since I wrote the Epilogue to the Second Edition in 1996, expectations amongst doctors who practise Sports Medicine in the UK have been raised by the formation of the Intercollegiate Academic Board (IAB) of Sport and Exercise Medicine. Membership of the Board has been drawn primarily from the colleges and faculties that constitute the Academy of Medical Royal Colleges to which the IAB in effect acts as a specialist advisory committee. A new UK diploma in Sport and Exercise Medicine has emerged, based on the Scottish Medical Royal Colleges examination, which will assess basic specialty training standards for the 'touch-line doctor' as well as doctors in 'for example, primary care and orthopaedics with a sub-speciality interest' (Macleod 1999). A higher specialty training programme that will satisfy the requirements of the Specialist Training Authority (STA) for CCST (Certificate of Completion of Specialist Training) status is envisaged: this will require the cooperation of a number of the Royal Colleges; flexibility and innovation are demanded.

Although new NHS specialties have emerged in recent years, and the STA has approved the award of CCST to doctors in 'emerging' specialties or sub-specialties (on the basis that de facto the particular specialty exists even though it is not an accepted NHS specialty), it seems that a further leap of faith is required by the appropriate authorities to establish career opportunities in Sports Medicine. Furthermore, the role within the NHS of the doctor with experience in sports injuries, whether at a basic level or at a higher accredited level, remains in doubt. The author envisages that approval will be given by community medicine for higher standards in exercise medicine for the benefit of the nation's health: the development of Centres of Excellence for diagnosis and management of soft tissue injuries, whether in professional sport (for which the argument for private medical care of a specialist nature remains strong) or for the millions of amateur sports people who benefit psychologically and physically from exercise, is a different matter.

Whatever the way forward in the Millennium, it is inescapable that:

- Sport will continue to be played; therefore, sports injuries will continue to occur.
- Patients with injuries sustained in sport will continue to swell the work-load of the general practitioner and junior traumatologist.

It is apparent that the IAB will have no responsibility for the inclusion of exercise physiology and pathophysiology in undergraduate medical training. Of equal disappointment is the slow progress made by the British Institute of Musculoskeletal Medicine (BIMM) in introducing basic science and clinical methods in musculoskeletal disorders to medical students. Accordingly, the views expressed by the author in a letter to the *British Medical Journal* (Hutson 1987) over a decade ago remain prescient.

An appreciable proportion of attendances at hospital accident departments, particularly at weekends, result from acute musculoskeletal injuries caused by sport. The numbers stretch the resources of junior emergency staff to a level at which their primary concern is to define whether (using conventional orthopaedic priorities) an injury requires referral to a fracture clinic. Patients with overuse injuries peculiar to sport also present to general practitioners, whose difficulties are often due to a lack of knowledge of biomechanics and techniques related to particular sports; decision-making and advice in consequence become arbitrary.

The only satisfactory remedy ultimately lies in an improved level of tuition in musculoskeletal examination techniques for medical students and an improved level of postgraduate education in recognizing and managing soft-tissue injuries. Such training would allow the doctor of first contact—the general practitioner and traumatologist—to cope adequately with most of the problems (however and wherever occurred) as part of primary health-care. The future generalist sports physician must inevitably come therefore from the ranks of general practice, and orthopaedic (physical) medical teaching needs to be an obligatory part of the general practitioner's vocational training scheme. Appropriate postgraduate education in sports medicine would then lead to the establishment of a satisfactory career structure for doctors in this specialty. With some two million sports injuries occurring every year this may well be inevitable.

Regrettably, there continues to be a body of opinion within the medical profession which considers sports injuries as self-imposed and therefore deserving of private treatment only. Soft-tissue trauma, however, may give rise to as much morbidity and loss of time from work as fractures, which have historically been accorded priority in orthopaedic practice. There is no point in attempting to gloss over the absence of fundamental training, but first there needs to be a radical revision of medical opinion in line with rising consumer demand in favour of accepting the need for the development of orthopaedic and sports medicine within the general framework of medicine in the United Kingdom.

As a final comment, the self-imposed or self-inflicted injury philosophy appears to be largely a medical argument. Will the National Lottery, by releasing funds to regional centres of excellence supported by the Sports Council, enable the development of sports medicine? Perhaps the more vocal element of the sporting community will be the final arbiter, by its support for, and hopefully its demand for, an appropriate level of service provision.

References

Hutson, M. A. (1987). Why sports injury clinics? *Br. Med. J.*, **295**, 1210.

Macleod, D. A. D. (1999). The Intercollegiate Academic Board of Sport and Exercise Medicine. *Br. J. Sports Med.*, **33**, 73–8.

INDEX